Optimization of Veterinary Antimicrobial Treatment in Companion and Food Animals

Optimization of Veterinary Antimicrobial Treatment in Companion and Food Animals

Editors

Nikola Puvača
Chantal Britt
Jonathan Gómez-Raja

MDPI • Basel • Beijing • Wuhan • Barcelona • Belgrade • Manchester • Tokyo • Cluj • Tianjin

Editors
Nikola Puvača
Department of Engineering
Management in Biotechnology
University BA in Novi Sad
Novi Sad
Serbia

Chantal Britt
Swiss 3R Competence Centre
University of Bern
Bern
Switzerland

Jonathan Gómez-Raja
Department of Health and Social
Services
Government of Extremadura
Badajoz
Spain

Editorial Office
MDPI
St. Alban-Anlage 66
4052 Basel, Switzerland

This is a reprint of articles from the Special Issue published online in the open access journal *Antibiotics* (ISSN 2079-6382) (available at: www.mdpi.com/journal/antibiotics/special_issues/anti_compa_animal).

For citation purposes, cite each article independently as indicated on the article page online and as indicated below:

LastName, A.A.; LastName, B.B.; LastName, C.C. Article Title. *Journal Name* **Year**, *Volume Number*, Page Range.

ISBN 978-3-0365-2130-5 (Hbk)
ISBN 978-3-0365-2129-9 (PDF)

Contents

About the Editors vii

Preface to "Optimization of Veterinary Antimicrobial Treatment in Companion and Food Animals" ix

Nikola Puvača and Rosa de Llanos Frutos
Antimicrobial Resistance in *Escherichia coli* Strains Isolated from Humans and Pet Animals
Reprinted from: *Antibiotics* **2021**, *10*, 69, doi:10.3390/antibiotics10010069 1

Erinda Lika, Nikola Puvača, Dejan Jeremić, Slobodan Stanojević, Tana Shtylla Kika, Sonila Cocoli and Rosa de Llanos Frutos
Antibiotic Susceptibility of *Staphylococcus* Species Isolated in Raw Chicken Meat from Retail Stores
Reprinted from: *Antibiotics* **2021**, *10*, 904, doi:10.3390/antibiotics10080904 21

Cesar Augusto Roque-Borda, Larissa Pires Pereira, Elisabete Aparecida Lopes Guastalli, Nilce Maria Soares, Priscilla Ayleen Bustos Mac-Lean, Douglas D'Alessandro Salgado, Andréia Bagliotti Meneguin, Marlus Chorilli and Eduardo Festozo Vicente
HPMCP-Coated Microcapsules Containing the Ctx(Ile^{21})-Ha Antimicrobial Peptide Reduce the Mortality Rate Caused by Resistant *Salmonella* Enteritidis in Laying Hens
Reprinted from: *Antibiotics* **2021**, *10*, 616, doi:10.3390/antibiotics10060616 31

Zorana Kovačević, Miodrag Radinović, Ivana Čabarkapa, Nebojša Kladar and Biljana Božin
Natural Agents against Bovine Mastitis Pathogens
Reprinted from: *Antibiotics* **2021**, *10*, 205, doi:10.3390/antibiotics10020205 47

Nikola Puvača, Jovana Milenković, Tamara Galonja Coghill, Vojislava Bursić, Aleksandra Petrović, Snežana Tanasković, Miloš Pelić, Dragana Ljubojević Pelić and Tatjana Miljković
Antimicrobial Activity of Selected Essential Oils against Selected Pathogenic Bacteria: In Vitro Study
Reprinted from: *Antibiotics* **2021**, *10*, 546, doi:10.3390/antibiotics10050546 63

Ning Xu, Miao Li, Xiaohui Ai and Zhoumeng Lin
Determination of Pharmacokinetic and Pharmacokinetic-Pharmacodynamic Parameters of Doxycycline against *Edwardsiella ictaluri* in Yellow Catfish (*Pelteobagrus fulvidraco*)
Reprinted from: *Antibiotics* **2021**, *10*, 329, doi:10.3390/antibiotics10030329 77

Stephen Little, Andrew Woodward, Glenn Browning and Helen Billman-Jacobe
In-Water Antibiotic Dosing Practices on Pig Farms
Reprinted from: *Antibiotics* **2021**, *10*, 169, doi:10.3390/antibiotics10020169 89

Anat Shnaiderman-Torban, Dror Marchaim, Shiri Navon-Venezia, Ori Lubrani, Yossi Paitan, Haya Arielly and Amir Steinman
Third Generation Cephalosporin Resistant *Enterobacterales* Infections in Hospitalized Horses and Donkeys: A Case–Case–Control Analysis
Reprinted from: *Antibiotics* **2021**, *10*, 155, doi:10.3390/antibiotics10020155 111

Muhammad Kashif Maan, Zhifei Weng, Menghong Dai, Zhenli Liu, Haihong Hao, Guyue Cheng, Yulian Wang, Xu Wang and Lingli Huang
The Spectrum of Antimicrobial Activity of Cyadox against Pathogens Collected from Pigs, Chicken, and Fish in China
Reprinted from: *Antibiotics* **2021**, *10*, 153, doi:10.3390/antibiotics10020153 125

Marília Salgado-Caxito, Andrea I. Moreno-Switt, Antonio Carlos Paes, Carlos Shiva, Jose M. Munita, Lina Rivas and Julio A. Benavides
Higher Prevalence of Extended-Spectrum Cephalosporin-Resistant *Enterobacterales* in Dogs Attended for Enteric Viruses in Brazil Before and After Treatment with Cephalosporins
Reprinted from: *Antibiotics* **2021**, *10*, 122, doi:10.3390/antibiotics10020122 . . . . **139**

Virpi Welling, Nils Lundeheim and Björn Bengtsson
A Pilot Study in Sweden on Efficacy of Benzylpenicillin, Oxytetracycline, and Florfenicol in Treatment of Acute Undifferentiated Respiratory Disease in Calves
Reprinted from: *Antibiotics* **2020**, *9*, 736, doi:10.3390/antibiotics9110736 . . . . **153**

Alexandru O. Doma, Roxana Popescu, Mihai Mitulețu, Delia Muntean, János Dégi, Marius V. Boldea, Isidora Radulov, Eugenia Dumitrescu, Florin Muselin, Nikola Puvača and Romeo T. Cristina
Comparative Evaluation of *qnrA*, *qnrB*, and *qnrS* Genes in *Enterobacteriaceae* Ciprofloxacin-Resistant Cases, in Swine Units and a Hospital from Western Romania
Reprinted from: *Antibiotics* **2020**, *9*, 698, doi:10.3390/antibiotics9100698 . . . . **165**

Máximo Petrocchi-Rilo, César-B. Gutiérrez-Martín, Esther Pérez-Fernández, Anna Vilaró, Lorenzo Fraile and Sonia Martínez-Martínez
Antimicrobial Resistance Genes in Porcine *Pasteurella multocida* Are Not Associated with Its Antimicrobial Susceptibility Pattern
Reprinted from: *Antibiotics* **2020**, *9*, 614, doi:10.3390/antibiotics9090614 . . . . **177**

Aude A. Ferran, Marlène Z. Lacroix, Alain Bousquet-Mélou, Ivain Duhil and Béatrice B. Roques
Levers to Improve Antibiotic Treatment of Lambs via Drinking Water in Sheep Fattening Houses: The Example of the Sulfadimethoxine/Trimethoprim Combination
Reprinted from: *Antibiotics* **2020**, *9*, 561, doi:10.3390/antibiotics9090561 . . . . **189**

Anat Shnaiderman-Torban, Shiri Navon-Venezia, Efrat Kelmer, Adar Cohen, Yossi Paitan, Haya Arielly and Amir Steinman
Extended-Spectrum -Lactamase-Producing *Enterobacterales* Shedding by Dogs and Cats Hospitalized in an Emergency and Critical Care Department of a Veterinary Teaching Hospital
Reprinted from: *Antibiotics* **2020**, *9*, 545, doi:10.3390/antibiotics9090545 . . . . **207**

Anna Vilaró, Elena Novell, Vicens Enrique-Tarancón, Jordi Balielles, Carles Vilalta, Sonia Martinez and Lorenzo José Fraile Sauce
Antimicrobial Susceptibility Pattern of Porcine Respiratory Bacteria in Spain
Reprinted from: *Antibiotics* **2020**, *9*, 402, doi:10.3390/antibiotics9070402 . . . . **223**

Rositsa Mileva, Manol Karadaev, Ivan Fasulkov, Tsvetelina Petkova, Nikolina Rusenova, Nasko Vasilev and Aneliya Milanova
Oxytetracycline Pharmacokinetics After Intramuscular Administration in Cows with Clinical Metritis Associated with *Trueperella Pyogenes* Infection
Reprinted from: *Antibiotics* **2020**, *9*, 392, doi:10.3390/antibiotics9070392 . . . . **237**

About the Editors

Nikola Puvača

Nikola Puvača is a Researcher and Associate Professor at the Department of Engineering Management in Biotechnology of the University Business Academy in Novi Sad, Serbia. He is a multidisciplinary scientist with Ph.D. diplomas in Biotechnology, Veterinary Medicine, and Human Medicine, and a postdoctoral diploma in Toxicology and Molecular Genetics. He has significant experience in animal and poultry science, with a major interest in nutrition, feed quality and safety, natural alternatives for antibiotics, and antimicrobial resistance. He is involved in many research collaborations in various science fields. He is serving as an Editorial Board Member and peer reviewer for many indexed journals, and he is the author of more than 200 scientific papers published in international journals and the proceedings of national and international conferences. He is a guest lecturer in several international universities, and has won many rewards for scientific and professional work.

Chantal Britt

Chantal Britt is Communications Officer at Swiss 3R Competence Centre in Switzerland. After graduation from the University of Geneva, Chantal learned her ropes as a journalist for more than 15 years at Bloomberg News and the English department of Swissinfo.ch, covering financial markets, the biotechnology industry, technology, research and medicine. She has worked as a communications specialist for the Swiss Group for Clinical Cancer Research (SAKK), Johnson & Johnson, and the European Society of Clinical Microbiology and Infectious Diseases. She was responsible for publications and communications at ESCMID and ECCMID for more than three years. Since 2018, Chantal has specialised in science communications at the Swiss 3R Competence Centre (3RCC), the Swiss Centre for Applied Human Toxicology (SCAHT) and Swiss Laboratory Animal Science Association (SGV). Chantal's goal is to help researchers explain their work and share their passion.

Jonathan Gómez-Raja

Jonathan Gómez-Raja is Chief Scientific Officer, FUNDESALUD, Government of Extremadura in Spain. Dr. Gomez-Raja has a Ph.D. in Microbiology from the University of Extremadura (Spain) and a Postdoc at the University of Minnesota (USA), and a Master's in International R&D programs management from the Polytechnic University of Madrid (Spain). He is an expert in Genetics and Molecular Biology, and his research has been focused on human fungal diseases and infectious diseases. He has developed his career in the USA, India, Germany, and Spain. Author of several articles published in scientific journals, as well as book chapters. Regular reviewer in European funding programs and relevant JCR-indexed journals. He has participated as a researcher and principal investigator in several research projects and coordinator in national and international scientific activities. He is an external expert for the Spanish Medicine Agency (AEMPS).

Preface to "Optimization of Veterinary Antimicrobial Treatment in Companion and Food Animals"

The global antimicrobial resistance crisis has been the driver of several international strategies on antimicrobial stewardship. Despite their good intentions, such broad strategies are only slowly being implemented in real life. Antimicrobial resistance bacteria flow among humans and animals and actions for fighting the problem must consider both sectors. Antimicrobial usage is one of the potential drivers for antimicrobial resistance. The usage of antibiotics concerning companion and food animals and antimicrobials is undoubtedly beneficial for the prevention of diseases and the improvement of livestock performance.

Unfortunately, in veterinary medicine, which is challenged by a shortage of experts in key disciplines related to antimicrobial stewardship, there are few antimicrobial treatment guidelines, and diagnostic tests are inferior compared to human microbiology, without providing enough valuable information, which makes it difficult to identify by whom, when, and how the antimicrobial products are used. The main aspects of antimicrobial resistance monitoring remain unsolved in both companion and food animals, the use of appropriate methods for collection of information at the animal and farm levels, and the choice of metrics of measurement of antimicrobial resistance and animal populations at risk.

This book is supported by COST Action CA18217 –European Network for Optimization of Veterinary Antimicrobial Treatment.

This book gathered researchers interested in antimicrobial resistance monitoring in animals, to optimize veterinary antimicrobial use with special emphasis to help in the development of antimicrobial treatment guidelines and refinement of microbiological diagnostic procedures, in both companion and food animals, and to use the gathered information to improve antimicrobial stewardship.

Nikola Puvača, Chantal Britt, Jonathan Gómez-Raja
Editors

antibiotics

MDPI

Review

Antimicrobial Resistance in *Escherichia coli* Strains Isolated from Humans and Pet Animals

Nikola Puvača [1,2,*] and Rosa de Llanos Frutos [1]

1 Faculty of Biomedical and Health Sciences, Jaume I University, Avinguda de Vicent Sos Baynat, s/n, 12071 Castelló de la Plana, Spain; al409850@uji.es

2 Department of Engineering Management in Biotechnology, Faculty of Economics and Engineering Management in Novi Sad, University Business Academy in Novi Sad, Cvećarska 2, 21000 Novi Sad, Serbia

* Correspondence: nikola.puvaca@fimek.edu.rs; Tel.: +381-65-219-1284

Abstract: Throughout scientific literature, we can find evidence that antimicrobial resistance has become a big problem in the recent years on a global scale. Public healthcare systems all over the world are faced with a great challenge in this respect. Obviously, there are many bacteria that can cause infections in humans and animals alike, but somehow it seems that the greatest threat nowadays comes from the *Enterobacteriaceae* members, especially *Escherichia coli*. Namely, we are witnesses to the fact that the systems that these bacteria developed to fight off antibiotics are the strongest and most diverse in *Enterobacteriaceae*. Our great advantage is in understanding the systems that bacteria developed to fight off antibiotics, so these can help us understand the connection between these microorganisms and the occurrence of antibiotic-resistance both in humans and their pets. Furthermore, unfavorable conditions related to the ease of *E. coli* transmission via the fecal–oral route among humans, environmental sources, and animals only add to the problem. For all the above stated reasons, it is evident that the epidemiology of *E. coli* strains and resistance mechanisms they have developed over time are extremely significant topics and all scientific findings in this area will be of vital importance in the fight against infections caused by these bacteria.

Keywords: antimicrobial resistance; antibiotics; public health; microbiology; *E. coli*

check for updates

Citation: Puvača, N.; de Llanos Frutos, R. Antimicrobial Resistance in *Escherichia coli* Strains Isolated from Humans and Pet Animals. *Antibiotics* **2021**, *10*, 69. https://doi.org/10.3390/antibiotics10010069

Received: 17 December 2020
Accepted: 12 January 2021
Published: 13 January 2021

1. Introduction

Scientists all over the world have studied *Escherichia coli* and it appears to be the most thoroughly investigated and best understood of all model microorganisms [1–4]. We already know that it is one of the first bacteria that colonizes the human gut immediately after birth [5–7]. On the other hand, *E. coli* is often the main culprit of infections in the gastrointestinal tract [8], as well as other parts of human and animal organisms [9,10]. In more precise terms, *E. coli* typically causes urinary infections [11,12], but it can also lead to many other serious infections and conditions, such as: appendicitis [13], pneumonia [14], meningitis [15], endocarditis [16], gastrointestinal infections [17], etc. Research findings have shown us that *E. coli* can cause infections in all age groups and those infections can be acquired in the general population, i.e., community-acquired, as well as related to healthcare institutions [18–20].

After Alexander Fleming had discovered penicillin in 1928, the whole course of medicine changed [21,22]. The revolutionary discovery of antibiotics made it possible for doctors to treat extremely severe cases of infectious diseases, which had previously been a very common cause of death [23,24]. That completely changed after antibiotics had been introduced and soon penicillin became the most widely used antibiotic in the world, saving millions of lives [25–27].

Unfortunately, only several years after doctors started using it in hospitals, the first cases of penicillin resistance by *Staphylococcus aureus* were identified [28]. Obviously, bacteria have managed to develop a system that can protect them and make them resistant to antibiotics [29]. Sadly, the situation with bacteria evolving resistance is getting worse day by day and we have literally come to a point when we can speak of the antimicrobial resistance presenting a worldwide problem [30–36].

When we speak about *E. coli*, the fact that it has been put on the World Health Organization's (WHO) list that contains 12 families of bacteria that present the biggest danger to human health [37,38]. Ever since the first reported cases, *E. coli's* resistance to antibiotic treatment has been continuously growing [39–42].

Scientific literature offers an abundance of research studies into the nature and behavior of *E. coli* [43–46]. The results point to several extremely interesting facts. This bacterium undoubtedly has considerable influence on human and animal lives [47,48], for the simple reason that it lives inside the gut and can very easily spread from fecal matter to the mouth [49,50]. Being the commensal bacteria of human and animal gut, it happens to be in close contact with numerous other bacteria [51]. However, perhaps the most fascinating thing about *E. coli* is its ability to pass on its genetic-resistant traits to microorganisms who share the same living environment, as well as to acquire resistance genes from them [52–54].

According to Poirel et al. [52] *E. coli* present a bacterium with a special place in the microbiological world since it can cause severe infections in humans and animals, and on the other hand represents a significant part of the autochthonous microbiota of the various hosts. The main apprehension is a transmission of virulent and resistant *E. coli* among animals and humans through various pathways. *E. coli* is a most important reservoir of resistance genes that may be accountable for treatment failures in both human and veterinary medicine [52]. An increasing number of resistance genes has been identified in *E. coli* isolates in the past 10 years, and many of these resistance genes were acquired by horizontal gene transfer. In the enterobacterial gene pool, *E. coli* acts as a donor and as a recipient of resistance genes and thereby can acquire resistance genes from other bacteria but can also pass on its resistance genes to other bacteria. Antimicrobial resistance in *E. coli* is considered one of the foremost disputes in both humans and animals at a global scale and needs to be considered as a real public health concern.

Barrios-Villa et al. [55] have observed increased evidence demonstrating the association between Crohn's Disease (CD), a type of Inflammatory Bowel Disease (IBD), and non-diarrheagenic Adherent/Invasive *E. coli* (AIEC) isolates. Genomes of five AIEC strains isolated from individuals without IBD were sequenced and compared with AIEC prototype strains (LF82 and NRG857c), and with extra-intestinal uropathogenic strain (UPEC CFT073). Non-IBD-AIEC strains showed an Average Nucleotide Identity up to 98% compared with control strains. Blast identities of the five non-IBD-AIEC strains were higher when compared to AIEC and UPEC reference strains than with another *E. coli* pathotypes, suggesting a relationship between them [55]. In the same study, Barrios-Villa et al. [55], an incomplete Type VI secretion system was found in non-IBD-AIEC strains; however, the Type II secretion system was complete. Several groups of genes reported in AIEC strains were searched in the five non-IBD-AIEC strains, and the presence of *fimA*, *fliC*, *fuhD*, *chuA*, *irp2*, and *cvaC* were confirmed. Other virulence factors were detected in non-IBD-AIEC strains, which were absent in AIEC reference strains, including EhaG, non-fimbrial adhesin 1, PapG, F17D-G, YehA/D, FeuC, IucD, CbtA, VgrG-1, Cnf1, and HlyE. Based on the differences in virulence determinants and single-nucleotide polymorphisms (SNPs), it is plausible to suggest that non-IBD AIEC strains belong to a different pathotype.

Meanwhile, genomic analysis of *E. coli* strains isolated from diseased chicken in the Czech Republic [56] showed that multiresistant phenotype was detected in most of the sequenced strains with the predominant resistance to β-lactams and quinolones being associated with TEM-type beta-lactamase genes and chromosomal *gyrA* mutations. The phylogenetic analysis proved a huge variety of isolates that were derived from all groups. Clusters of closely related isolates within ST23 and ST429 indicated a possible local spread of these clones. Moreover, the ST429 cluster carried $bla_{\text{CMY-2,}-59}$ genes for AmpC β-lactamase and isolates of both clusters were well-equipped with virulence-associated genes, with significant variations in allocation of specific virulence-associated genes among phylogenetically distant lineages. Zoonotic APEC STs were also identified, such as ST117, ST354, and ST95, showing numerous molecular elements typical for human ExPEC [56].

As already stated, antibiotic resistance found in microorganisms presents a big challenge for medical practice in the whole world [57–61]. This is to a great extent the consequence of wrong or uncritical consumption of antibiotics.

In a study by Abdelhalim et al. [62], from 17 Crohn's disease patients and 14 healthy controls *E. coli* strains were isolated, 59% and 50% of them were identified as AIEC strains. It was discovered that *chuA* and *ratA* genes were the most significant genetic markers associated with AIEC compared to non-AIEC strains isolated from Crohn's disease patients and healthy controls $p = 0.0119, 0.0094$, respectively. Most *E. coli* strains obtained from Crohn's disease patients showed antibiotic resistance (71%) compared to healthy controls (29%) against at least one antibiotic. Investigation have demonstrated significant differences between AIEC strains and non-AIEC strains in terms of the prevalence of *chuA* and *ratA* virulence genes and the antibiotic resistance profiles. Furthermore, AIEC strains isolated from Crohn's disease patients were found to be more resistant to β-lactam and aminoglycoside antibiotics than AIEC strains isolated from healthy controls [62].

E. coli strains isolated from animals in Tunisia [63] revealed occurrence of plasmid-mediated quinolone resistance between themselves. With 51 nalidixic acid-resistant isolates, 9 PMQR genes were harbored (5 co-harbored *qnrS1* and *qnrB1*, 3 harbored *qnrS1* and 1 harbored *qnrB1*). Two types of mutation in the QRDR of GyrA were observed: S83L and D87N. For the QRDR of ParC, the substitution S80I was observed as well, while A class 1 integron was found in isolates, respectively. The *tetA* or *tetB* gene was observed and both were co-harbored by two isolates. The *sul1*, *sul2*, and *sul3* genes were discovered, respectively. According to the presence of specific virulence genes, the nine strains were classified as UPEC, EAEC, and EPEC [63]. All mentioned highlight the plausible role of the avian industry as a reservoir of human pathogenic *E. coli* strains.

Yu et al. [64] have investigated the prevalence and antimicrobial-resistance phenotypes and genotypes of *E. coli* isolated from raw milk samples from mastitis cases in four regions of China. A total of 83 strains of *E. coli* were isolated and identified, but without any significant differences in the number of *E. coli* isolates detected among the two sampling seasons in the same regions. Nevertheless, a significant difference in *E. coli* prevalence was found among the four different regions. The isolates were most frequently resistant to penicillin (100%), acetylspiramycin (100%), lincomycin (98.8%), oxacillin (98.8%), and sulphamethoxazole (53%). All the *E. coli* strains were multiresistant to three antimicrobial classes, and the most frequent multidrug-resistance patterns for the isolates were resistant to three or four classes of drugs simultaneously [64].

In Egypt, Farhat et al. [65] have investigated the antimicrobial resistance patterns, the distribution of phylogenetic groups, and the prevalence and characteristics of integron-bearing *E. coli* isolates from outpatients with community-acquired urinary tract infections. A total of 134 human urine samples were positive for *E. coli*, from which a total of 80 samples were selected for further analyses. Most of the isolates (62.5%) proved multidrug resistance profiles. Group B2 was the most predominant phylogenetic group (52.5%), followed by group F (21.25%), Clade I or II (12.5%), and finally isolates of unknown phylogroup (13.75%). Of the 80 selected isolates, 7 of them carried class 1 integrons, which contained 3 different types of integrated gene cassettes, conferring resistance to streptomycin, trimethoprim, and some open reading frames of unknown function [65].

Low hygiene levels, lack of clean water, or poor sanitary conditions can create perfect conditions for the development and transmission of infections [66]. In addition to that, Farhani et al. [67] have total of 80 *E. coli* isolates, separated into 51 different genotypes. Using the Multi Locus VNTR Analysis (MLVA) profiles, a minimum spanning tree (MST) algorithm showed two clonal complexes with 71 isolates and only 9 isolates were stayed out of clonal complexes in the form of a singleton. High genotypic diversity was seen among *E. coli* strains isolated from hospital wastewaters; however, many isolates showed a close genetic relationship. Authors have concluded that MLVA as a rapid, inexpensive, and useful tool could be used for analysis of the phylogenetic relationships between *E. coli* strains [67].

Extended-spectrum beta-lactamases (ESBLs) are specific enzymes, which show resistance to almost all beta-lactam antibiotics [68], including penicillin [69], cephalosporin [70], etc. [71]. Cases of infections in which ESBLs are produced usually have quite an unpredictable course. *E. coli* is an example of a multidrug-resistant and ESBL-producing bacterium that can be the source of extremely severe infections [72–74]. As has previously been stated, some strains of *E. coli* can also cause very serious medical conditions connected with urinary and gastrointestinal tract and central nervous system [75]. On the other hand, the side effects of a prolonged usage of antibiotics include the occurrence of antibiotic resistance [76–78]. Today we have evidence that people can get antibiotic-resistant *E. coli* directly or indirectly from the environment [79,80]. Therefore, it is very important that we first evaluate the existence of drug-resistant *E. coli* in our surroundings and based on such findings try to outline the human and veterinary healthcare guidelines [81–86].

This paper aims to describe how people have facilitated the evolution of *E. coli's* antibiotic resistance, while also presenting the specific mechanisms that this bacterium has developed over time to protect itself from the most typically prescribed and consumed antibiotics.

2. Usage of Antibiotics in Different Countries of EU Region and Spread of *E. coli* Resistance to Antibiotics

It is absolutely clear to us today that the antibiotic resistance of *E. coli* and some other bacteria involves a combination of different factors [87,88]. Research results indicate that *E. coli* exhibits the strongest resistance to the longest used and most commonly prescribed antibiotics [89–91]. This is exactly the case with sulfonamides, which were first used in humans around 1930s [92]. Some twenty years later, the first resistant strains of *E. coli* appeared and with time this resistance only grew stronger. It has also been found that low-income [93] and mid-income countries (Table 1) are regions with the highest antibiotic-resistance rates and it is precisely in these regions that we see the highest consumption of antibiotics [94]. On the other hand, high-income nations show a lower rate of antibiotic resistance, resulting from lower usage of antibiotics. In some high-income countries the consumption is high, for example in Belgium, France, and Italy. This is even more complex when comparing to low-income countries where on one hand the consumption may be high but the availability of many of the more advanced antimicrobials is limited [95].

In the 2017 revision of the WHO Model List of Essential Medicines, antibiotics in the list were grouped into three AWaRe categories: Access, Watch, and Reserve. According to the WHO AWaRe categories [96], the classification showed that the Access group antibiotics accounted for more than 50% of total consumption both in Serbia and Spain [93]. The size of the population (in thousands) living in the European Region in 2015 was 912,984, respectively. Of the 53 Member States of the region, none is a low-income country, 20 are middle-income countries, and 33 are high-income countries. The median proportional consumption of the Access group values ranged between 61% in Spain to 64% in Serbia. The median proportion of Watch group antibiotics related to total consumption values ranging from less than 34% in Serbia and 28.5% in Spain. Reserve group antibiotics were only rarely used. The most widely used Reserve group antibiotics were intravenous fosfomycin, followed by cefepime, colistin, linezolid, and daptomycin. The antibiotics assigned to the Other group varied from 1.5% in Serbia to 9.5% in Spain (Figure 1). Overall consumption of antibiotics in these 46 countries ranged from 7.66 to 38.18 DDD per 1000 inhabitants per day. The overall absolute weight (not adjusted by population size) varied from 2.18 ton (Iceland) to 1195.69 tons (Turkey) per year.

Table 1. The consumption of total antibiotics in Defined Daily Doses, in DDD per 1000 inhabitants per day in countries of European region based on WHO database [93].

Country	DDD/1000 Inhabitants Per Day	Country	DDD/1000 Inhabitants Per Day
Albania	16.41	Kosovo	20.18
Armenia	10.31	Kyrgyzstan	17.94
Austria	12.17	Latvia	13.30
Azerbaijan	7.66	Lithuania	15.83
Belarus	17.48	Luxemburg	22.31
Belgium	25.57	Malta	21.88
Bosnia and Herzegovina	17.85	Montenegro	29.33
Bulgaria	20.25	Netherlands	9.78
Croatia	20.28	Norway	16.97
Cyprus	27.14	Poland	24.30
Czech Republic	17.18	Portugal	17.72
Denmark	17.84	North Macedonia	13.42
Estonia	12.13	Romania	28.50
Finland	18.52	Russia	14.82
France	25.92	Serbia	31.57
Georgia	24.44	Slovakia	24.34
Germany	11.49	Slovenia	13.48
Greece	33.85	Spain	17.96
Hungary	16.31	Sweden	13.73
Iceland	17.87	Tajikistan	21.95
Ireland	23.27	Turkey	38.18
Italy	26.62	United Kingdom	20.47
Kazakhstan	17.89	Uzbekistan	8.56

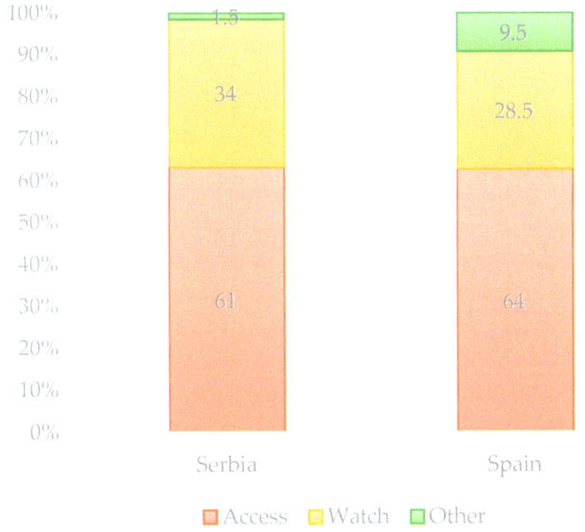

Figure 1. Proportional consumption of antibiotics by AWaRe categorization, % [93,96].

It is a widespread opinion among scientists that antibiotic resistance has developed as the result of human activity and commonly applied treatment with antibiotics [97]. On the other hand, studies of bacteria living inside human body and other environmental bacteria helped us discover many other resistance factors that did not develop over time as a reaction to antibiotics, but were probably part of bacteria genomes in the first place [98–100]. Scientists often refer to those characteristics as the intrinsic resistance of bacteria [101]. It presents a great advantage of that particular bacteria strain, as its main task is to inhibit or eliminate other bacteria that live in the same environment and compete for food [102–104]. Hence, intrinsic resistance is different from the extrinsic antibiotic resistance, which was triggered primarily by human action [105]. In times of constantly growing antibiotic resistance and in a situation when we seem not to have any readily available antibacterial agents, it is extremely important to thoroughly study the intrinsic resistance of bacteria. That could lead to the development of a new method of fight against bacterial resistance [106]. If we could manage somehow to inhibit the factors that intrinsic resistance is composed of, perhaps bacteria would then become highly sensitive to antibiotics again. *E. coli* and other gram-negative bacteria have two important characteristics, which are the foundations of their intrinsic resistance. Namely, they have a protective impermeable membrane and a large number of efflux pumps, which successfully remove all unwanted substances from inside the cell [107–109].

Antibiotic resistance is an ecosystem problem threatening the interrelated human–animal–environment health under the "One Health" framework. Resistant bacteria arising in one geographical area can spread via cross-reservoir transmission to other areas worldwide either by direct exposure or through the food chain and the environment. Drivers of antibiotic resistance are complex and multisectoral particularly in lower- and middle-income countries. These include inappropriate socio-ecological behaviors; poverty; overcrowding; lack of surveillance systems; food supply chain safety issues; highly contaminated waste effluents; and loose rules and regulations. Iskandar et al. [110] have investigated the drivers of antibiotic resistance from a "One Health" perspective. They have summarized the results from many researches that have been conducted over the years and shown that the market failures are the leading cause for the negative externality of antibiotic resistance that extends in scope from the individual to the global ecosystem. Iskandar et al. [110] highlighted that the problem will continue to prevail if governments do not prioritize the "One Health" approach and if individual's accountability is still denied in a world struggling with profound socio-economic problems.

Dsani et al. [111] investigated the spread of *E. coli* isolates from raw meat in Greater Accra region in Ghana, to antibiotics resistance, respectively. Usually, raw meat can be contaminated with antibiotic resistant pathogens and consumption of meat contaminated with antibiotic resistant *E. coli* is associated with grave health care consequences. In their research, *E. coli* was detected in half of raw meat samples. Isolates were resistant to ampicillin (57%), tetracycline (45%), sulfamethoxazole-trimethoprim (21%), and cefuroxime (17%). Multidrug resistance (MDR) was identified in 22% of the isolates. The $bla_{TEM\ gene}$ was detected in 4% of *E. coli* isolates [111]. Dsani et al. [111] concluded that levels of microbial contamination of raw meat in their research were unacceptable and highlighted that meat handlers and consumers are at risk of foodborne infections from *E. coli* including ESBL producing *E. coli*, which is resistant to nearly all antibiotics in use.

According to Hassan et al. [112], a last resort antibiotic is colistin. Colistin is crucial for managing infections with carbapenem-resistant *Enterobacteriaceae*. The recent emergence of mobile-colistin-resistance (*mcr*) genes has jeopardized the efficiency of this antibiotic. Aquaculture is a foremost contributor to the evolution and dissemination of *mcr*. Nevertheless, data on *mcr* in aquaculture are narrow. In Lebanon, a country with developed antimicrobial stewardship the occurrence of *mcr-1* was evaluated in fish. Mobile-colistin-resistance-*1* was detected in 5 *E. coli* isolated from fish intestines. The isolates were classified as multidrug-resistant and their colistin minimum inhibitory concentration ranged between 16 and 32 μg/mL. Whole genome sequencing analysis showed that *mcr-1* was carried on transmissible IncX4 plasmids and that the isolates harbored more than 14 antibiotic resistance genes. The isolates belonged to ST48 and ST101, which have been associated with *mcr* and can occur in humans and fish and help in spreading of antibiotic resistance of *E. coli*.

While, Montealegre et al. [113] have showed how high genomic diversity and heterogeneous origins of pathogenic and antibiotic-resistant *E. coli* in household settings represent a challenge to reducing transmission in low-income settings. Transmission of *E. coli* between hosts and with the environment is believed to happen more frequently in regions with poor sanitation. Montealegre et al. [113] performed whole-genome comparative analyses on 60 *E. coli* isolates from soils and fecal from cattle, chickens, and humans, in households in rural Bangladesh. Results suggest that in rural Bangladesh, a high level of *E. coli* in soil is possible led by contributions from multiple and diverse *E. coli* sources (human and animal) that share an accessory gene pool relatively unique to previously published *E. coli* genomes. Thus, interventions to reduce environmental pathogen or antimicrobial resistance transmission should adopt integrated "One Health" approaches that consider heterogeneous origins and high diversity to improve effectiveness and reduce prevalence and transmission [113].

It has been confirmed that wastewater treatment plant effluents are influenced by hospital wastewaters [114] in Germany. Alexander et al. [114] quantified the abundances of antibiotic resistance genes and facultative pathogenic bacteria as well as one mobile genetic element in genomic DNA via qPCR from 23 different wastewater treatment plant effluents in Germany. Total of 12 clinically relevant antibiotic resistance genes were categorized into frequently, intermediately, and rarely occurring genetic parameters of communal wastewaters. Taxonomic PCR quantifications of 5 facultative pathogenic bacteria targeting *E. coli, P. aeruginosa, K. pneumoniae, A. baumannii,* and enterococci were performed.

Since communal wastewater treatment plants are the direct link to the aquatic environment, wastewater treatment plants should be monitored according to their antibiotic resistance genes and facultative pathogenic bacteria abundances and discharges to decide about the need of advanced treatment options. Critical threshold volumes of hospital wastewaters should be defined to discuss the effect of a decentralized wastewater treatment, because they can serve as an excellent reservoir in spreading of *E. coli* resistance to antibiotic.

3. Inappropriate Prescribing of Antibiotics

According to scientific literature, we are now witnessing a rapid evolution of bacteria and a tremendous increase in multidrug-resistant strains largely due to selective pressure and a long-term interaction between the applied antibiotics and bacteria [115–117]. It seems that antibiotics have been prescribed too often and many times perhaps even inappropriately. When a person has bacterial infection and has been prescribed antibiotic treatment, what normally happens is that all susceptible bacteria get killed. However, together with the pathogenic microorganisms that caused the infection, many other microorganisms found in that specific environment will get eliminated too. On the other hand, if there are some resistant microorganisms in that environment, whether they are pathogenic or not, they will be the ones who will survive, quickly spread and outnumber all others [98,105,107].

We are all aware of the fact that millions of lives have been saved thanks to the discovery of antibiotics [118]. No wonder that this revolutionary medicine has often been considered as the "miracle drug" [118]. Unfortunately, antibiotics have been prescribed too often and sometimes even when it was not absolutely necessary [119]. Nowadays, we have a global problem, which presents an enormous threat to healthcare systems around the world. What is even more alarming is that in many countries there has not been an adequate response to this crisis. The abuse of antibiotics is still a major issue. According to the global antibiotic sales database, when we compare antibiotic consumption for the years 2000 and 2015, we can see an evident increase from around 11 doses per 1000 inhabitants per day to almost 16, which is an increase of almost 40% for the period of five years [120]. Having analyzed the statistics, together with research findings, it seems that the mean value for antibiotic consumption was largely influenced by low-income and mid-income countries [121]. These countries appear to have the largest number of multidrug-resistant bacterial infections. An even bigger problem is that studies show a considerable increase in the consumption of antibiotics such as carbapenems and colistin, which should be prescribed when everything else fails [122,123]. This could perhaps explain the emergence of *E. coli* strains resistant to precisely these antibiotics. Scientists claim that in the past there were some only very rare cases of resistance of *E. coli* to carbapenems (depending on the part of the world in question), but that in the future we may see a great increase of resistance to carbapenems [124,125]. This is mainly because of the existence of the enzymes called carbapenemases, which break down carbapenems and make them ineffective [126]. These enzymes with versatile hydrolytic capacities are plasmid-encoded and easily transmitted [127].

Medicines including vaccines are a critical component in the management of both infectious diseases and noncommunicable diseases reflected in global sales of medicines likely to exceed 1.5 trillion € by the end of 2023 and currently growing at a compounded annual growth rate of 3 to 6% [128]. Medicines also play a critical role in lower- and middle-income countries, which is in accordance with previously findings of Iskandar et al. [110]. Because usually these costs are "out-of-pocket", there can be devastating outcomes for families when some of the members turn out to be sick. These outcomes and apprehensions are aggravated by the WHO assessing that more than half of all medicines are prescribed inappropriately, with approximately half of all patients failing to take them correctly [128].

Antibiotic resistance poses a great threat to human, animal, and environmental health. Beta-Lactam antibiotics have been successful in combating bacterial infections. Still, the overuse, inappropriate prescribing, unavailability of new antibiotics, and regulation barriers have exacerbated bacterial resistance to these antibiotics. 1,4,7-Triazacyclononane (TACN) is a cyclic organic tridentate inhibitor with strong metal-chelating abilities that has been shown to inhibit β-lactamase enzymes and may represent an important breakthrough in the treatment of drug-resistant *E. coli* bacterial strains. However, its cytotoxicity in the liver is unknown [129].

Antimicrobial stewardship is a foundation of endeavors to reduce antimicrobial resistance. To determine factors potentially influencing probability of prescribing antimicrobials for pet animals, Singleton et al. [130] analyzed electronic health records for unwell dogs (n = 155,732 unique dogs, 281,543 consultations) and cats (n = 69,236 unique cats, 111,139 consultations) voluntarily contributed by 173 UK veterinary practices. Results of their pet animal study demonstrate the potential of preventive healthcare and client engagement to encourage responsible antimicrobial drug use [130].

Robbins et al. [131] investigated the antimicrobial prescribing practices in small animal emergency and critical care. According to authors antimicrobial use contributes to emergence of antimicrobial resistance [131]. They have assumed that antimicrobial prescribing behavior varies between the emergency and critical care services in a veterinary teaching hospital, so they tried to investigate antimicrobial prescribing patterns, assess adherence to stewardship principles, and to evaluate the prevalence of multidrug-resistant (MDR) bacterial isolates. Robbins et al. [131] after investigation, which showed that the most prescribed antibiotics in emergence was amoxicillin, metronidazole, and ampicillin with the most common reasons for antimicrobial prescriptions being skin disease, gastrointestinal disease, and respiratory disease. Regarding the critical care, authors have recorded most prescribed ampicillin, enrofloxacin, and metronidazole, with the most common reasons for antimicrobial prescriptions such as gastrointestinal disease, respiratory diseases, and sepsis. Robbins et al. [131] concluded that antimicrobial prescription was common with comparable patterns. However, devotion to guidelines for urinary and respiratory infections was poor.

Lehner et al. [132] conducted the study with the objective to investigate antimicrobial prescriptions by Swiss veterinarians before and after introduction of the online ASP AntibioticScout.ch in December 2016. In the methodology, authors have used a retrospective study, where the prescriptions of antimicrobials in 2016 and 2018 were compared and their appropriateness was assessed by a justification score. The results of the study revealed that percentage of dogs prescribed antimicrobials decreased significantly between 2016 and 2018, which led to a conclusion that antimicrobials were used more carefully. The study highlights the continued need for ASPs in veterinary medicine [132].

Not only the regular hospitals and veterinary clinics have a problem with inappropriate prescribing of antibiotics, but the dentist's clinics also have the same problem. Antibiotic resistance is a global public health problem. Around 55% of dental antibiotic prescribing is deemed inappropriate [133]. Evidence to that issue can be seen from an experiment where a total of 26 dentists were recruited for the 12-week study using a pre–post design. For six weeks, dentists self-recorded their prescription of antibiotics, analgesics, and anxiolytics. After dentists were provided education and website access, they recorded their prescription for a further six weeks. Results of the experiment reveled a substantial reduction of 44.6% in the number of inappropriate indications for which antibiotics were prescribed after the intervention and a decrease of 40.5% in the total number of antibiotics. Paracetamol with codeine substantially reduced by 56.8%. For the highly prescribed antibiotics amoxicillin, phenoxymethylpenicillin, and metronidazole, there was an improvement in the accuracy of the prescriptions ranging from 0–64.7 to 74.2–100% [133].

It is especially important that such a type of experiment showed the intervention of targeted education and the prescribing tool was effective in improving dental prescribing, knowledge, and confidence of practitioners, as well as providing an effective antibiotic stewardship tool. This context-specific intervention shows substantial promise for implementation into not only in dental practice, but veterinary and other medical practices as well.

One of the main factors that contribute to the growing antibiotic-resistance is the over-prescription of antibiotics [134]. Unfortunately, research shows that in more than 70% of cases, doctors in the US prescribed the wrong antibiotics [135]. Evidently, it is both the overuse and the inappropriate choice of antibiotics that we can blame for the antibiotic resistance that bacteria have evolved over the years [136]. In many cases, the prescribed antibiotics are suitable for acute respiratory tract infections [137–140], while for example ciprofloxacin is one of the antibiotics that is prescribed too often and inappropriately, and no wonder that *E. coli* is highly resistant to it [141,142]. Another very interesting finding shows that humans and animals with diarrhea used antibiotics quite frequently before they started experiencing the mentioned symptoms [143–145]. This could lead us to the conclusion that perhaps the previously used antibiotics had potentially disrupted the gut microbiota and resulted in the excessive number of pathogenic organisms resistant to drugs [117].

4. Mechanisms of β-Lactams Resistance towards *E. coli*

The Gram-negative bacteria called *Enterobacteriaceae* is known for its amazing capacity to become resistant to many different types of antibiotics [146,147]. *Klebsiella* and *E. coli* are the bacteria that cause the largest number of infections in humans [148], and are most often mentioned when speaking of multidrug-resistant bacteria [74,127,149]. Unfortunately, we are witnesses to the fact that *E. coli* has been increasingly developing strains that are insusceptible to the most common types of antibiotics, such as β-lactams, sulfonamides, fosfomycin, etc. [70,71,88,150]. What presents an even greater concern for doctors and scientists these days is that *E. coli* reveals resistance even to carbapenems and polymyxins, which are considered by many as the last resort antibiotics [151].

If we analyze the molecular structure of beta-lactams, we can see that they consist of the so-called β-lactam ring, which is supposed to inhibit the synthesis of the bacterial cell wall [70]. Beta-lactam antibiotics are specially targeted at bacterial enzymes called penicillin-binding proteins (PBPs) [152]. Unfortunately for us, bacteria have developed several methods of protection against β-lactams [153]:

1. Production of β-lactamases, which render β-lactams ineffective
2. Inhibited penetration of antibiotics to the intended location
3. Modification of the target site PBPs
4. Activation of efflux pumps

In more concrete terms, *E. coli* produces enzymes that are called "beta-lactamases" [154]. They are quite old compounds with over 2800 unique proteins [155]. The classification of β-lactamases is based on their function and structure [156]. Throughout literature, the most frequently used classification of beta-lactamases is the Ambler classification [157]. It focuses on the similarity of structure and according to this classification we can divide proteins into four main groups: the classes A, C, and D of serine-β-lactamases and the class B of metallo-β-lactamases [157].

Gram-negative bacteria are capable of producing different β-lactamases [156]. From the scientific point of view, the most important beta-lactamases that *E. coli* produces are carbapenemases [158], the extended-spectrum beta-lactamases (ESBL) [159], and AmpC beta-lactamases (AmpC) [160].

4.1. *Prevalence of Antibiotic Resistance in E. coli Isolates by Disk Diffusion Method*

Prevalence of selected antibiotic resistance in *E. coli* strains isolated from humans and pet animals is shown in Figures 2 and 3.

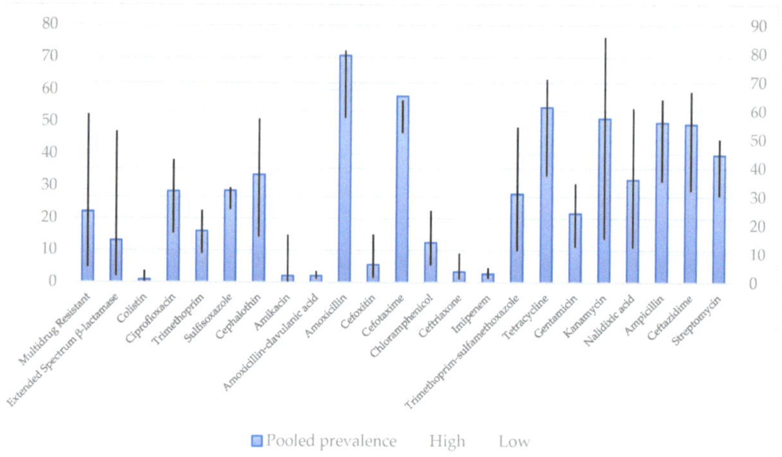

Figure 2. Pooled prevalence of antibiotic resistance isolates in humans by disk diffusion method, % [161].

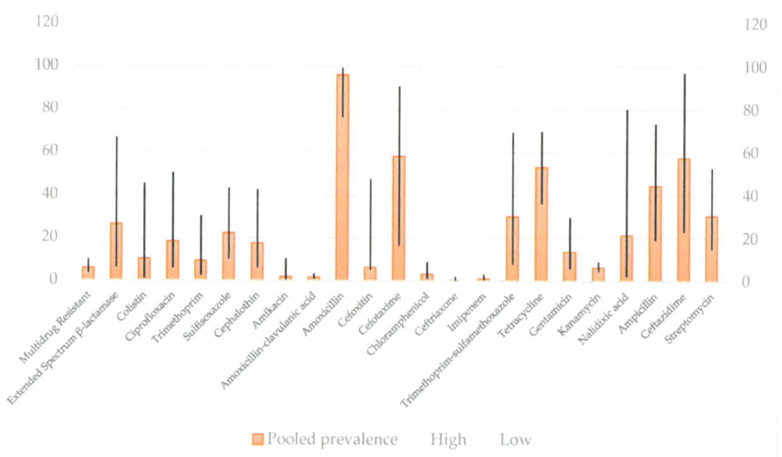

Figure 3. Pooled prevalence of antibiotic resistance isolates in pet animals by disk diffusion method, % [161].

As shown in Figure 2, highest rate of resistance of *E. coli* to amoxicillin were observed while the lowest rate of resistance was observed in colistin.

The same case as in Figure 2 was shown in Figure 3 regarding the resistance of *E. coli* to amoxicillin in pet animals, while the lowest rate of resistance was observed in ceftriaxone, respectively. This analysis nicely illustrates the evolution of antibiotic resistance and can be used for describing drug-resistance prevalence in the most recent *E. coli* strains. What is more, it shows a significantly higher prevalence of extended-spectrum beta-lactamase in pet animal isolates than in human isolates.

4.2. *Prevalence of Antibiotic Resistance in E. coli Isolates by Minimum Inhibitory Concentration*

Prevalence of selected antibiotic resistance in *E. coli* strains isolated from humans and pet animals by minimum inhibitory concentration (MIC) method is shown in Figures 4 and 5.

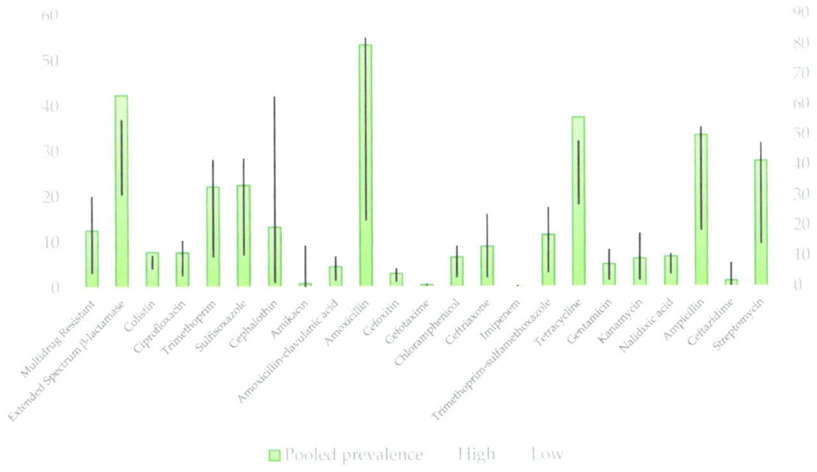

Figure 4. Pooled prevalence of antibiotic resistance isolates in humans by minimum inhibitory concentration, % [161].

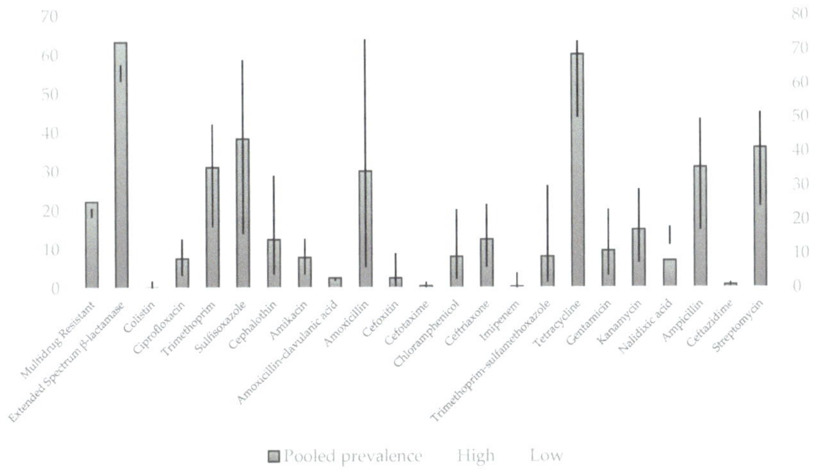

Figure 5. Pooled prevalence of antibiotic resistance isolates in pet animals by minimum inhibitory concentration, % [161].

As shown in Figure 4, in *E. coli* strains obtained from humans, the bacterium showed the lowest resistance to imipenem, while it exhibited the highest resistance to amoxicillin. These data are not completely in accordance with the data shown in Figure 2, where the lowest rate of resistance was observed in colistin, compared to those ones recorded for imipenem, respectively [161].

When pet animal isolates were analyzed, the lowest resistance rate was found for colistin, while the highest resistance was exhibited to tetracycline. Compared to isolates in pet animals by disk diffusion method (Figure 3), the lowest resistance identified was to ceftriaxone, while the highest resistance was found to amoxicillin, which is in accordance with data showed in Figure 5 obtained by the MIC method.

5. Conclusions

E. coli colonizes human and animals' gut, which facilitates its spreading from fecal matter to the mouth. Due to its fascinating capacity to transfer drug resistance to other microorganisms and also acquire it from others that share the same environment, we can speak of *E. coli's* huge evolutionary advantage. The antibiotic resistance genes are located on plasmids, which enables the easy horizontal spread of antibiotic resistance among different bacteria and, thus, poses a serious threat to medicine. With time, *E. coli* has developed several methods for neutralizing the power of antibiotics. Unfortunately, only one strain of *E. coli* can possess resistance genes that can fight off several different types of antibiotics, which makes the whole situation even more complicated for patients with bacterial infections.

The phenomenon of antibiotic resistance in bacteria is multifactorial and depends on an interplay of a number of factors, but the common denominator is clearly the overuse of antibiotics, both in humans and animals. Therefore, the whole world is seriously in need of antibiotic or antimicrobial stewardship programs, which are supposed to prevent the overuse of antibiotics and, thus, reduce antibiotic resistance. On the other hand, all that is not enough if some socioeconomic issues remain unresolved, such as poor hygiene, lack of drinking water, or bad living conditions and overcrowded households. These factors only add to the severity of the problem of antibiotic resistance and go beyond simply restricting the consumption of antibiotics. Obviously, knowing all of the above-mentioned facts, the solution to the problem of antibiotic or multidrug resistance is not a simple one, but requires integrated efforts on all sides. It is of vital importance to closely and continuously monitor hygiene conditions in hospitals as well as waste disposal methods. As far as the treatment of patients with bacterial infections is concerned, such patients need to be carefully examined in order to bring the right decision regarding the choice of antibiotic to be given. We need to continue evaluating antibiotic-sensitivity in humans and animals while also working on the development and implementation of reliable antibiotic strategies.

If we tackle this issue seriously and responsibly and undertake all the necessary corrective actions, we may regain control over *E. coli* infections, both in Europe and the whole world.

Author Contributions: Conceptualization, N.P.; methodology, N.P.; software, N.P.; validation, N.P.; formal analysis, N.P.; investigation, N.P.; resources, N.P.; data curation, N.P.; writing—original draft preparation, N.P.; writing—review and editing, R.d.L.F.; visualization, N.P.; supervision, R.d.L.F.; project administration, N.P.; funding acquisition, N.P. All authors have read and agreed to the published version of the manuscript.

Funding: This research was funded by the Ministry for Education, Science and Technological Development of the Republic of Serbia.

Data Availability Statement: Data is contained within the article.

Acknowledgments: This research is supported by COST Action CA18217—European Network for Optimization of Veterinary Antimicrobial Treatment.

Conflicts of Interest: The authors declare no conflict of interest. The funders had no role in the design of the study; in the collection, analyses, or interpretation of data; in the writing of the manuscript, or in the decision to publish the results.

References

1. Hill, R.A.; Hunt, J.; Sanders, E.; Tran, M.; Burk, G.A.; Mlsna, T.E.; Fitzkee, N.C. Effect of Biochar on Microbial Growth: A Metabolomics and Bacteriological Investigation in *E. Coli*. *Environ. Sci. Technol.* **2019**, *53*, 2635–2646. [CrossRef] [PubMed]
2. Lovley, D.R.; Holmes, D.E. Protein Nanowires: The Electrification of the Microbial World and Maybe Our Own. *J. Bacteriol.* **2020**, *202*, e00331-20. [CrossRef] [PubMed]
3. Ranganathan, S.; Smith, E.M.; Abel, J.D.F.; Barry, E.M. Research in a Time of Enteroids and Organoids: How the Human Gut Model Has Transformed the Study of Enteric Bacterial Pathogens. *Gut Microbes* **2020**, *12*, 1795492. [CrossRef] [PubMed]
4. Macklin, D.N.; Horst, T.A.A.; Choi, H.; Ruggero, N.A.; Carrera, J.; Mason, J.C.; Sun, G.; Agmon, E.; DeFelice, M.M.; Maayan, I.; et al. Simultaneous Cross-Evaluation of Heterogeneous *E. Coli* Datasets via Mechanistic Simulation. *Science* **2020**, *369*, eaav3751. [CrossRef] [PubMed]
5. Micenková, L.; Bosák, J.; Smatana, S.; Novotný, A.; Budinská, E.; Šmajs, D. Administration of the Probiotic Escherichia Coli Strain A0 34/86 Resulted in a Stable Colonization of the Human Intestine During the First Year of Life. *Probiot. Antimicrob. Prot.* **2020**, *12*, 343–350. [CrossRef] [PubMed]
6. Bittinger, K.; Zhao, C.; Li, Y.; Ford, E.; Friedman, E.S.; Ni, J.; Kulkarni, C.V.; Cai, J.; Tian, Y.; Liu, Q.; et al. Bacterial Colonization Reprograms the Neonatal Gut Metabolome. *Nat. Microbiol.* **2020**, *5*, 838–847. [CrossRef]
7. Secher, T.; Brehin, C.; Oswald, E. Early Settlers: Which *E. Coli* Strains Do You Not Want at Birth? *Am. J. Physiol. Gastrointest. Liver Physiol.* **2016**, *311*, G123–G129. [CrossRef]
8. Rossi, E.; Cimdins, A.; Lüthje, P.; Brauner, A.; Sjöling, Å.; Landini, P.; Römling, U. "It's a Gut Feeling"—*Escherichia Coli* Biofilm Formation in the Gastrointestinal Tract Environment. *Crit. Rev. Microbiol.* **2018**, *44*, 1–30. [CrossRef]
9. Zhang, S.; Abbas, M.; Rehman, M.U.; Huang, Y.; Zhou, R.; Gong, S.; Yang, H.; Chen, S.; Wang, M.; Cheng, A. Dissemination of Antibiotic Resistance Genes (ARGs) via Integrons in Escherichia Coli: A Risk to Human Health. *Environ. Pollut.* **2020**, *266*, 115260. [CrossRef]
10. Abebe, E.; Gugsa, G.; Ahmed, M. Review on Major Food-Borne Zoonotic Bacterial Pathogens. *J. Trop. Med.* **2020**, *2020*, 4674235. [CrossRef]
11. Isla, A.L.; Polo, J.M.; Isa, M.A.; Sala, R.B.; Sutil, R.S.; Quintas, J.J.; Moradillo, J.G.; Padilla, D.A.G.; Rojo, E.G.; Martínez, J.B.P.; et al. Urinary Infections in Patients with Catheters in the Upper Urinary Tract: Microbiological Study. *Urol. Int.* **2017**, *98*, 442–448. [CrossRef] [PubMed]
12. Rodrigues, W.; Miguel, C.; Nogueira, A.; Vieira, C.U.; Paulino, T.; Soares, S.; De Resende, E.; Chica, J.L.; Araújo, M.; Oliveira, C. Antibiotic Resistance of Bacteria Involved in Urinary Infections in Brazil: A Cross-Sectional and Retrospective Study. *Int. J. Environ. Res. Public Health* **2016**, *13*, 918. [CrossRef]
13. Song, D.W.; Park, B.K.; Suh, S.W.; Lee, S.E.; Kim, J.W.; Park, J.-M.; Kim, H.R.; Lee, M.-K.; Choi, Y.S.; Kim, B.G.; et al. Bacterial Culture and Antibiotic Susceptibility in Patients with Acute Appendicitis. *Int. J. Colorectal Dis.* **2018**, *33*, 441–447. [CrossRef] [PubMed]
14. Park, J.; Kim, S.; Lim, H.; Liu, A.; Hu, S.; Lee, J.; Zhuo, H.; Hao, Q.; Matthay, M.A.; Lee, J.-W. Therapeutic Effects of Human Mesenchymal Stem Cell Microvesicles in an Ex Vivo Perfused Human Lung Injured with Severe *E. Coli* Pneumonia. *Thorax* **2019**, *74*, 43–50. [CrossRef]
15. Zhao, W.-D.; Liu, D.-X.; Wei, J.-Y.; Miao, Z.-W.; Zhang, K.; Su, Z.-K.; Zhang, X.-W.; Li, Q.; Fang, W.-G.; Qin, X.-X.; et al. Caspr1 Is a Host Receptor for Meningitis-Causing Escherichia Coli. *Nat. Commun.* **2018**, *9*, 2296. [CrossRef] [PubMed]
16. Akuzawa, N.; Kurabayashi, M. Native Valve Endocarditis Due to Escherichia Coli Infection: A Case Report and Review of the Literature. *BMC Cardiovasc. Disord.* **2018**, *18*, 195. [CrossRef]
17. Sarowska, J.; Koloch, B.F.; Kmiecik, A.J.; Madrzak, M.F.; Ksiazczyk, M.; Ploskonska, G.B.; Krol, I.C. Virulence Factors, Prevalence and Potential Transmission of Extraintestinal Pathogenic Escherichia Coli Isolated from Different Sources: Recent Reports. *Gut Pathog.* **2019**, *11*, 10. [CrossRef]
18. Poolman, J.T.; Anderson, A.S. Escherichia Coli and Staphylococcus Aureus: Leading Bacterial Pathogens of Healthcare Associated Infections and Bacteremia in Older-Age Populations. *Expert Rev. Vaccines* **2018**, *17*, 607–618. [CrossRef]
19. Kubone, P.Z.; Mlisana, K.P.; Govinden, U.; Abia, A.L.K.; Essack, S.Y. Antibiotic Susceptibility and Molecular Characterization of Uropathogenic Escherichia Coli Associated with Community-Acquired Urinary Tract Infections in Urban and Rural Settings in South Africa. *Trop. Med. Infect. Dis.* **2020**, *5*, 176. [CrossRef]
20. Djordjevic, Z.; Folic, M.; Jankovic, S. Community-Acquired Urinary Tract Infections: Causative Agents and Their Resistance to Antimicrobial Drugs. *Vojnosanit. Pregl.* **2016**, *73*, 1109–1115. [CrossRef]
21. Gaynes, R. The Discovery of Penicillin—New Insights After More Than 75 Years of Clinical Use. *Emerg. Infect. Dis.* **2017**, *23*, 849–853. [CrossRef]
22. Hutchings, M.I.; Truman, A.W.; Wilkinson, B. Antibiotics: Past, Present and Future. *Curr. Opin. Microbiol.* **2019**, *51*, 72–80. [CrossRef] [PubMed]
23. Dodds, D.R. Antibiotic Resistance: A Current Epilogue. *Biochem. Pharmacol.* **2017**, *134*, 139–146. [CrossRef] [PubMed]

24. Aminov, R. History of Antimicrobial Drug Discovery: Major Classes and Health Impact. *Biochem. Pharmacol.* **2017**, *133*, 4–19. [CrossRef] [PubMed]
25. de Opitz, C.L.M.; Sass, P. Tackling Antimicrobial Resistance by Exploring New Mechanisms of Antibiotic Action. *Future Microbiol.* **2020**, *15*, 703–708. [CrossRef]
26. Gajdács, M.; Albericio, F. Antibiotic Resistance: From the Bench to Patients. *Antibiotics* **2019**, *8*, 129. [CrossRef]
27. Coates, A.R.M.; Hu, Y.; Holt, J.; Yeh, P. Antibiotic Combination Therapy against Resistant Bacterial Infections: Synergy, Rejuvenation and Resistance Reduction. *Expert Rev. Anti Infect. Ther.* **2020**, *18*, 5–15. [CrossRef]
28. Wong, J.W.; Ip, M.; Tang, A.; Wei, V.W.; Wong, S.Y.; Riley, S.; Read, J.M.; Kwok, K.O. Prevalence and Risk Factors of Community-Associated Methicillin-Resistant Staphylococcus Aureus Carriage in Asia-Pacific Region from 2000 to 2016: A Systematic Review and Meta-Analysis. *Clin. Epidemiol.* **2018**, *10*, 1489–1501. [CrossRef]
29. Adeiza, S.S.; Onaolapo, J.A.; Olayinka, B.O. Prevalence, Risk-Factors, and Antimicrobial Susceptibility Profile of Methicillin-Resistant Staphylococcus Aureus (MRSA) Obtained from Nares of Patients and Staff of Sokoto State-Owned Hospitals in Nigeria. *GMS Hyg. Infect. Control* **2020**, *15*, Doc25. [CrossRef]
30. Queenan, K.; Häsler, B.; Rushton, J. A One Health Approach to Antimicrobial Resistance Surveillance: Is There a Business Case for It? *Int. J. Antimicrob. Agents* **2016**, *48*, 422–427. [CrossRef]
31. Tillotson, G.S.; Zinner, S.H. Burden of Antimicrobial Resistance in an Era of Decreasing Susceptibility. *Expert Rev. Anti Infect. Ther.* **2017**, *15*, 663–676. [CrossRef] [PubMed]
32. Heward, E.; Cullen, M.; Hobson, J. Microbiology and Antimicrobial Susceptibility of Otitis Externa: A Changing Pattern of Antimicrobial Resistance. *J. Laryngol. Otol.* **2018**, *132*, 314–317. [CrossRef]
33. Cillóniz, C.; Ardanuy, C.; Vila, J.; Torres, A. What Is the Clinical Relevance of Drug-Resistant Pneumococcus? *Curr. Opin. Pulm. Med.* **2016**, *22*, 227–234. [CrossRef] [PubMed]
34. Roman, A.C.; Roman, J.V.; Flores, M.A.V.; Villaseñor, H.F.; Vidal, J.E.; Amador, S.M.; Llanos, A.M.G.; Nuñez, E.G.; Serrano, J.M.; Pastrana, G.T.; et al. Detection of Antimicrobial-Resistance Diarrheagenic Escherichia Coli Strains in Surface Water Used to Irrigate Food Products in the Northwest of Mexico. *Int. J. Food Microbiol.* **2019**, *304*, 1–10. [CrossRef] [PubMed]
35. Relhan, N.; Pathengay, A.; Schwartz, S.G.; Flynn, H.W. Emerging Worldwide Antimicrobial Resistance, Antibiotic Stewardship and Alternative Intravitreal Agents for the Treatment of Endophthalmitis. *Retina* **2017**, *37*, 811–818. [CrossRef] [PubMed]
36. Tomičić, Z.; Čabarkapa, I.; Čolović, R.; Đuragić, O.; Tomičić, R. Salmonella in the Feed Industry: Problems and Potential Solutions. *J. Agron. Technol. Eng. Manag.* **2019**, *2*, 130–137.
37. Serwecińska, L.; Kiedrzyńska, E.; Kiedrzyński, M. A Catchment-Scale Assessment of the Sanitary Condition of Treated Wastewater and River Water Based on Fecal Indicators and Carbapenem-Resistant Acinetobacter Spp. *Sci. Total Environ.* **2021**, *750*, 142266. [CrossRef] [PubMed]
38. Tagliabue, A.; Rappuoli, R. Changing Priorities in Vaccinology: Antibiotic Resistance Moving to the Top. *Front. Immunol.* **2018**, *9*, 1068. [CrossRef] [PubMed]
39. Mutairi, R.A.; Tovmasyan, A.; Haberle, I.B.; Benov, L. Sublethal Photodynamic Treatment Does Not Lead to Development of Resistance. *Front. Microbiol.* **2018**, *9*, 1699. [CrossRef] [PubMed]
40. Hong, J.; Hu, J.; Ke, F. Experimental Induction of Bacterial Resistance to the Antimicrobial Peptide Tachyplesin I and Investigation of the Resistance Mechanisms. *Antimicrob. Agents Chemother.* **2016**, *60*, 6067–6075. [CrossRef]
41. van den Bergh, B.; Michiels, J.E.; Fauvart, M.; Michiels, J. Should We Develop Screens for Multi-Drug Antibiotic Tolerance? *Expert Rev. Anti Infect. Ther.* **2016**, *14*, 613–616. [CrossRef] [PubMed]
42. Spagnolo, F.; Rinaldi, C.; Sajorda, D.R.; Dykhuizen, D.E. Evolution of Resistance to Continuously Increasing Streptomycin Concentrations in Populations of Escherichia Coli. *Antimicrob. Agents Chemother.* **2016**, *60*, 1336–1342. [CrossRef] [PubMed]
43. Iakovides, I.C.; Kordatou, I.M.; Moreira, N.F.F.; Ribeiro, A.R.; Fernandes, T.; Pereira, M.F.R.; Nunes, O.C.; Manaia, C.M.; Silva, A.M.T.; Kassinos, D.F. Continuous Ozonation of Urban Wastewater: Removal of Antibiotics, Antibiotic-Resistant Escherichia Coli and Antibiotic Resistance Genes and Phytotoxicity. *Water Res.* **2019**, *159*, 333–347. [CrossRef] [PubMed]
44. Dass, S.C.; Bosilevac, J.M.; Weinroth, M.; Elowsky, C.G.; Zhou, Y.; Anandappa, A.; Wang, R. Impact of Mixed Biofilm Formation with Environmental Microorganisms on *E. Coli* O157:H7 Survival against Sanitization. *NPJ Sci. Food* **2020**, *4*, 16. [CrossRef]
45. Khan, S.; Imran, A.; Malik, A.; Chaudhary, A.A.; Rub, A.; Jan, A.T.; Syed, J.B.; Rolfo, C. Bacterial Imbalance and Gut Pathologies: Association and Contribution of *E. Coli* in Inflammatory Bowel Disease. *Crit. Rev. Clin. Lab. Sci.* **2019**, *56*, 1–17. [CrossRef] [PubMed]
46. Danson, A.E.; McStea, A.; Wang, L.; Pollitt, A.Y.; Fernandez, M.L.M.; Moraes, I.; Walsh, M.A.; MacIntyre, S.; Watson, K.A. Super-Resolution Fluorescence Microscopy Reveals Clustering Behaviour of Chlamydia Pneumoniae's Major Outer Membrane Protein. *Biology* **2020**, *9*, 344. [CrossRef]
47. Pereira, R.V.; Altier, C.; Siler, J.D.; Mann, S.; Jordan, D.; Warnick, L.D. Longitudinal Effects of Enrofloxacin or Tulathromycin Use in Preweaned Calves at High Risk of Bovine Respiratory Disease on the Shedding of Antimicrobial-Resistant Fecal Escherichia Coli. *J. Dairy Sci.* **2020**, *103*, 10547–10559. [CrossRef]
48. Ellis, S.J.; Crossman, L.C.; McGrath, C.J.; Chattaway, M.A.; Hölken, J.M.; Brett, B.; Bundy, L.; Kay, G.L.; Wain, J.; Schüller, S. Identification and Characterisation of Enteroaggregative Escherichia Coli Subtypes Associated with Human Disease. *Sci. Rep.* **2020**, *10*, 7475. [CrossRef]

49. Kwong, L.H.; Ercumen, A.; Pickering, A.J.; Arsenault, J.E.; Islam, M.; Parvez, S.M.; Unicomb, L.; Rahman, M.; Davis, J.; Luby, S.P. Ingestion of Fecal Bacteria along Multiple Pathways by Young Children in Rural Bangladesh Participating in a Cluster-Randomized Trial of Water, Sanitation, and Hygiene Interventions (WASH Benefits). *Environ. Sci. Technol.* **2020**, *54*, 13828–13838. [CrossRef]
50. Lauridsen, H.C.M.; Vallance, B.A.; Krogfelt, K.A.; Petersen, A.M. *Escherichia Coli* Pathobionts Associated with Inflammatory Bowel Disease. *Clin. Microbiol. Rev.* **2019**, *32*, e00060-18. [CrossRef]
51. Lopes, J.G.; Sourjik, V. Chemotaxis of Escherichia Coli to Major Hormones and Polyamines Present in Human Gut. *ISME J.* **2018**, *12*, 2736–2747. [CrossRef] [PubMed]
52. Poirel, L.; Madec, J.-Y.; Lupo, A.; Schink, A.-K.; Kieffer, N.; Nordmann, P.; Schwarz, S. Antimicrobial Resistance in *Escherichia coli*. In *Antimicrobial Resistance in Bacteria from Livestock and Companion Animals*; Schwarz, S., Cavaco, L.M., Shen, J., Eds.; ASM Press: Washington, DC, USA, 2018; pp. 289–316. ISBN 978-1-68367-052-0.
53. Card, R.M.; Cawthraw, S.A.; Garcia, J.N.; Ellis, R.J.; Kay, G.; Pallen, M.J.; Woodward, M.J.; Anjum, M.F. An In Vitro Chicken Gut Model Demonstrates Transfer of a Multidrug Resistance Plasmid from Salmonella to Commensal Escherichia Coli. *mBio* **2017**, *8*, e00777-17. [CrossRef] [PubMed]
54. Ramiro, R.S.; Durão, P.; Bank, C.; Gordo, I. Low Mutational Load and High Mutation Rate Variation in Gut Commensal Bacteria. *PLoS Biol.* **2020**, *18*, e3000617. [CrossRef] [PubMed]
55. Villa, E.B.; de la Peña, C.F.M.; Zaraín, P.L.; Cevallos, M.A.; Torres, C.; Torres, A.G.; Gracia, R.d.C.R. Comparative Genomics of a Subset of Adherent/Invasive Escherichia Coli Strains Isolated from Individuals without Inflammatory Bowel Disease. *Genomics* **2020**, *112*, 1813–1820. [CrossRef] [PubMed]
56. Papouskova, A.; Masarikova, M.; Valcek, A.; Senk, D.; Cejkova, D.; Jahodarova, E.; Cizek, A. Genomic Analysis of Escherichia Coli Strains Isolated from Diseased Chicken in the Czech Republic. *BMC Vet. Res.* **2020**, *16*, 189. [CrossRef]
57. Aslam, B.; Wang, W.; Arshad, M.I.; Khurshid, M.; Muzammil, S.; Rasool, M.H.; Nisar, M.A.; Alvi, R.F.; Aslam, M.A.; Qamar, M.U.; et al. Antibiotic Resistance: A Rundown of a Global Crisis. *Infect. Drug Resist.* **2018**, *11*, 1645–1658. [CrossRef]
58. Mihankhah, A.; Khoshbakht, R.; Raeisi, M.; Raeisi, V. Prevalence and Antibiotic Resistance Pattern of Bacteria Isolated from Urinary Tract Infections in Northern Iran. *J. Res. Med. Sci.* **2017**, *22*, 108. [CrossRef]
59. Millan, A.S. Evolution of Plasmid-Mediated Antibiotic Resistance in the Clinical Context. *Trends Microbiol.* **2018**, *26*, 978–985. [CrossRef]
60. Ljubojević, D.; Velhner, M.; Todorović, D.; Pajić, M.; Milanov, D. Tetracycline Resistance in Escherichia Coli Isolates from Poultry. *Arch. Vet. Med.* **2016**, *9*, 61–81. [CrossRef]
61. Puvača, N.; Lika, E.; Tufarelli, V.; Bursić, V.; Ljubojević Pelić, D.; Nikolova, N.; Petrović, A.; Prodanović, R.; Vuković, G.; Lević, J.; et al. Influence of Different Tetracycline Antimicrobial Therapy of Mycoplasma (Mycoplasma Synoviae) in Laying Hens Compared to Tea Tree Essential Oil on Table Egg Quality and Antibiotics Residues. *Foods* **2020**, *9*, 612. [CrossRef]
62. Abdelhalim, K.A.; Uzel, A.; Ünal, N.G. Virulence Determinants and Genetic Diversity of Adherent-Invasive Escherichia Coli (AIEC) Strains Isolated from Patients with Crohn's Disease. *Microb. Pathog.* **2020**, *145*, 104233. [CrossRef] [PubMed]
63. Kilani, H.; Ferjani, S.; Mansouri, R.; Benboubaker, I.B.; Abbassi, M.S. Occurrence of Plasmid-Mediated Quinolone Resistance Determinants among Escherichia Coli Strains Isolated from Animals in Tunisia: Specific Pathovars Acquired Qnr Genes. *J. Glob. Antimicrob. Resist.* **2020**, *20*, 50–55. [CrossRef] [PubMed]
64. Yu, Z.N.; Wang, J.; Ho, H.; Wang, Y.T.; Huang, S.N.; Han, R.W. Prevalence and Antimicrobial-Resistance Phenotypes and Genotypes of Escherichia Coli Isolated from Raw Milk Samples from Mastitis Cases in Four Regions of China. *J. Glob. Antimicrob. Resist.* **2020**, *22*, 94–101. [CrossRef] [PubMed]
65. Farahat, E.M.; Hassuna, N.A.; Hammad, A.M.; Abdel Fattah, M.; Khairalla, A.S. Distribution of Integrons and Phylogenetic Groups among *Escherichia Coli* Causing Community-acquired Urinary Tract Infection in Upper Egypt. *Can. J. Microbiol.* **2020**, cjm-2020-0292. [CrossRef] [PubMed]
66. Ramay, B.M.; Caudell, M.A.; Rosales, C.C.; Archila, L.D.; Palmer, G.H.; Jarquin, C.; Moreno, P.; McCracken, J.P.; Rosenkrantz, L.; Amram, O.; et al. Antibiotic Use and Hygiene Interact to Influence the Distribution of Antimicrobial-Resistant Bacteria in Low-Income Communities in Guatemala. *Sci. Rep.* **2020**, *10*, 13767. [CrossRef]
67. Farahani, O.; Ranjbar, R.; Jahromy, S.H.; Arabzadeh, B. Multilocus Variable-Number Tandem-Repeat Analysis for Genotyping of Escherichia Coli Strains Isolated from Hospital Wastewater, Tehran, Iran. *Iran J. Public Health* **2020**, *49*, 4829. [CrossRef]
68. Riquelme, F.M.; Hernández, E.C.; Soto, M.G.; Ruiz, M.E.; Marí, J.M.N.; Fernández, J.G. Clinical Relevance of Antibiotic Susceptibility Profiles for Screening Gram-Negative Microorganisms Resistant to Beta-Lactam Antibiotics. *Microorganisms* **2020**, *8*, 1555. [CrossRef]
69. Kapoor, G.; Saigal, S.; Elongavan, A. Action and Resistance Mechanisms of Antibiotics: A Guide for Clinicians. *J. Anaesthesiol. Clin. Pharmacol.* **2017**, *33*, 300–305. [CrossRef]
70. Rahman, S.U.; Ali, T.; Ali, I.; Khan, N.A.; Han, B.; Gao, J. The Growing Genetic and Functional Diversity of Extended Spectrum Beta-Lactamases. *BioMed Res. Int.* **2018**, *2018*, 9519718. [CrossRef]
71. Doma, A.O.; Popescu, R.; Mitulețu, M.; Muntean, D.; Dégi, J.; Boldea, M.V.; Radulov, I.; Dumitrescu, E.; Muselin, F.; Puvača, N.; et al. Comparative Evaluation of QnrA, QnrB, and QnrS Genes in Enterobacteriaceae Ciprofloxacin-Resistant Cases, in Swine Units and a Hospital from Western Romania. *Antibiotics* **2020**, *9*, 698. [CrossRef]

72. Rilo, M.P.; Martín, C.-B.G.; Fernández, E.P.; Vilaró, A.; Fraile, L.; Martínez, S.M. Antimicrobial Resistance Genes in Porcine Pasteurella Multocida Are Not Associated with Its Antimicrobial Susceptibility Pattern. *Antibiotics* **2020**, *9*, 614. [CrossRef] [PubMed]
73. Torban, A.S.; Venezia, S.N.; Kelmer, E.; Cohen, A.; Paitan, Y.; Arielly, H.; Steinman, A. Extended-Spectrum β-Lactamase-Producing Enterobacterles Shedding by Dogs and Cats Hospitalized in an Emergency and Critical Care Department of a Veterinary Teaching Hospital. *Antibiotics* **2020**, *9*, 545. [CrossRef] [PubMed]
74. Falgenhauer, L.; Schwengers, O.; Schmiedel, J.; Baars, C.; Lambrecht, O.; Heß, S.; Berendonk, T.U.; Falgenhauer, J.; Chakraborty, T.; Imirzalioglu, C. Multidrug-Resistant and Clinically Relevant Gram-Negative Bacteria Are Present in German Surface Waters. *Front. Microbiol.* **2019**, *10*, 2779. [CrossRef] [PubMed]
75. Santos, A.C.d.M.; Santos, F.F.; Silva, R.M.; Gomes, T.A.T. Diversity of Hybrid- and Hetero-Pathogenic Escherichia Coli and Their Potential Implication in More Severe Diseases. *Front. Cell Infect. Microbiol.* **2020**, *10*, 339. [CrossRef] [PubMed]
76. Qiu, W.; Sun, J.; Fang, M.; Luo, S.; Tian, Y.; Dong, P.; Xu, B.; Zheng, C. Occurrence of Antibiotics in the Main Rivers of Shenzhen, China: Association with Antibiotic Resistance Genes and Microbial Community. *Sci. Total Environ.* **2019**, *653*, 334–341. [CrossRef]
77. Sanganyado, E.; Gwenzi, W. Antibiotic Resistance in Drinking Water Systems: Occurrence, Removal, and Human Health Risks. *Sci. Total Environ.* **2019**, *669*, 785–797. [CrossRef]
78. Mölstad, S.; Löfmark, S.; Carlin, K.; Erntell, M.; Aspevall, O.; Blad, L.; Hanberger, H.; Hedin, K.; Hellman, J.; Norman, C.; et al. Lessons Learnt during 20 Years of the Swedish Strategic Programme against Antibiotic Resistance. *Bull. World Health Organ.* **2017**, *95*, 764–773. [CrossRef]
79. Osińska, A.; Korzeniewska, E.; Harnisz, M.; Niestępski, S. The Prevalence and Characterization of Antibiotic-Resistant and Virulent Escherichia Coli Strains in the Municipal Wastewater System and Their Environmental Fate. *Sci. Total Environ.* **2017**, *577*, 367–375. [CrossRef]
80. Montealegre, M.C.; Roy, S.; Böni, F.; Hossain, M.I.; Daneshmand, T.N.; Caduff, L.; Faruque, A.S.G.; Islam, M.A.; Julian, T.R. Risk Factors for Detection, Survival, and Growth of Antibiotic-Resistant and Pathogenic *Escherichia Coli* in Household Soils in Rural Bangladesh. *Appl. Environ. Microbiol.* **2018**, *84*, e01978-18. [CrossRef]
81. Kaesbohrer, A.; Lebl, K.B.; Irrgang, A.; Fischer, J.; Kämpf, P.; Schiffmann, A.; Werckenthin, C.; Busch, M.; Kreienbrock, L.; Hille, K. Diversity in Prevalence and Characteristics of ESBL/PAmpC Producing *E. Coli* in Food in Germany. *Vet. Microbiol.* **2019**, *233*, 52–60. [CrossRef]
82. Marano, R.B.M.; Fernandes, T.; Manaia, C.M.; Nunes, O.; Morrison, D.; Berendonk, T.U.; Kreuzinger, N.; Tenson, T.; Corno, G.; Kassinos, D.F.; et al. A Global Multinational Survey of Cefotaxime-Resistant Coliforms in Urban Wastewater Treatment Plants. *Environ. Int.* **2020**, *144*, 106035. [CrossRef] [PubMed]
83. Gardy, J.L.; Loman, N.J. Towards a Genomics-Informed, Real-Time, Global Pathogen Surveillance System. *Nat. Rev. Genet* **2018**, *19*, 9–20. [CrossRef] [PubMed]
84. Ferran, A.A.; Lacroix, M.Z.; Mélou, A.B.; Duhil, I.; Roques, B.B. Levers to Improve Antibiotic Treatment of Lambs via Drinking Water in Sheep Fattening Houses: The Example of the Sulfadimethoxine/Trimethoprim Combination. *Antibiotics* **2020**, *9*, 561. [CrossRef] [PubMed]
85. Vilaró, A.; Novell, E.; Tarancón, V.E.; Balielles, J.; Vilalta, C.; Martinez, S.; Fraile Sauce, L.J. Antimicrobial Susceptibility Pattern of Porcine Respiratory Bacteria in Spain. *Antibiotics* **2020**, *9*, 402. [CrossRef] [PubMed]
86. Mileva, R.; Karadaev, M.; Fasulkov, I.; Petkova, T.; Rusenova, N.; Vasilev, N.; Milanova, A. Oxytetracycline Pharmacokinetics After Intramuscular Administration in Cows with Clinical Metritis Associated with Trueperella Pyogenes Infection. *Antibiotics* **2020**, *9*, 392. [CrossRef]
87. Martens, E.; Demain, A.L. The Antibiotic Resistance Crisis, with a Focus on the United States. *J. Antibiot.* **2017**, *70*, 520–526. [CrossRef]
88. Padmini, N.; Ajilda, A.A.K.; Sivakumar, N.; Selvakumar, G. Extended Spectrum β-Lactamase Producing *Escherichia Coli* and *Klebsiella Pneumoniae*: Critical Tools for Antibiotic Resistance Pattern. *J. Basic Microbiol.* **2017**, *57*, 460–470. [CrossRef]
89. Sharaha, U.; Diaz, E.R.; Riesenberg, K.; Bigio, I.J.; Huleihel, M.; Salman, A. Using Infrared Spectroscopy and Multivariate Analysis to Detect Antibiotics' Resistant *Escherichia Coli* Bacteria. *Anal. Chem.* **2017**, *89*, 8782–8790. [CrossRef]
90. Moradigaravand, D.; Palm, M.; Farewell, A.; Mustonen, V.; Warringer, J.; Parts, L. Prediction of Antibiotic Resistance in Escherichia Coli from Large-Scale Pan-Genome Data. *PLoS Comput. Biol.* **2018**, *14*, e1006258. [CrossRef]
91. Lukačišinová, M.; Fernando, B.; Bollenbach, T. Highly Parallel Lab Evolution Reveals That Epistasis Can Curb the Evolution of Antibiotic Resistance. *Nat. Commun.* **2020**, *11*, 3105. [CrossRef]
92. Swain, S.S.; Paidesetty, S.K.; Padhy, R.N. Phytochemical Conjugation as a Potential Semisynthetic Approach toward Reactive and Reuse of Obsolete Sulfonamides against Pathogenic Bacteria. *Drug Dev. Res.* **2020**, ddr.21746. [CrossRef] [PubMed]
93. World Health Organization. *WHO Report on Surveillance of Antibiotic Consumption: 2016–2018 Early Implementation*; World Health Organization: Geneva, Switzerland, 2018; p. 128.
94. Colson, A.R.; Megiddo, I.; Uria, G.A.; Gandra, S.; Bedford, T.; Morton, A.; Cooke, R.M.; Laxminarayan, R. Quantifying Uncertainty about Future Antimicrobial Resistance: Comparing Structured Expert Judgment and Statistical Forecasting Methods. *PLoS ONE* **2019**, *14*, e0219190. [CrossRef] [PubMed]

95. Sartelli, M.C.; Hardcastle, T.; Catena, F.; Mefire, A.C.; Coccolini, F.; Dhingra, S.; Haque, M.; Hodonou, A.; Iskandar, K.; Labricciosa, F.M.; et al. Antibiotic Use in Low and Middle-Income Countries and the Challenges of Antimicrobial Resistance in Surgery. *Antibiotics* **2020**, *9*, 497. [CrossRef]
96. Hsia, Y.; Sharland, M.; Jackson, C.; Wong, I.C.K.; Magrini, N.; Bielicki, J.A. Consumption of Oral Antibiotic Formulations for Young Children According to the WHO Access, Watch, Reserve (AWaRe) Antibiotic Groups: An Analysis of Sales Data from 70 Middle-Income and High-Income Countries. *Lancet Infect. Dis.* **2019**, *19*, 67–75. [CrossRef]
97. Yan, W.; Xiao, Y.; Yan, W.; Ding, R.; Wang, S.; Zhao, F. The Effect of Bioelectrochemical Systems on Antibiotics Removal and Antibiotic Resistance Genes: A Review. *Chem. Eng. J.* **2019**, *358*, 1421–1437. [CrossRef]
98. Xie, J.; Jin, L.; He, T.; Chen, B.; Luo, X.; Feng, B.; Huang, W.; Li, J.; Fu, P.; Li, X. Bacteria and Antibiotic Resistance Genes (ARGs) in $PM_{2.5}$ from China: Implications for Human Exposure. *Environ. Sci. Technol.* **2019**, *53*, 963–972. [CrossRef]
99. Palme, J.B.; Kristiansson, E.; Larsson, D.G.J. Environmental Factors Influencing the Development and Spread of Antibiotic Resistance. *FEMS Microbiol. Rev.* **2018**, *42*, fux053. [CrossRef]
100. Merrikh, H.; Kohli, R.M. Targeting Evolution to Inhibit Antibiotic Resistance. *FEBS J.* **2020**, *287*, 4341–4353. [CrossRef]
101. Marine, J.-C.; Dawson, S.-J.; Dawson, M.A. Non-Genetic Mechanisms of Therapeutic Resistance in Cancer. *Nat. Rev. Cancer* **2020**, *20*, 743–756. [CrossRef]
102. Heir, E.; Møretrø, T.; Simensen, A.; Langsrud, S. Listeria Monocytogenes Strains Show Large Variations in Competitive Growth in Mixed Culture Biofilms and Suspensions with Bacteria from Food Processing Environments. *Int. J. Food Microbiol.* **2018**, *275*, 46–55. [CrossRef]
103. Stubbendieck, R.M.; May, D.S.; Chevrette, M.G.; Temkin, M.I.; Pienkowski, E.W.; Cagnazzo, J.; Carlson, C.M.; Gern, J.E.; Currie, C.R. Competition among Nasal Bacteria Suggests a Role for Siderophore-Mediated Interactions in Shaping the Human Nasal Microbiota. *Appl. Environ. Microbiol.* **2018**, *85*, e02406-18. [CrossRef] [PubMed]
104. de Filippis, F.; Pasolli, E.; Ercolini, D. The Food-Gut Axis: Lactic Acid Bacteria and Their Link to Food, the Gut Microbiome and Human Health. *FEMS Microbiol. Rev.* **2020**, *44*, 454–489. [CrossRef] [PubMed]
105. Iwu, C.D.; Korsten, L.; Okoh, A.I. The Incidence of Antibiotic Resistance within and beyond the Agricultural Ecosystem: A Concern for Public Health. *Microbiol. Open* **2020**, *9*, e1035. [CrossRef] [PubMed]
106. Calap, P.D.; Martínez, J.D. Bacteriophages: Protagonists of a Post-Antibiotic Era. *Antibiotics* **2018**, *7*, 66. [CrossRef]
107. Reygaert, W.C. An Overview of the Antimicrobial Resistance Mechanisms of Bacteria. *AIMS Microbiol.* **2018**, *4*, 482–501. [CrossRef]
108. Wang, Y.; Alenazy, R.; Gu, X.; Polyak, S.W.; Zhang, P.; Sykes, M.J.; Zhang, N.; Venter, H.; Ma, S. Design and Structural Optimization of Novel 2H-Benzo[h]Chromene Derivatives That Target AcrB and Reverse Bacterial Multidrug Resistance. *Eur. J. Med. Chem.* **2020**, 113049. [CrossRef]
109. Impey, R.E.; Hawkins, D.A.; Sutton, J.M.; da Costa, T.P.S. Overcoming Intrinsic and Acquired Resistance Mechanisms Associated with the Cell Wall of Gram-Negative Bacteria. *Antibiotics* **2020**, *9*, 623. [CrossRef]
110. Iskandar, K.; Molinier, L.; Hallit, S.; Sartelli, M.; Catena, F.; Coccolini, F.; Craig Hardcastle, T.; Roques, C.; Salameh, P. Drivers of Antibiotic Resistance Transmission in Low- and Middle-Income Countries from a "One Health" Perspective—A Review. *Antibiotics* **2020**, *9*, 372. [CrossRef]
111. Dsani, E.; Afari, E.A.; Appiah, A.D.; Kenu, E.; Kaburi, B.B.; Egyir, B. Antimicrobial Resistance and Molecular Detection of Extended Spectrum β-Lactamase Producing Escherichia Coli Isolates from Raw Meat in Greater Accra Region, Ghana. *BMC Microbiol.* **2020**, *20*, 253. [CrossRef]
112. Hassan, J.; Eddine, R.Z.; Mann, D.; Li, S.; Deng, X.; Saoud, I.P.; Kassem, I.I. The Mobile Colistin Resistance Gene, Mcr-1.1, Is Carried on IncX4 Plasmids in Multidrug Resistant E. Coli Isolated from Rainbow Trout Aquaculture. *Microorganisms* **2020**, *8*, 1636. [CrossRef]
113. Montealegre, M.C.; Rodríguez, A.T.; Roy, S.; Hossain, M.I.; Islam, M.A.; Lanza, V.F.; Julian, T.R. High Genomic Diversity and Heterogenous Origins of Pathogenic and Antibiotic-Resistant *Escherichia Coli* in Household Settings Represent a Challenge to Reducing Transmission in Low-Income Settings. *mSphere* **2020**, *5*, e00704-19. [CrossRef] [PubMed]
114. Alexander, J.; Hembach, N.; Schwartz, T. Evaluation of Antibiotic Resistance Dissemination by Wastewater Treatment Plant Effluents with Different Catchment Areas in Germany. *Sci. Rep.* **2020**, *10*, 8952. [CrossRef] [PubMed]
115. Pang, X.; Li, D.; Zhu, J.; Cheng, J.; Liu, G. Beyond Antibiotics: Photo/Sonodynamic Approaches for Bacterial Theranostics. *Nano Micro Lett.* **2020**, *12*, 144. [CrossRef]
116. Durão, P.; Balbontín, R.; Gordo, I. Evolutionary Mechanisms Shaping the Maintenance of Antibiotic Resistance. *Trends Microbiol.* **2018**, *26*, 677–691. [CrossRef]
117. Ivanov, I.I.; Frutos, R.d.L.; Manel, N.; Yoshinaga, K.; Rifkin, D.B.; Sartor, R.B.; Finlay, B.B.; Littman, D.R. Specific Microbiota Direct the Differentiation of IL-17-Producing T-Helper Cells in the Mucosa of the Small Intestine. *Cell Host Microbe.* **2008**, *4*, 337–349. [CrossRef]
118. Lobanovska, M.; Pilla, G. Penicillin's Discovery and Antibiotic Resistance: Lessons for the Future? *Yale J. Biol. Med.* **2017**, *90*, 135–145.
119. Lartey, S.F.; Yee, M.; Gaarslev, C.; Khan, R. Why Do General Practitioners Prescribe Antibiotics for Upper Respiratory Tract Infections to Meet Patient Expectations: A Mixed Methods Study. *BMJ Open* **2016**, *6*, e012244. [CrossRef]
120. Chui, C.S.L.; Cowling, B.J.; Lim, W.W.; Hui, C.K.M.; Chan, E.W.; Wong, I.C.K.; Wu, P. Patterns of Inpatient Antibiotic Use Among Public Hospitals in Hong Kong from 2000 to 2015. *Drug Saf.* **2020**, *43*, 595–606. [CrossRef]

121. Osoro, A.A.; Atitwa, E.B.; Moturi, J.K. Universal Health Coverage. *WJSSR* **2020**, *7*, p14. [CrossRef]
122. Tsao, L.-H.; Hsin, C.-Y.; Liu, H.-Y.; Chuang, H.-C.; Chen, L.-Y.; Lee, Y.-J. Risk Factors for Healthcare-Associated Infection Caused by Carbapenem-Resistant Pseudomonas Aeruginosa. *J. Microbiol. Immunol. Infect.* **2018**, *51*, 359–366. [CrossRef]
123. Dhesi, Z.; Enne, V.I.; O'Grady, J.; Gant, V.; Livermore, D.M. Rapid and Point-of-Care Testing in Respiratory Tract Infections: An Antibiotic Guardian? *ACS Pharmacol. Transl. Sci.* **2020**, *3*, 401–417. [CrossRef] [PubMed]
124. David, S.; Reuter, S.; Harris, S.R.; Glasner, C.; Feltwell, T.; Argimon, S.; Abudahab, K.; Goater, R.; Giani, T.; Errico, G.; et al. Epidemic of Carbapenem-Resistant Klebsiella Pneumoniae in Europe Is Driven by Nosocomial Spread. *Nat. Microbiol.* **2019**, *4*, 1919–1929. [CrossRef] [PubMed]
125. Codjoe, F.; Donkor, E. Carbapenem Resistance: A Review. *Med. Sci.* **2017**, *6*, 1. [CrossRef]
126. Pitout, J.D.D.; Peirano, G.; Kock, M.M.; Strydom, K.-A.; Matsumura, Y. The Global Ascendency of OXA-48-Type Carbapenemases. *Clin. Microbiol. Rev.* **2019**, *33*, e00102-19. [CrossRef] [PubMed]
127. Paterson, D.L.; Bonomo, R.A. Multidrug-Resistant Gram-Negative Pathogens: The Urgent Need for 'Old' Polymyxins. In *Polymyxin Antibiotics: From Laboratory Bench to Bedside*; Li, J., Nation, R.L., Kaye, K.S., Eds.; Advances in Experimental Medicine and Biology; Springer International Publishing: Cham, The Netherlands, 2019; Volume 1145, pp. 9–13. ISBN 978-3-030-16371-6.
128. Godman, B. Ongoing Initiatives to Improve the Prescribing of Medicines across Sectors and the Implications. *Adv. Hum. Biol.* **2020**, *10*, 85. [CrossRef]
129. Mcoyi, S.; Amoako, D.G.; Somboro, A.M.; Khumalo, H.M.; Khan, R.B. The Molecular Effect of 1,4,7-triazacyclononane on Oxidative Stress Parameters in Human Hepatocellular Carcinoma (HepG2) Cells. *J. Biochem. Mol. Toxicol.* **2020**, *34*, e22607. [CrossRef] [PubMed]
130. Singleton, D.A.; Pinchbeck, G.L.; Radford, A.D.; Arsevska, E.; Dawson, S.; Jones, P.H.; Noble, P.-J.M.; Williams, N.J.; Sánchez-Vizcaíno, F. Factors Associated with Prescription of Antimicrobial Drugs for Dogs and Cats, United Kingdom, 2014–2016. *Emerg. Infect. Dis.* **2020**, *26*, 1778–1791. [CrossRef]
131. Robbins, S.N.; Goggs, R.; Lhermie, G.; Paul, D.F.L.; Menard, J. Antimicrobial Prescribing Practices in Small Animal Emergency and Critical Care. *Front. Vet. Sci.* **2020**, *7*, 110. [CrossRef]
132. Lehner, C.; Hubbuch, A.; Schmitt, K.; Regula, G.S.; Willi, B.; Mevissen, M.; Peter, R.; Muentener, C.R.; Naegeli, H.; Schuller, S. Effect of Antimicrobial Stewardship on Antimicrobial Prescriptions for Selected Diseases of Dogs in Switzerland. *J. Vet. Intern. Med.* **2020**, *34*, 2418–2431. [CrossRef]
133. Teoh, L.; Stewart, K.; Marino, R.J.; McCullough, M.J. Improvement of Dental Prescribing Practices Using Education and a Prescribing Tool: A Pilot Intervention Study. *Br. J. Clin. Pharmacol.* **2020**, 4373. [CrossRef]
134. Bansal, R.; Jain, A.; Goyal, M.; Singh, T.; Sood, H.; Malviya, H.S. Antibiotic Abuse during Endodontic Treatment: A Contributing Factor to Antibiotic Resistance. *J. Fam. Med. Prim Care* **2019**, *8*, 3518–3524. [CrossRef]
135. Nadeem, S.F.; Gohar, U.F.; Tahir, S.F.; Mukhtar, H.; Pornpukdeewattana, S.; Nukthamna, P.; Moula Ali, A.M.; Bavisetty, S.C.B.; Massa, S. Antimicrobial Resistance: More than 70 Years of War between Humans and Bacteria. *Crit. Rev. Microbiol.* **2020**, *46*, 578–599. [CrossRef] [PubMed]
136. Podolsky, S.H. The Evolving Response to Antibiotic Resistance (1945–2018). *Palgrave Commun.* **2018**, *4*, 124. [CrossRef]
137. Choez, X.S.; Acurio, M.L.A.; Sotomayor, R.E.J. Appropriateness and Adequacy of Antibiotic Prescription for Upper Respiratory Tract Infections in Ambulatory Health Care Centers in Ecuador. *BMC Pharmacol. Toxicol.* **2018**, *19*, 46. [CrossRef]
138. Brink, A.J.; van Wyk, J.; Moodley, V.M.; Corcoran, C.; Ekermans, P.; Nutt, L.; Boyles, T.; Perovic, O.; Feldman, C.; Richards, G.; et al. The Role of Appropriate Diagnostic Testing in Acute Respiratory Tract Infections: An Antibiotic Stewardship Strategy to Minimise Diagnostic Uncertainty in Primary Care. *S. Afr. Med. J.* **2016**, *106*, 554. [CrossRef] [PubMed]
139. Teratani, Y.; Hagiya, H.; Koyama, T.; Adachi, M.; Ohshima, A.; Zamami, Y.; Tanaka, H.Y.; Tatebe, Y.; Tasaka, K.; Mikami, N.; et al. Pattern of Antibiotic Prescriptions for Outpatients with Acute Respiratory Tract Infections in Japan, 2013–15: A Retrospective Observational Study. *Fam. Pract.* **2019**, *36*, 402–409. [CrossRef]
140. Stuart, B.; Brotherwood, H.; van't Hoff, C.; Brown, A.; van den Bruel, A.; Hay, A.D.; Moore, M.; Little, P. Exploring the Appropriateness of Antibiotic Prescribing for Common Respiratory Tract Infections in UK Primary Care. *J. Antimicrob. Chemother.* **2019**, *75*, dkz410. [CrossRef]
141. Pouwels, K.B.; Pebody, B.M.; Smieszek, T.; Hopkins, S.; Robotham, J.V. Selection and Co-Selection of Antibiotic Resistances among Escherichia Coli by Antibiotic Use in Primary Care: An Ecological Analysis. *PLoS ONE* **2019**, *14*, e0218134. [CrossRef]
142. Shively, N.R.; Buehrle, D.J.; Clancy, C.J.; Decker, B.K. Prevalence of Inappropriate Antibiotic Prescribing in Primary Care Clinics within a Veterans Affairs Health Care System. *Antimicrob. Agents Chemother.* **2018**, *62*, e00337-18. [CrossRef]
143. Roess, A.; Leibler, J.H.; Graham, J.P.; Lowenstein, C.; Waters, W.F. Animal Husbandry Practices and Perceptions of Zoonotic Infectious Disease Risks Among Livestock Keepers in a Rural Parish of Quito, Ecuador. *Am. J. Trop. Med. Hyg.* **2016**, *95*, 1450–1458. [CrossRef]
144. Riddle, M.S.; Connor, B.A.; Beeching, N.J.; DuPont, H.L.; Hamer, D.H.; Kozarsky, P.; Libman, M.; Steffen, R.; Taylor, D.; Tribble, D.R.; et al. Guidelines for the Prevention and Treatment of Travelers' Diarrhea: A Graded Expert Panel Report. *J. Travel Med.* **2017**, *24*, S63–S80. [CrossRef] [PubMed]
145. Giallourou, N.; Medlock, G.L.; Bolick, D.T.; Medeiros, P.H.; Ledwaba, S.E.; Kolling, G.L.; Tung, K.; Guerry, P.; Swann, J.R.; Guerrant, R.L. A Novel Mouse Model of Campylobacter Jejuni Enteropathy and Diarrhea. *PLoS Pathog.* **2018**, *14*, e1007083. [CrossRef] [PubMed]

146. Vergalli, J.; Bodrenko, I.V.; Masi, M.; Moynié, L.; Gutiérrez, S.A.; Naismith, J.H.; Regli, A.D.; Ceccarelli, M.; van den Berg, B.; Winterhalter, M.; et al. Porins and Small-Molecule Translocation across the Outer Membrane of Gram-Negative Bacteria. *Nat. Rev. Microbiol.* **2020**, *18*, 164–176. [CrossRef] [PubMed]
147. Arzanlou, M.; Chai, W.C.; Venter, H. Intrinsic, Adaptive and Acquired Antimicrobial Resistance in Gram-Negative Bacteria. *Essays Biochem.* **2017**, *61*, 49–59. [CrossRef] [PubMed]
148. Dunn, S.J.; Connor, C.; McNally, A. The Evolution and Transmission of Multi-Drug Resistant Escherichia Coli and Klebsiella Pneumoniae: The Complexity of Clones and Plasmids. *Curr. Opin. Microbiol.* **2019**, *51*, 51–56. [CrossRef]
149. Kayastha, K.; Dhungel, B.; Karki, S.; Adhikari, B.; Banjara, M.R.; Rijal, K.R.; Ghimire, P. Extended-Spectrum β-Lactamase-Producing *Escherichia Coli* and *Klebsiella* Species in Pediatric Patients Visiting International Friendship Children's Hospital, Kathmandu, Nepal. *Infect. Dis. (Auckl.)* **2020**, *13*, 117863372090979. [CrossRef]
150. Feria, C. Patterns and Mechanisms of Resistance to Beta-Lactams and Beta-Lactamase Inhibitors in Uropathogenic Escherichia Coli Isolated from Dogs in Portugal. *J. Antimicrob. Chemother.* **2002**, *49*, 77–85. [CrossRef]
151. Liu, J.; Huang, Z.; Ruan, B.; Wang, H.; Chen, M.; Rehman, S.; Wu, P. Quantitative Proteomic Analysis Reveals the Mechanisms of Polymyxin B Toxicity to Escherichia Coli. *Chemosphere* **2020**, *259*, 127449. [CrossRef]
152. Sharifzadeh, S.; Dempwolff, F.; Kearns, D.B.; Carlson, E.E. Harnessing β-Lactam Antibiotics for Illumination of the Activity of Penicillin-Binding Proteins in *Bacillus Subtilis*. *ACS Chem. Biol.* **2020**, *15*, 1242–1251. [CrossRef]
153. Decuyper, L.; Jukič, M.; Sosič, I.; Žula, A.; D'hooghe, M.; Gobec, S. Antibacterial and β-Lactamase Inhibitory Activity of Monocyclic β-Lactams. *Med. Res. Rev.* **2018**, *38*, 426–503. [CrossRef]
154. Hameed, A.S.H.; Louis, G.; Karthikeyan, C.; Thajuddin, N.; Ravi, G. Impact of L-Arginine and l-Histidine on the Structural, Optical and Antibacterial Properties of Mg Doped ZnO Nanoparticles Tested against Extended-Spectrum Beta-Lactamases (ESBLs) Producing Escherichia Coli. *Spectrochim. Acta Part A Mol. Biomol. Spectrosc.* **2019**, *211*, 373–382. [CrossRef] [PubMed]
155. Andersson, D.I.; Balaban, N.Q.; Baquero, F.; Courvalin, P.; Glaser, P.; Gophna, U.; Kishony, R.; Molin, S.; Tønjum, T. Antibiotic Resistance: Turning Evolutionary Principles into Clinical Reality. *FEMS Microbiol. Rev.* **2020**, *44*, 171–188. [CrossRef] [PubMed]
156. Bush, K. Past and Present Perspectives on β-Lactamases. *Antimicrob. Agents Chemother.* **2018**, *62*, e01076-18. [CrossRef] [PubMed]
157. Silveira, M.C.; da Silva, R.A.; da Mota, F.F.; Catanho, M.; Jardim, R.; Guimarães, A.C.R.; de Miranda, A.B. Systematic Identification and Classification of β-Lactamases Based on Sequence Similarity Criteria: β-Lactamase Annotation. *Evol. Bioinform. Online* **2018**, *14*, 117693431879735. [CrossRef] [PubMed]
158. Both, A.; Huang, J.; Kaase, M.; Hezel, J.; Wertheimer, D.; Fenner, I.; Günther, T.; Grundhoff, A.; Büttner, H.; Aepfelbacher, M.; et al. First Report of Escherichia Coli Co-Producing NDM-1 and OXA-232. *Diagn. Microbiol. Infect. Dis.* **2016**, *86*, 437–438. [CrossRef]
159. Montso, K.P.; Dlamini, S.B.; Kumar, A.; Ateba, C.N. Antimicrobial Resistance Factors of Extended-Spectrum Beta-Lactamases Producing *Escherichia Coli* and *Klebsiella Pneumoniae* Isolated from Cattle Farms and Raw Beef in North-West Province, South Africa. *BioMed Res. Int.* **2019**, *2019*, 4318306. [CrossRef]
160. Aguirre, L.; Vidal, A.; Seminati, C.; Tello, M.; Redondo, N.; Darwich, L.; Martín, M. Antimicrobial Resistance Profile and Prevalence of Extended-Spectrum Beta-Lactamases (ESBL), AmpC Beta-Lactamases and Colistin Resistance (Mcr) Genes in Escherichia Coli from Swine between 1999 and 2018. *Porc. Health Manag.* **2020**, *6*, 8. [CrossRef]
161. Pormohammad, A.; Nasiri, M.J.; Azimi, T. Prevalence of Antibiotic Resistance in Escherichia Coli Strains Simultaneously Isolated from Humans, Animals, Food, and the Environment: A Systematic Review and Meta-Analysis. *Infect. Drug Resist.* **2019**, *12*, 1181–1197. [CrossRef]

antibiotics

Article

Antibiotic Susceptibility of *Staphylococcus* Species Isolated in Raw Chicken Meat from Retail Stores

Erinda Lika [1], Nikola Puvača [2,3,*], Dejan Jeremić [4], Slobodan Stanojević [5], Tana Shtylla Kika [1], Sonila Cocoli [1] and Rosa de Llanos Frutos [2]

1 Faculty of Veterinary Medicine, Agricultural University of Tirana, Koder Kamez, 1029 Tirana, Albania; elika@ubt.edu.al (E.L.); tana.shtylla@ubt.edu.al (T.S.K.); scocoli@ubt.edu.al (S.C.)
2 Faculty of Health, Jaume I University, Avinguda de Vicent Sos Baynat, s/n, 12071 Castelló de la Plana, Spain; dellanos@uji.es
3 Department of Engineering Management in Biotechnology, Faculty of Economics and Engineering Management in Novi Sad, University Business Academy in Novi Sad, Cvećarska 2, 21000 Novi Sad, Serbia
4 Faculty of Business and Financial Studies, University of Business Studies in Banja Luka, Jovana Dučića 23a, 78000 Banja Luka, Bosnia and Herzegovina; djeremic@sequestergroup.com
5 Faculty of Applied Management, Economics and Finance, University Business Academy in Novi Sad, Jevrejska 24/1, 11000 Belgrade, Serbia; slobodan.stanojevic@mef.edu.rs
* Correspondence: nikola.puvaca@fimek.edu.rs; Tel.: +381-65-219-1284

Abstract: The study was aimed at evaluating the presence of antibiotic-resistant *Staphylococcus aureus* in retailed raw chicken meat from retail stores intended for human consumption. The presence, characterization, and antibiotic susceptibility of *S. aureus* from 38 retail raw chicken meat samples was performed using a standard microbiological method involving mannitol salt agar (MSA) and Mueller-Hinton agar (MHA). All the samples were positive for *Staphylococcus* species, of which 34 (89.5%) were positive for *S. aureus*. The *S. aureus* isolates were most resistant to tetracycline (88.24%), erythromycin (82.35%), and chloramphenicol (61.77%). Nevertheless, decreased resistance towards gentamycin (23.53%) and cotrimoxazole (38.24%) were recorded. All the *S. aureus* isolates in this study were resistant to cloxacillin, amoxicillin, and augmentin (amoxicillin + clavulanic acid). The present findings show how the raw chicken meat samples could be a potential source of multidrug-resistant *S. aureus* strains dissemination. Therefore, this study suggests high-level contamination of meat with multidrug-resistant *S. aureus* and highlights the public health consequences of consuming such products. Undoubtedly, uncontrolled drugs in food animal production as growth stimulators or medicinal treatment present a possible consequence to people's health. Having the aforementioned in mind, there is a necessity to control the use of drugs and monitor any residues left in the food intended for human consumption.

Keywords: antibiotic resistance; microbes; raw meat; foodborne pathogens; retail stores; *S. aureus*

Citation: Lika, E.; Puvača, N.; Jeremić, D.; Stanojević, S.; Shtylla Kika, T.; Cocoli, S.; de Llanos Frutos, R. Antibiotic Susceptibility of *Staphylococcus* Species Isolated in Raw Chicken Meat from Retail Stores. *Antibiotics* **2021**, *10*, 904. https://doi.org/10.3390/antibiotics10080904

Academic Editors: Nicholas Dixon and Anna Psaroulaki

Received: 16 June 2021
Accepted: 21 July 2021
Published: 23 July 2021

1. Introduction

Meat and meat products are among the most consumed foods and are important sources of all the B-complex vitamins, as well as minerals, proteins, and amino acids in humans.

Meat of animal origin is the primary source of protein and valuable qualities of vitamins for most people in many parts of the world, thus it is essential for the growth, repair, and maintenance of body cells and necessary for our everyday activities [1,2]. Meat is the main source of iron in heme form, which is one of the most deficient micronutrients in humans [3]. Due to the chemical composition and biological characteristics, meats are highly perishable foods providing an excellent source of nutrients for the growth of several hazardous microorganisms that can cause infection in humans, resulting in spoilage of the meat and, therefore, economic loss [4,5]. The microbial pathogens found in meat microorganisms are *Listeria monocytogenes* [6], *Micrococcus* spp. [7], *Staphylococcus* spp. [8],

Clostridium spp. [9], *Bacillus* spp. [10], *Brochotrix thermophacta* [11], *Salmonella* spp. [12], *Escherichia coli* [13], *Serratia* spp. [14] and *Pseudomonas* spp. [15]. Growth of foodborne pathogens such as *Salmonella,* and toxin-producing strains of *E. coli, L. monocytogenes, C. perfringens,* and *S. aureus* are the main concern with meat and poultry products [16–18]. These bacteria are the most common cause of foodborne illnesses. Besides poultry meat, *S. aureus* as well as Methicillin-resistant *S. aureus* can be found in swine [19] and cattle [20] meat.

The most significant Gram-positive organism that has gained attention because of its associated hospital- and community-acquired infections is *S. aureus* [21–23]. This bacterium multiplies quickly at room temperature to produce toxins that cause food poisoning [24]. Naturally, its distribution is very common globally, but the most important infection origin of *S. aureus* is food [25]. According to Scallan et al. [26], *S. aureus* has come into the spotlight as a foodborne pathogen with more than 200,000 estimated yearly infections domestically acquired within the US. The number of cases may actually be higher than this, however the lower known incidences of *S. aureus* foodborne disease could be due to misdiagnosis, inadequate sample collection and laboratory analyses, lack of seeking medical health care by the affected persons (complicating the laboratory confirmation), and lack of routine surveillance of clinical stool specimens for *S. aureus* [27].

Staphylococcal food contamination represents the greatest economically significant foodborne illness [28] and produces gastrointestinal illness through a wide variety of toxins [29], including staphylococcal enterotoxins characterized by vomiting and diarrhea within 2 to 6 h after the consumption of contaminated food [30–32]. A large number of daily consumed foods serve as an optimum growth medium for *S. aureus* [27], and this varies from country to country, especially due to different habits in food consumption [33]. *S. aureus* and other pathogens in meat result from improper hygienic practices at the point of handling by slaughter personnel during meat processing, and other faulty abattoir processes such as improper evisceration of animals which increases the chances of cross-contamination of gut pathogens to meat [34,35].

Residues from medicines, insecticides, herbicides, and other compounds used in daily agricultural practice could be detected in minor quantities in food of animal origin. A few hundred compounds, mainly antibiotics, have been used to cure animals and protect their health, however, some of them have also been used to enhance food animal production. Among many unethically used compounds, the most often used are antimicrobials, β-adrenoreceptor blocking agents, ivermectin, sedatives, coccidiostats, vasodilatory drugs, and painkillers. Residues from such compounds in food products are a major public health concern, especially with rising interest and increased awareness of the potential deposits of drugs and their metabolites in the meat and meat products consumed by humans, as well as the development of antimicrobial resistance (AMR). Treatment of *S. aureus* infections involves the use of antibiotics [36]. However, the use and misuse of antibiotics prophylactically or sub-therapeutically to prevent bacterial infections in livestock and the resultant residue, in general have been responsible for the development of multidrug-resistant bacterial isolates and a significant public health issue. Several microorganisms have developed resistance to various antibiotics, which have triggered the expansion of novel antibiotics with a higher resistance level [37–39].

Numerous studies have shown the presence of *S. aureus* in raw meat and meat products from retail stores with a prevalence below 1% in Asia [40], up to around 12% in Europe [41].

The study was aimed at evaluating the antimicrobial resistance profile of *S. aureus* isolates in retail raw chicken meat intended for human consumption.

2. Results and Discussion

We examined a total of 38 samples of raw chicken meat from retail stores for the presence of *Staphylococcus* spp. Our results showed that all 38 samples were positive for *Staphylococcus* spp. of which 89.5% (34 samples) of the confirmed isolates were *S. aureus*. All the isolates fermented mannitol salt agar and appeared golden yellow, showing the biochemical characteristics previously reported by Konuku et al. [42] for *Staphylococcus* spp. Our results of the occurrence of *Staphylococcus* spp. in meat samples is in agreement with previously reported results that describe *S. aureus* as a common pathogen of raw meats [41,43].

The presence of antimicrobial-resistant bacteria in meat has been widely reported from different parts of the world. The use of antibiotics in livestock and the resultant residue contribute to high antibiotic resistance levels of *S. aureus* found in meat products. All the *S. aureus* isolates in this study were resistant to cloxacillin, amoxicillin, and augmentin (Figure 1). In accordance with the findings of our research, Waters et al. [44] also reported strains of *S. aureus* in US meat and poultry resistant to ciprofloxacin, quinupristin/dalfopristin, clindamycin, erythromycin, oxacillin, and daptomycin. Varying resistance of *S. aureus* from raw meat has been reported by many authors, ranging from 25.00% to 73.30% [34,43,45,46].

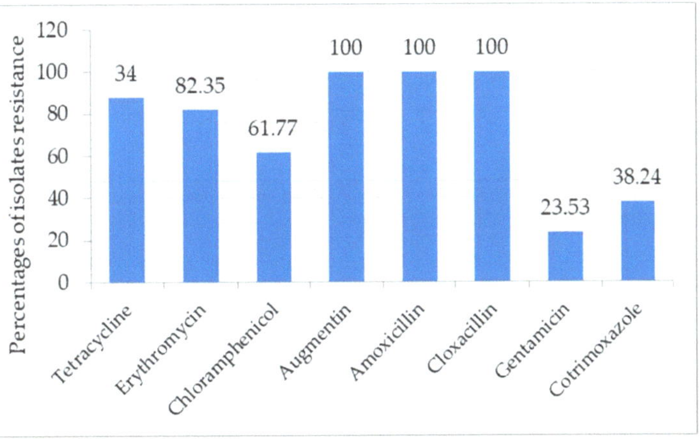

Figure 1. Percentage of *S. aureus* isolates resistant to common antibiotics (number of positive samples; $n = 34$), %.

S. aureus strains were least resistant to gentamycin (23.53%) and cotrimoxazole (38.24%). Some authors have reported that *S. aureus* gentamicin-resistant isolates from raw meat can range up to 19.40% [34,47–49]. This may lower percentage may be because it is in injection form and hardly used, unlike a vast majority of antibiotics that come in capsule or tablet forms. For cotrimoxazole, contrary to the findings of this study, Effah et al. [50] reported a 57.80% resistance of Methicillin-resistant *S. aureus* isolated from raw meat. Other authors, however, reported varying resistances (8.00 to 34.2%) to Methicillin-resistant *S. aureus* (MRSA) from humans [51,52].

S. aureus is among the most prevalent cause of clinical infections globally and has garnered substantial public attention due to the increased mortality associated with the multidrug resistance phenomenon. Our findings also show the potential dissemination of multidrug-resistant *S. aureus* strains in the raw chicken meat samples examined. *S. aureus* isolates were multidrug-resistant to at least three antibiotics tested (Table 1). Consistent with the findings of our research, Effah et al. [50] reported multidrug resistance of MRSA to 16 antibiotics, of which 6 of those antibiotics were among those herein tested. The presence of multidrug-resistant strains poses a severe public health risk, as well as other emerging novel diseases [53].

Table 1. Multidrug resistance of *S. aureus* isolates in raw chicken meat samples.

Antibiotics	Isolate's Resistance (n)
AUG-AMX-CXC-TET-ERY	8
AUG-AMX-CXC-TET-ERY-CHL	6
AUG-AMX-CXC-TET-ERY-CHL-COT	8
AUG-AMX-CXC-TET-ERY-CHL-COT-GEN	6

AUG—augmentin; AMX—amoxicillin; ERY—erythromycin; TET—tetracycline; CXC—cloxacillin; GEN—gentamicin; COT—cotrimoxazole; CHL—chloramphenicol; n—number of isolates.

Antibiotic susceptibility patterns for the raw chicken meat associated bacteria identified in this study are presented in Table 2. Antibiotics included in the testing were augmentin, amoxicillin, erythromycin, tetracycline, cloxacillin, gentamicin, cotrimoxazole, and chloramphenicol. According to Kovačević et al. [54], the most used antibiotics in inflammation therapy in food animals are penicillin, streptomycin, gentamicin, tetracycline, cephalexin, sulfonamides, and enrofloxacin.

Table 2. Antibiotic susceptibility patterns for the raw chicken meat associated bacteria.

Bacteria	AUG	AMX	ERY	TET	CXC	GEN	COT	CHL
Staphylococcus spp.	R	R	R	R	R	R	I	R

AUG—augmentin; AMX—amoxicillin; ERY—erythromycin; TET—tetracycline; CXC—cloxacillin; GEN—gentamicin; COT—cotrimoxazole; CHL—chloramphenicol; I—intermediate; R—resistant.

Correspondence analysis was used to describe the bactericidal potential of different antibiotics on bacteria isolated from the raw chicken meat samples and shows associations of different bacteria and the evaluated antibiotics in terms of bacteria resistance (R) or sensitivity (S). As previously stated, *Staphylococcus* spp. have shown resistance toward all investigated antibiotics, with intermediate (I) resistance towards COT and GEN. As in our findings, Regecová et al. [55] investigated antimicrobial resistance of coagulase-negative Staphylococci isolated from sea fish meat. They observed that all isolates showed antimicrobial resistance to seven antibiotics, with most isolates resistant to ampicillin (AMP) and GEN. Ljubojević et al. [56] pointed out significant problems of widespread use of tetracyclines in poultry farming. Irregular and unprescribed usage of antibiotics may have resulted in the development and transmission of resistant strains from poultry to humans via the food chain. Furthermore, Puvača and de Llanos [57] have explained mechanisms of transmission and resistance via the fecal-oral route between humans, environmental sources, and food and pet animals in their review. The significant impact on drug resistance could also be due to inappropriate antibiotic medical decision therapy [58].

The minimum inhibitory concentrations (MICs) and minimal bactericidal concentrations (MBCs) of *S. aureus* and *Staphylococcus* spp. to augmentin, amoxicillin, and cloxacillin antibiotics are shown in Table 3. Our results show that all isolates of *S. aureus* and *Staphylococcus* spp. found in raw chicken meat samples were multidrug resistant to these three antibiotics. Recorded MIC/BMC concentration in our study regarding *S. aureus* was as follows: AMX > CXC > AUG (8.2/16.4 mg/L > 6.4/12.8 mg/L > 5.8/11.6 mg/L); while *Staphylococcus* spp. recorded a similar trend (7.6/15.4 mg/L > 7.3/14.6 mg/L > 4.6/9.2 mg/L).

In the research of Thorburn et al. [59], post-antibiotic and post-β-lactamase inhibitor effects of amoxicillin were investigated. The effects of AMX were investigated on several bacteria including *S. aureus* and *E. coli* and a necessity for antibiotic dosage reduction was observed. Also, Sader et al. [60] highlighted that the usage of third-generation antibiotics exhibits more balanced spectrums of activity against pathogens and infections when compared with other antibiotics, but only in strictly controlled therapy.

Table 3. Minimum inhibitory concentrations (MICs) and minimal bactericidal concentrations (MBCs) of *S. aureus* and *Staphylococcus* spp. to augmentin, amoxicillin, and cloxacillin antibiotics.

Sample		AUG			AMX			CXC	
	MIC, mg/L	MBC, mg/L	Cutoff, mg/L	MIC, mg/L	MBC, mg/L	Cutoff, mg/L	MIC, mg/L	MBC, mg/L	Cutoff, mg/L
S. aureus	5.8	11.6	1.45	8.2	16.4	2.05	6.4	12.8	1.6
Staphylococcus spp.	4.6	9.2	1.15	7.6	15.4	1.9	7.3	14.6	1.83

AUG—augmentin; AMX—amoxicillin; CXC—cloxacillin.

3. Materials and Methods

The fresh raw chicken meat samples (thighs, breasts, and wings of the same chicken) were randomly purchased in January 2021, from a total of 38 different retail meat stores originating from different producers in a territory of the Autonomous Province of Vojvodina located in the Republic of Serbia. Chickens came from independent processing plants. Meat samples were packed in a protective atmosphere and transferred in sterile flask coolers at +4 °C, upon which samples were sent to the laboratory for further analysis.

A total of 25 g of mixture of meat samples were ground and aseptically weighed into a stomacher bag containing 225 mL of sterile saline solution. This was followed by homogenization in a stomacher (Lab. Lemco 400, Worthing, West Sussex, UK) for about 100 s. To prepare decimal dilutions, 1.0 mL of the initial suspension (10^{-1}) to 9.0 mL of peptone saline diluent (PSD) (to a tolerance of $\pm 2\%$ at ambient temperature), avoiding contact between the pipette tip and the diluent, was transferred and mixed carefully using a vortex mixer (Drawell, Chongqing, China) for 5–10 s. PSD was prepared by suspending 15 g of Peptone Water in 1000 mL of distilled water, followed by the addition of the test carbohydrate until completely dissolved, and then dispensed into inverted Durham's tubes and sterilized by autoclaving at 121 °C for 15 min. The time lapse between preparation of the initial suspension and the beginning of preparation of the further dilutions did not exceed 30 min, and the overall time lapse between preparation of the initial suspension and inoculation of the plating media did not exceed 45 min. After a ten-fold serial dilution, 0.1 mL of diluted homogenate was spread-plated in duplicates on mannitol salt agar (MSA) supplemented with egg yolk-tellurite emulsion (Oxoid Limited, Basingstoke, Hampshire, UK), and incubated at 35 °C for 24 h.

From each plate, typical colonies of *Staphylococcus* spp. with similar morphologies were isolated and cultured separately on MSA before storing in Nutrient Agar Slant for confirmation. Identification of bacterial isolates was confirmed using the Cowan and Steel [61] manual for the Identification of Medical Bacteria, and Bergey and Holt [62] manual of Determinative Bacteriology.

Antibiotic sensitivity patterns of all the confirmed *Staphylococcus* spp. were performed using the standard disk diffusion method on Mueller-Hinton agar (Titan, Biotech Ltd.) following the procedures recommended by the Clinical and Laboratory Standards Institute (CLSI) [63]. Ten commonly used antibiotics (µg/disc) such as augmentin (30 µg) (amoxicillin + clavulanic acid), amoxycillin (25 µg), erythromycin (5 µg), tetracycline (10 µg), cloxacillin (5 µg), gentamycin (10 µg), cotrimoxazole (25 µg), chloramphenicol (30 µg) were tested. From an overnight culture in Brain Heart Infusion Broth, a 10^8 cell/mL (0.5 MacFarland turbidity standards) bacterial culture was prepared in sterile saline solution, from which 0.1 mL was inoculated onto Mueller-Hinton agar, after which antibiotic discs were carefully and aseptically placed on the surface of the agar. The plates were incubated at 37 °C for 24 h. Inhibition zones for various isolates were measured and interpreted as sensitive, intermediate, or resistant according to the CLSI [64,65]. When a single isolate was resistant to one key antimicrobial agent, multidrug resistance was registered [66].

The Brain Heart Infusion (BHI) Broth microdilution method was used to establish the minimal inhibitory concentrations (MIC) corresponding to the Clinical and Laboratory Standards Institute guideline [67]. The 180 µL aliquots of Tryptone soya broth were added to 96-well microtiter plates. As the final step, 20 μL of the standardized bacterial suspension (10^8 cell/mL) was inoculated into each well. The assay was performed in a total volume of 200 μL with final antimicrobial concentrations ranging from 100 to 0.09 mg/L, while the final microbial concentration was 10^5 CFU/mL. Plates were incubated at 37 °C, during 6 h in darkness. After visual examination, the plates were additionally incubated for 18 h. Change of color from blue (oxidized) to pink (reduced) indicated the growth of bacteria. MIC was defined as the lowest concentration at which the color change occurred [68]. Bacterial growth was determined by measuring absorbance at 600 nm.

To determine the minimum bactericidal concentration (MBC), known as the lowest concentration that reduces the bacterial population 99.9% after incubation at 35 °C for 24 h, 100 μL of the microtiter wells with no visible growth in the MIC determination assay was transferred to count agar plates (Lab M, International Diagnostics Group Plc, Bury, Lancashire, UK), which were incubated at 37 °C for 24 h. Those wells that yielded plates with no visible colonies were considered to be the MBC.

4. Conclusions

The role of food in the spread of pathogens cannot be over-emphasized in public health. Based on our results, raw chicken meat from retail stores remains a potential source in transmitting pathogenic foodborne bacteria. All the samples were positive for *Staphylococcus* species, of which 34 (89.5%) were positive for *S. aureus*. The *S. aureus* isolates were most resistant to tetracycline (88.24%), erythromycin (82.35%), and chloramphenicol (61.77%), while decreased resistance toward gentamycin (23.53%) and cotrimoxazole (38.24%) was recorded. All the *S. aureus* isolates in this study were resistant to cloxacillin, amoxicillin, and augmentin (amoxicillin + clavulanic acid). Therefore, there is the need for adequate food processing, especially at a suitable temperature, to reduce the possible microbial contamination in the food products, as well as surveillance of and good hygiene practice by meat handlers in the face of an increasing threat of multidrug-resistant *S. aureus* both in animals and humans. From our findings, it was determined that raw chicken meat from retail stores can be classified as "very high additional risk" or even as "high additional risk". This highlights the importance of continued surveillance and the need to take measures in the primary sector to minimize the risk for the consumer.

Author Contributions: Conceptualization, N.P. and E.L.; methodology, S.C.; software, N.P.; validation, S.C., and T.S.K.; formal analysis, N.P.; investigation, E.L.; resources, D.J.; data curation, S.S.; writing—original draft preparation, N.P.; writing—review and editing, R.d.L.F.; visualization, N.P.; supervision, T.S.K.; project administration, N.P.; funding acquisition, N.P. All authors have read and agreed to the published version of the manuscript.

Funding: This research was funded by Ministry of Education, Science and Technological Development of the Republic of Serbia.

Institutional Review Board Statement: Not applicable.

Informed Consent Statement: Not applicable.

Data Availability Statement: Data is contained within the article.

Acknowledgments: This research was supported by Ministry of Education, Science and Technological Development of the Republic of Serbia, and through a Beatriz Galindo Fellowship of the Ministerio de Educacion y Formacion Profesional, Spanish Government (BGP18/00062).

Conflicts of Interest: The authors declare no conflict of interest. The funders had no role in the design of the study; in the collection, analyses, or interpretation of data; in the writing of the manuscript, or in the decision to publish the results.

References

1. de Castro Cardoso Pereira, P.M.; dos Reis Baltazar Vicente, A.F. Meat Nutritional Composition and Nutritive Role in the Human Diet. *Meat Sci.* **2013**, *93*, 586–592. [CrossRef]

2. Olmedilla-Alonso, B.; Jiménez-Colmenero, F.; Sánchez-Muniz, F.J. Development and Assessment of Healthy Properties of Meat and Meat Products Designed as Functional Foods. *Meat Sci.* **2013**, *95*, 919–930. [CrossRef] [PubMed]
3. Shubham, K.; Anukiruthika, T.; Dutta, S.; Kashyap, A.V.; Moses, J.A.; Anandharamakrishnan, C. Iron Deficiency Anemia: A Comprehensive Review on Iron Absorption, Bioavailability and Emerging Food Fortification Approaches. *Trends Food Sci. Technol.* **2020**, *99*, 58–75. [CrossRef]
4. Doulgeraki, A.I.; Ercolini, D.; Villani, F.; Nychas, G.-J.E. Spoilage Microbiota Associated to the Storage of Raw Meat in Different Conditions. *Int. J. Food Microbiol.* **2012**, *157*, 130–141. [CrossRef] [PubMed]
5. Lika, E. Sustainable Rural Development in Albania Through Agriculture and Livestock: Challenges in the European Union Perspective. *J. Agron. Technol. Eng. Manag.* **2021**, *4*, 577–582.
6. Moretro, T.; Langsrud, S.; Heir, E. Bacteria on Meat Abattoir Process Surfaces after Sanitation: Characterisation of Survival Properties of *Listeria Monocytogenes* and the Commensal Bacterial Flora. *Adv. Microbiol.* **2013**, *3*, 10. [CrossRef]
7. Møretrø, T.; Langsrud, S. Residential Bacteria on Surfaces in the Food Industry and Their Implications for Food Safety and Quality. *Compr. Rev. Food Sci. Food Saf.* **2017**, *16*, 1022–1041. [CrossRef]
8. Lavilla Lerma, L.; Benomar, N.; Gálvez, A.; Abriouel, H. Prevalence of Bacteria Resistant to Antibiotics and/or Biocides on Meat Processing Plant Surfaces throughout Meat Chain Production. *Int. J. Food Microbiol.* **2013**, *161*, 97–106. [CrossRef]
9. Nørrung, B.; Andersen, J.K.; Buncic, S. Main Concerns of Pathogenic Microorganisms in Meat. In *Safety of Meat and Processed Meat*; Toldrá, F., Ed.; Food Microbiology and Food Safety; Springer: New York, NY, USA, 2009; pp. 3–29, ISBN 978-0-387-89026-5.
10. Van Ba, H.; Seo, H.-W.; Pil-Nam, S.; Kim, Y.-S.; Park, B.Y.; Moon, S.-S.; Kang, S.-J.; Choi, Y.-M.; Kim, J.-H. The Effects of Pre-and Post-Slaughter Spray Application with Organic Acids on Microbial Population Reductions on Beef Carcasses. *Meat Sci.* **2018**, *137*, 16–23. [CrossRef]
11. Breuch, R.; Klein, D.; Siefke, E.; Hebel, M.; Herbert, U.; Wickleder, C.; Kaul, P. Differentiation of Meat-Related Microorganisms Using Paper-Based Surface-Enhanced Raman Spectroscopy Combined with Multivariate Statistical Analysis. *Talanta* **2020**, *219*, 121315. [CrossRef] [PubMed]
12. Visvalingam, J.; Zhang, P.; Ells, T.C.; Yang, X. Dynamics of Biofilm Formation by Salmonella Typhimurium and Beef Processing Plant Bacteria in Mono- and Dual-Species Cultures. *Microb. Ecol.* **2019**, *78*, 375–387. [CrossRef]
13. Huang, L.; Hwang, C.-A.; Fang, T. Improved Estimation of Thermal Resistance of *Escherichia coli* O157:H7, *Salmonella* spp., and *Listeria monocytogenes* in Meat and Poultry—The Effect of Temperature and Fat and A Global Analysis. *Food Control* **2019**, *96*, 29–38. [CrossRef]
14. Odeyemi, O.A.; Alegbeleye, O.O.; Strateva, M.; Stratev, D. Understanding Spoilage Microbial Community and Spoilage Mechanisms in Foods of Animal Origin. *Compr. Rev. Food Sci. Food Saf.* **2020**, *19*, 311–331. [CrossRef] [PubMed]
15. Ríos-Castillo, A.G.; Ripolles-Avila, C.; Rodríguez-Jerez, J.J. Evaluation of Bacterial Population Using Multiple Sampling Methods and the Identification of Bacteria Detected on Supermarket Food Contact Surfaces. *Food Control* **2021**, *119*, 107471. [CrossRef]
16. Schirone, M.; Visciano, P.; Tofalo, R.; Suzzi, G. Editorial: Foodborne Pathogens: Hygiene and Safety. *Front. Microbiol.* **2019**, *10*, 1974. [CrossRef] [PubMed]
17. Sosnowski, M.; Osek, J. Microbiological Safety of Food of Animal Origin from Organic Farms. *J. Vet. Res.* **2021**, *65*, 87–92. [CrossRef] [PubMed]
18. Charlermroj, R.; Makornwattana, M.; Phuengwas, S.; Meerak, J.; Pichpol, D.; Karoonuthaisiri, N. DNA-Based Bead Array Technology for Simultaneous Identification of Eleven Foodborne Pathogens in Chicken Meat. *Food Control* **2019**, *101*, 81–88. [CrossRef]
19. Smith, T.C.; Male, M.J.; Harper, A.L.; Kroeger, J.S.; Tinkler, G.P.; Moritz, E.D.; Capuano, A.W.; Herwaldt, L.A.; Diekema, D.J. Methicillin-Resistant Staphylococcus Aureus (MRSA) Strain ST398 Is Present in Midwestern U.S. Swine and Swine Workers. *PLoS ONE* **2009**, *4*, e4258. [CrossRef]
20. Hasman, H.; Moodley, A.; Guardabassi, L.; Stegger, M.; Skov, R.L.; Aarestrup, F.M. Spa Type Distribution in Staphylococcus Aureus Originating from Pigs, Cattle and Poultry. *Vet. Microbiol.* **2010**, *141*, 326–331. [CrossRef]
21. Wu, D.; Chen, Y.; Sun, L.; Qu, T.; Wang, H.; Yu, Y. Prevalence of Fosfomycin Resistance in Methicillin-Resistant *Staphylococcus Aureus* Isolated from Patients in a University Hospital in China from 2013 to 2015. *JPN J. Infect. Dis.* **2018**, *71*, 312–314. [CrossRef]
22. Mendes, R.E.; Sader, H.S.; Castanheira, M.; Flamm, R.K. Distribution of Main Gram-Positive Pathogens Causing Bloodstream Infections in United States and European Hospitals during the SENTRY Antimicrobial Surveillance Program (2010–2016): Concomitant Analysis of Oritavancin in Vitro Activity. *J. Chemother.* **2018**, *30*, 280–289. [CrossRef] [PubMed]
23. Bush, K.; Bradford, P.A. Epidemiology of β-Lactamase-Producing Pathogens. *Clin. Microbiol. Rev.* **2020**, *33*. [CrossRef] [PubMed]
24. Hennekinne, J.-A. Chapter 7—Staphylococcus aureus as a Leading Cause of Foodborne Outbreaks Worldwide. In *Staphylococcus Aureus*; Fetsch, A., Ed.; Academic Press: Cambridge, MA, USA, 2018; pp. 129–146, ISBN 978-0-12-809671-0.
25. Ebert, M. Chapter 11—Hygiene Principles to Avoid Contamination/Cross-Contamination in the Kitchen and During Food Processing. In *Staphylococcus Aureus*; Fetsch, A., Ed.; Academic Press: Cambridge, MA, USA, 2018; pp. 217–234, ISBN 978-0-12-809671-0.
26. Scallan, E.; Hoekstra, R.M.; Angulo, F.J.; Tauxe, R.V.; Widdowson, M.-A.; Roy, S.L.; Jones, J.L.; Griffin, P.M. Foodborne Illness Acquired in the United States—Major Pathogens. *Emerg. Infect. Dis.* **2011**, *17*, 7–15. [CrossRef] [PubMed]
27. Kadariya, J.; Smith, T.C.; Thapaliya, D. Staphylococcus Aureus and Staphylococcal Food-Borne Disease: An Ongoing Challenge in Public Health. *BioMed Res. Int.* **2014**, *2014*, e827965. [CrossRef] [PubMed]

28. Chen, J.; Lü, Z.; An, Z.; Ji, P.; Liu, X. Antibacterial Activities of Sophorolipids and Nisin and Their Combination against Foodborne Pathogen Staphylococcus Aureus. *Eur. J. Lipid Sci. Technol.* **2020**, *122*, 1900333. [CrossRef]
29. Abril, G.A.; Villa, G.T.; Barros-Velázquez, J.; Cañas, B.; Sánchez-Pérez, A.; Calo-Mata, P.; Carrera, M. Staphylococcus Aureus Exotoxins and Their Detection in the Dairy Industry and Mastitis. *Toxins* **2020**, *12*, 537. [CrossRef]
30. Umeda, K.; Nakamura, H.; Yamamoto, K.; Nishina, N.; Yasufuku, K.; Hirai, Y.; Hirayama, T.; Goto, K.; Hase, A.; Ogasawara, J. Molecular and Epidemiological Characterization of Staphylococcal Foodborne Outbreak of Staphylococcus Aureus Harboring Seg, Sei, Sem, Sen, Seo, and Selu Genes without Production of Classical Enterotoxins. *Int. J. Food Microbiol.* **2017**, *256*, 30–35. [CrossRef]
31. Denayer, S.; Delbrassinne, L.; Nia, Y.; Botteldoorn, N. Food-Borne Outbreak Investigation and Molecular Typing: High Diversity of Staphylococcus Aureus Strains and Importance of Toxin Detection. *Toxins* **2017**, *9*, 407. [CrossRef]
32. Le, H.H.T.; Dalsgaard, A.; Andersen, P.S.; Nguyen, H.M.; Ta, Y.T.; Nguyen, T.T. Large-Scale Staphylococcus Aureus Foodborne Disease Poisoning Outbreak among Primary School Children. *Microbiol. Res.* **2021**, *12*, 5. [CrossRef]
33. Argudín, M.Á.; Mendoza, M.C.; Rodicio, M.R. Food Poisoning and Staphylococcus Aureus Enterotoxins. *Toxins* **2010**, *2*, 1751–1773. [CrossRef]
34. Jaja, I.F.; Jaja, C.-J.I.; Chigor, N.V.; Anyanwu, M.U.; Maduabuchi, E.K.; Oguttu, J.W.; Green, E. Antimicrobial Resistance Phenotype of *Staphylococcus aureus* and *Escherichia coli* Isolates Obtained from Meat in the Formal and Informal Sectors in South Africa. *BioMed Res. Int.* **2020**, *2020*, 3979482. [CrossRef] [PubMed]
35. Puvača, N.; Milenković, J.; Galonja Coghill, T.; Bursić, V.; Petrović, A.; Tanasković, S.; Pelić, M.; Ljubojević Pelić, D.; Miljković, T. Antimicrobial Activity of Selected Essential Oils against Selected Pathogenic Bacteria: In Vitro Study. *Antibiotics* **2021**, *10*, 546. [CrossRef] [PubMed]
36. Leong, H.N.; Kurup, A.; Tan, M.Y.; Kwa, A.L.H.; Liau, K.H.; Wilcox, M.H. Management of Complicated Skin and Soft Tissue Infections with a Special Focus on the Role of Newer Antibiotics. *Infect. Drug Resist.* **2018**, *11*, 1959–1974. [CrossRef] [PubMed]
37. Wellington, E.M.; Boxall, A.B.; Cross, P.; Feil, E.J.; Gaze, W.H.; Hawkey, P.M.; Johnson-Rollings, A.S.; Jones, D.L.; Lee, N.M.; Otten, W.; et al. The Role of the Natural Environment in the Emergence of Antibiotic Resistance in Gram-Negative Bacteria. *Lancet Infect. Dis.* **2013**, *13*, 155–165. [CrossRef]
38. Omwenga, I.; Aboge, G.O.; Mitema, E.S.; Obiero, G.; Ngaywa, C.; Ngwili, N.; Wamwere, G.; Wainaina, M.; Bett, B. Antimicrobial Usage and Detection of Multidrug-Resistant Staphylococcus Aureus, Including Methicillin-Resistant Strains in Raw Milk of Livestock from Northern Kenya. *Microb. Drug Resist.* **2020**. [CrossRef] [PubMed]
39. Kimera, Z.I.; Mgaya, F.X.; Misinzo, G.; Mshana, S.E.; Moremi, N.; Matee, M.I.N. Multidrug-Resistant, Including Extended-Spectrum Beta Lactamase-Producing and Quinolone-Resistant, *Escherichia coli* Isolated from Poultry and Domestic Pigs in Dar Es Salaam, Tanzania. *Antibiotics* **2021**, *10*, 406. [CrossRef]
40. Lim, S.-K.; Nam, H.-M.; Park, H.-J.; Lee, H.-S.; Choi, M.-J.; Jung, S.-C.; Lee, J.-Y.; Kim, Y.-C.; Song, S.-W.; Wee, S.-H. Prevalence and Characterization of Methicillin-Resistant Staphylococcus Aureus in Raw Meat in Korea. *J. Microbiol. Biotechnol.* **2010**, *20*, 775–778. [CrossRef] [PubMed]
41. de Boer, E.; Zwartkruis-Nahuis, J.T.M.; Wit, B.; Huijsdens, X.W.; de Neeling, A.J.; Bosch, T.; van Oosterom, R.A.A.; Vila, A.; Heuvelink, A.E. Prevalence of Methicillin-Resistant Staphylococcus Aureus in Meat. *Int. J. Food Microbiol.* **2009**, *134*, 52–56. [CrossRef]
42. Konuku, S.; Rajan, M.M.; Muruhan, S. Morphological and Biochemical Characteristics and Antibiotic Resistance Pattern of Staphylococcus Aureus Isolated from Grapes. *Int. J. Nutr. Pharmacol. Neurol. Dis.* **2012**, *2*, 70. [CrossRef]
43. Pesavento, G.; Ducci, B.; Comodo, N.; Nostro, A.L. Antimicrobial Resistance Profile of Staphylococcus Aureus Isolated from Raw Meat: A Research for Methicillin Resistant Staphylococcus Aureus (MRSA). *Food Control* **2007**, *18*, 196–200. [CrossRef]
44. Waters, A.E.; Contente-Cuomo, T.; Buchhagen, J.; Liu, C.M.; Watson, L.; Pearce, K.; Foster, J.T.; Bowers, J.; Driebe, E.M.; Engelthaler, D.M.; et al. Multidrug-Resistant Staphylococcus Aureus in US Meat and Poultry. *Clin. Infect. Dis.* **2011**, *52*, 1227–1230. [CrossRef]
45. Yucel, N.; Citak, S.; Bayhün, S. Antimicrobial Resistance Profile of Staphylococcus Aureus Isolated from Clinical Samples and Foods of Animal Origin. *Foodborne Pathog. Dis.* **2010**, *8*, 427–431. [CrossRef] [PubMed]
46. Pekana, A.; Green, E. Antimicrobial Resistance Profiles of Staphylococcus Aureus Isolated from Meat Carcasses and Bovine Milk in Abattoirs and Dairy Farms of the Eastern Cape, South Africa. *Int. J. Environ. Res. Public Health* **2018**, *15*, 2223. [CrossRef]
47. Wu, S.; Huang, J.; Wu, Q.; Zhang, J.; Zhang, F.; Yang, X.; Wu, H.; Zeng, H.; Chen, M.; Ding, Y.; et al. Staphylococcus Aureus Isolated From Retail Meat and Meat Products in China: Incidence, Antibiotic Resistance and Genetic Diversity. *Front. Microbiol.* **2018**, *9*, 2767. [CrossRef]
48. Kim, Y.B.; Seo, K.W.; Jeon, H.Y.; Lim, S.-K.; Lee, Y.J. Characteristics of the Antimicrobial Resistance of Staphylococcus Aureus Isolated from Chicken Meat Produced by Different Integrated Broiler Operations in Korea. *Poult. Sci.* **2018**, *97*, 962–969. [CrossRef] [PubMed]
49. Adzitey, F.; Ekli, R.; Abu, A. Prevalence and Antibiotic Susceptibility of Staphylococcus Aureus Isolated from Raw and Grilled Beef in Nyankpala Community in the Northern Region of Ghana. *Cogent Food Agric.* **2019**, *5*, 1671115. [CrossRef]
50. Effah, C.Y.; Otoo, B.A.F.; Ntiefo, R.A. Prevalence and Phenotypic Antibiotic Bioassay of Methicillin-Resistant Staphylococcus Aureus in Raw Meats Sold at Various Retail Outlets in the Cape Coast Metropolis of Ghana. *J. Food Microbiol.* **2018**, *2*, 7–11.

51. Goldberg, E.; Paul, M.; Talker, O.; Samra, Z.; Raskin, M.; Hazzan, R.; Leibovici, L.; Bishara, J. Co-Trimoxazole versus Vancomycin for the Treatment of Methicillin-Resistant Staphylococcus Aureus Bacteraemia: A Retrospective Cohort Study. *J. Antimicrob. Chemother.* **2010**, *65*, 1779–1783. [CrossRef]
52. Marwa, K.J.; Mushi, M.F.; Konje, E.; Alele, P.E.; Kidola, J.; Mirambo, M.M. Resistance to Cotrimoxazole and Other Antimicrobials among Isolates from HIV/AIDS and Non-HIV/AIDS Patients at Bugando Medical Centre, Mwanza, Tanzania. *AIDS Res. Treat.* **2015**, *2015*, 103874. [CrossRef]
53. Puvača, N.; Lika, E.; Brkanlić, S.; Esteve, E.B.; Ilić, D.; Kika, S.; Brkić, I. The Pandemic of SARS-CoV-2 as a Worldwide Health Safety Risk. *J. Agron. Technol. Eng. Manag.* **2021**, *4*, 10.
54. Kovačević, Z.; Radinović, M.; Čabarkapa, I.; Kladar, N.; Božin, B. Natural Agents against Bovine Mastitis Pathogens. *Antibiotics* **2021**, *10*, 205. [CrossRef]
55. Regecová, I.; Pipová, M.; Jevinová, P.; Marušková, K.; Kmeť, V.; Popelka, P. Species Identification and Antimicrobial Resistance of Coagulase-Negative Staphylococci Isolated from the Meat of Sea Fish. *J. Food Sci.* **2014**, *79*, M898–M902. [CrossRef]
56. Ljubojević, D.; Pelić, M.; Puvača, N.; Milanov, D. Resistance to Tetracycline in *Escherichia coli* Isolates from Poultry Meat: Epidemiology, Policy and Perspective. *Worlds Poult. Sci. J.* **2017**, *73*, 409–417. [CrossRef]
57. Puvača, N.; de Llanos Frutos, R. Antimicrobial Resistance in *Escherichia coli* Strains Isolated from Humans and Pet Animals. *Antibiotics* **2021**, *10*, 69. [CrossRef] [PubMed]
58. Puvača, N.; Britt, C. Welfare and Legal Aspects of Making Decisions on Medical Treatments of Pet Animals. *Pravo—Teorija I Praksa* **2020**, *37*, 55–64. [CrossRef]
59. Thorburn, C.E.; Molesworth, S.J.; Sutherland, R.; Rittenhouse, S. Postantibiotic and Post-Beta-Lactamase Inhibitor Effects of Amoxicillin plus Clavulanate. *Antimicrob. Agents Chemother.* **1996**, *40*, 2796–2801. [CrossRef] [PubMed]
60. Sader, H.S.; Jacobs, M.R.; Fritsche, T.R. Review of the Spectrum and Potency of Orally Administered Cephalosporins and Amoxicillin/Clavulanate. *Diagn. Microbiol. Infect. Dis.* **2007**, *57*, S5–S12. [CrossRef]
61. Cowan, S.T.; Steel, K.J. Manual for the Identification of Medical Bacteria. *Man. Identif. Med. Bacteria.* **1965**, *149*, 852.
62. Bergey, D.H.; Holt, J.G. *Bergey's Manual of Determinative Bacteriology*; Lippincott Williams & Wilkins (LWW): Philadelphia, PA, USA, 1994; ISBN 978-0-683-00603-2.
63. *Methods for Dilution Antimicrobial Susceptibility Tests for Bacteria That Grow Aerobically*; Approved Standards—Ninth Edition; Clinical and Laboratory Standards Institute: Wayne, PA, USA, 2012.
64. *Performance Standards for Antimicrobial Disk and Dilution Susceptibility Tests for Bacteria Isolated from Animals*; Clinical and Laboratory Standards Institute: Wayne, PA, USA, 2008.
65. *Performance Standards for Antimicrobial Disk Susceptibility Tests*; Approved Standard M02-A12 2007; Clinical and Laboratory Standards Institute: Wayne, PA, USA, 2007.
66. Magiorakos, A.-P.; Srinivasan, A.; Carey, R.B.; Carmeli, Y.; Falagas, M.E.; Giske, C.G.; Harbarth, S.; Hindler, J.F.; Kahlmeter, G.; Olsson-Liljequist, B.; et al. Multidrug-Resistant, Extensively Drug-Resistant and Pandrug-Resistant Bacteria: An International Expert Proposal for Interim Standard Definitions for Acquired Resistance. *Clin. Microbiol. Infect.* **2012**, *18*, 268–281. [CrossRef]
67. CLSI. *Performance Standards for Antimicrobial Susceptibility Testing*; 25th Informational Supplement; Clinical and Laboratory Standards Institute: Wayne, PA, USA, 2018.
68. Elshikh, M.; Ahmed, S.; Funston, S.; Dunlop, P.; McGaw, M.; Marchant, R.; Banat, I.M. Resazurin-Based 96-Well Plate Microdilution Method for the Determination of Minimum Inhibitory Concentration of Biosurfactants. *Biotechnol. Lett.* **2016**, *38*, 1015–1019. [CrossRef]

antibiotics

MDPI

Article

HPMCP-Coated Microcapsules Containing the Ctx(Ile^{21})-Ha Antimicrobial Peptide Reduce the Mortality Rate Caused by Resistant *Salmonella* Enteritidis in Laying Hens

Cesar Augusto Roque-Borda [1], Larissa Pires Pereira [2], Elisabete Aparecida Lopes Guastalli [3], Nilce Maria Soares [3], Priscilla Ayleen Bustos Mac-Lean [2], Douglas D'Alessandro Salgado [2], Andréia Bagliotti Meneguin [4], Marlus Chorilli [4] and Eduardo Festozo Vicente [2,*]

[1] School of Agricultural and Veterinarian Sciences, São Paulo State University (Unesp), Jaboticabal, São Paulo 14884-900, Brazil; cesar.roque@unesp.br

[2] School of Sciences and Engineering, São Paulo State University (Unesp), Tupã, São Paulo 17602-496, Brazil; larissa.pereira@unipac.com.br (L.P.P.); priscilla.mac-lean@unesp.br (P.A.B.M.-L.); douglas.salgado@unesp.br (D.D.S.)

[3] Poultry Health Specialized Laboratory, Biological Institute, Bastos, São Paulo 17690-000, Brazil; elisabete.guastalli@sp.gov.br (E.A.L.G.); updbastos@biologico.sp.gov.br (N.M.S.)

[4] School of Pharmaceutical Sciences, São Paulo State University (Unesp), Araraquara, São Paulo 14801-902, Brazil; andreia.meneguin@unesp.br (A.B.M.); marlus.chorilli@unesp.br (M.C.)

* Correspondence: eduardo.vicente@unesp.br; Tel.: +55-143-404-4262

check for updates

Citation: Roque-Borda, C.A.; Pereira, L.P.; Guastalli, E.A.L.; Soares, N.M.; Mac-Lean, P.A.B.; Salgado, D.D.; Meneguin, A.B.; Chorilli, M.; Vicente, E.F. HPMCP-Coated Microcapsules Containing the Ctx(Ile^{21})-Ha Antimicrobial Peptide Reduce the Mortality Rate Caused by Resistant *Salmonella* Enteritidis in Laying Hens. *Antibiotics* **2021**, *10*, 616. https://doi.org/10.3390/antibiotics10060616

Academic Editors: Nikola Puvača, Chantal Britt and Jonathan Gómez-Raja

Received: 28 April 2021
Accepted: 19 May 2021
Published: 21 May 2021

Abstract: The constant use of synthetic antibiotics as growth promoters can cause bacterial resistance in chicks. Consequently, the use of these drugs has been restricted in different countries. In recent years, antimicrobial peptides have gained relevance due to their minimal capacity for bacterial resistance and does not generate toxic residues that harm the environment and human health. In this study, a Ctx(Ile^{21})-Ha antimicrobial peptide was employed, due to its previously reported great antimicrobial potential, to evaluate its application effects in laying chicks challenged with *Salmonella* Enteritidis, resistant to nalidixic acid and spectinomycin. For this, Ctx(Ile^{21})-Ha was synthesized, microencapsulated and coated with hypromellose phthalate (HPMCP) to be released in the intestine. Two different doses (20 and 40 mg of Ctx(Ile^{21})-Ha per kg of isoproteic and isoenergetic poultry feed) were included in the chick's food and administered for 28 days. Antimicrobial activity, effect and response as treatment were evaluated. Statistical results were analyzed in detail and indicate that the formulated Ctx(Ile^{21})-Ha peptide had a positive and significant effect in relation to the reduction of chick mortality in the first days of life. However, there was moderate evidence (p = 0.07), not considered statistically significant, in the differences in laying chick weight between the control and microencapsulation treatment groups as a function of time. Therefore, the microencapsulated Ctx(Ile^{21})-Ha antimicrobial peptide can be an interesting and promising option in the substitution of conventional antibiotics.

Keywords: AMP; HPMCP; chicks; microencapsulation; mortality rate

1. Introduction

Salmonella is a bacterium of public health importance and can contaminate food or spaces due to its high risk of transmission, mainly by its common host, the poultry [1]. The frequent transmission, as well as in attempts to control *Salmonella*, allowed this microorganism to generate or acquire resistance to several commercial drugs. *Salmonella*-accelerated proliferation would be related to the immunity alteration by stress factors, products of excessive manipulation or environmental conditions [2]. In 2017, in the last update of the WHO global warning about bacterial resistance, a list of global priorities of resistant bacteria to antibiotics was declared and published, in which *Salmonella* sp. fluoroquinolone-resistant was classified in the high priority group (number 2). Therefore, based on public health policies, there is a very high degree of concern about these aggressive pathogenic bacteria species. In this scenario, antibiotics used in the poultry industry are increasingly restricted and discovery of new drugs is becoming essential and in urgent demand [3,4].

In recent years, antimicrobial peptides (AMPs) have been a central object of study, attributable to their great capacity to control bacterial pathogens, including viruses and fungi [5,6]. Specifically, the Ctx(Ile^{21})-Ha antimicrobial peptide is an amphipathic and cationic peptide, isolated from an Brazilian amphibian skin (*Hypsiboas albopunctatus*) [7], which has a high antimicrobial capacity, demonstrated in pathogens of public health interest [8]. Thus, Ctx(Ile^{21})-Ha and others AMPs are considered natural antibiotics, as they are part of a biological defense innate immune system. In addition, they are biocompatible, can modulate immune systems and have high biological activities with minimal concentrations [9]. An interesting feature of AMPs is that they can generate a minimal level of bacterial resistance [10]. As a result of these attractive characteristics, AMP application in poultry as a feed additive is promising, but challenging [11–14].

Although there is optimistic application, the use of these molecules is limited due to instability factors, such as denaturation or acid hydrolysis degradation, produced by gastric acids in the stomach of monogastric animals. To overcome these issues, coated bioformulations to protect bioactive molecules are demanded. Microencapsulation, a standard pharmacotechnical methodology and a very well-established technique in the literature, is used to control, protect and maintain compounds' biological activities [15].

Some types of encapsulations were developed to improve poultry production. For example, spray drying is employed to microencapsulated probiotics and can maintain 90% of stability, allowing them to be installed in the chicken intestine [16]. Enteric coating is a protection method widely used in pharmaceuticals, which permits the targeted transport of biomolecules or drugs to be released at a specific site, depending on the conditions of the polymer used, such as hydroxypropyl methylcellulose phthalate (HPMCP) [17]. This is a modified polymer, derived from cellulose and is pH dependent, which it tends to dissolve in liquid solutions at pH > 6.5, playing an excellent role as a drug carrier against intestinal pathogens [18].

These parameters allowed us to design an innovative product based on microencapsulates and enteric coating of a biocompatible molecule with potential antimicrobial activity. The Ctx(Ile^{21})-Ha AMP was chosen due to its properties, previously reported by our research group [8]. In this way, the objective of this study was to evaluate the in vivo effect of HPMCP-coated microcapsules containing the Ctx(Ile^{21})-Ha antimicrobial peptide application against *Salmonella* Enteritidis in chickens, to demonstrate its great potential as an innovative natural feed additive in poultry production.

2. Material and Methods

2.1. Chemical Reagents

HPMCP (Grade HP-55, Nominal Phthalyl Content 31%) was kindly donated by Shin-Etsu Chemical (Tokyo, Japan), and the other chemical reagents were obtained in HPLC grade (Sigma-Aldrich Co., Missouri, USA). *N,N*-dimethylformamide (DMF) was purchased from Neon Comercial (São Paulo, Brazil), dichloromethane (DCM) was purchased from Anidrol Products Laboratories (São Paulo, Brazil), sodium alginate with low molecular weight (12,000–40,000 g mol^{-1}, M/G ratio of 0.8) and aluminum chloride were obtained from Êxodo Científica (São Paulo, Brazil). Fmoc-amino acids were purchased from AAPPTEC (Kentucky, USA). Brain Heart Infusion (BHI) broth, Mueller Hinton (MH) agar, Bright Green Agar (BG), selenite broth (SB), nutrient broth (NB), and other microbiological reagents were purchased from SPLABOR (São Paulo, Brazil).

2.2. Ctx(Ile^{21})-Ha Antimicrobial Peptide Synthesis

The antimicrobial peptide Ctx(Ile^{21})-Ha was synthesized manually using solid phase peptide synthesis (SPPS) with a Fmoc strategy protocol. The complete methodology is described according to Roque Borda et al. [19] Briefly, peptide was assembled at a

0.2 mmol scale on a Fmoc-Rink Amide resin of 0.68 mmol g^{-1} substitution, using threefold excess and preconditioned for 15 min in DMF and DCM as main SPPS solvents. 4-methylpiperidine/DMF (1:4, v/v) was used to remove the Fmoc amino group protectors from amino acids. Having finished the entire peptide primary sequence, Ctx(Ile^{21})-Ha peptide was separated from the resin using a solution containing trifluoroacetic acid/ultrapure water/triisopropylsilane (95:2.5:2.5, *v*/*v*/*v*), at 160 rpm for 2 h at room temperature. Next, samples were freeze-dried (Liotop model K108, Sao Paulo, Brazil) to obtain the peptide in a white and flocculent powder material.

The peptide purity degree was determined by analytical HPLC (Shimadzu, model Prominence with membrane degasser DGU-20A5R, UV detector SPD-20A, column oven CTO-20A, automatic sampler SIL-10AF, fraction collector FRC-10A and LC-20AT dual-pump, C18 column) at a flow rate of 1 mL min^{-1} and a detection at wavelength of 220 nm, using as mobile phases 0.045% aqueous TFA (eluent A) and 0.036% TFA in acetonitrile (eluent B) for 30 min. Subsequently, samples were lyophilized and stored until use. The Ctx(Ile^{21})-Ha peptide was employed only if the purity degree was higher than 95%. After that, the peptide was confirmed and characterized by ESI-MS (Electron Spray Injection Mass Spectrometry), employing a mass spectrometer (Bruker, CA, USA). Pure Ctx(Ile^{21})-Ha peptide concentrations were determined by UV spectroscopy, considering tryptophan extinction coefficient of 5600 M^{-1} cm^{-1} at a wavelength of 220 nm.

2.3. Development of Ctx(Ile^{21})-Ha Coated Microcapsules (ERCtx)

Ctx(Ile^{21})-Ha was encapsulated by an ionotropic gelation method, following the method described in Roque-Borda et al. [19] Summarily, the peptide-alginate solution was prepared with an initial concentration of 14 (PEP1) and 28 µmol L^{-1} (PEP2) of Ctx(Ile^{21})-Ha peptide in 2% (w/w) sodium alginate, homogenized using an UltraTurrax-T18 (IKA-Labortechnik, Staufen, Germany) at 25,000 rpm min^{-1} and sonicated with an ultrasound probe (Hilscher, Hesse, Germany) for 15 min. Therefore, a crosslinking solution was prepared with 5% aluminum chloride. Capsules were obtained using a syringe pump (NE-1000, New Era Pump System Inc., New York, USA) with a feed flow rate of 1.5 µL h^{-1} at room temperature. After that, they were dried and stored in darkness.

Ctx(Ile^{21})-Ha microcapsules were coated by the fluidized-bed method, preparing a coating solution with 10% w/w HPMCP, 25% w/w ammonium hydroxide, 2.5% w/v triethylcitrate and 62.5% of water. The microcapsules were placed on a fluidized-bed (LabMaq MLF 100, Sao Paulo, Brazil) at 40 °C, 0.25 L min^{-1} blower, 0.4 mL min^{-1} peristaltic pump and 100% vibration as a system condition and yielded a 75% of peptide microencapsulation.

2.4. In Vivo Experiment in Chicks

Animal experiments were approved by the local Animal Ethics Committee-School of Sciences and Engineering, UNESP, Tupã, Brazil (Number process. 06/2018-CEUA). The mortality rate of the chicks was the guiding variable for the calculation of the sample size [20].

To perform the in vivo assays, 135 commercials female chicks from Hy-lines Brown, Brazil, were acquired from a commercial hatchery. Chick swabs were taken at random, and a box swab sample, to detect *Salmonella* Enteritidis (*S.* Enteritidis) in newborn chickens and verify that they were free of infection. Thus, confirming that all the chicks used in this experiment were negative for this bacterium, the samples were cultured in SB 2X for 24 h at 37 °C. For the inoculum, *Salmonella* Enteritidis resistant to nalidixic acid and spectinomycin (SE $Nal^{R}Spc^{R}$, code P125109-bacterial strain from donated by the Laboratory of Ornithopathology FCAV/UNESP), was grown in a nutrient broth (NB) for 24 h at 37 °C. All chicks challenge was carried out with using 0.2 mL of 10^9 CFU mL^{-1} of *S.* Enteritidis.

Chicks were randomly distributed into three groups, separated into 45 chicks for each treatment. They were identified with enumerated tape around the right leg. From the first day of the experiment, animals received water and powder feed ad libitum and doses of antimicrobial peptide Ctx(Ile^{21})-Ha microencapsulated were added to the feed and administered to chicks from the first day of life. Control treatment (CTRL) was defined as that which received only the initial commercial feed for chicks without any additives; the PEP1 treatment received the ERCtx with 20 mg of Ctx(Ile^{21})-Ha microencapsulated per kg of poultry feed and the PEP2 treatment received the ERCtx with 40 mg of Ctx(Ile^{21})-Ha microencapsulated per kg of poultry feed. Both microparticles were added to the initial commercial feed of the control treatment (isoproteic and isoenergetic for chicks, in the first 28 days of life, considering a mean of total amount of accumulated poultry feed of 598.5 g consumed, according to the management guide of Hy-line Brown commercial laying hens).

For the chick cloacal swab, 15 chicks were selected for each group. A collection of the fecal excretion was performed two times each week. The collected samples were incubated in 3 mL of SB and Novobiocin (Nov) at 37 °C for 24 h, to later be seeded in BG Nal/Spec and incubated again. This procedure was repeated throughout the experiment. The results were expressed as presence/absence of *S.* Enteritidis, depending on their being positive or negative for the pathogen, respectively [21,22]. In addition, chicks were weighed alive from 12 days of age until the end of the experiment. For the microbiological analyses, five chicks were used for each treatment for the day of the analyses (total of 30 chicks per treatment). Likewise, the chicks were weighed in triplicate for each treatment.

For the evaluation of intestinal infection, five chickens from each group were sacrificed for the count of *S.* Enteritidis in the cecal content, carried out on days 2, 5, 7, 14, 21 and 28 post-infection (dpi). The samples were collected aseptically, with the help of sterilized forceps and individual scissors for each chick. The previously weighed tubes were conditioned in PBS pH 7.4 in the ratio 1:10, w/v, and were homogenized in vortex. The samples were seeded and cultured on a BG Nal/Spec agar plate at 37 °C for 24 h and counted in colony-forming units (CFU).

2.5. Statistical Analysis

To perform the total count of *S.* Enteritidis in CFU/mL, the data were transformed into a Napierian logarithm (Ln) to adapt the model recommended in ANOVA. Mortality was analyzed using the Chi-square test. The results were analyzed by software R package version 3.6.0 (R Foundation for Statistical Computing: Vienna, Austria).

3. Results

3.1. Peptide Analysis

Ctx(Ile^{21})-Ha AMP was synthesized successfully by SPPS methodology. In the initial analysis, 590 mg of crude mass of AMP was obtained, which was subsequently purified. The purification yield was 20% with a total pure mass of 120 mg. The characterization analysis was carried out by HPLC and Mass Spectrometry, confirmed the obtaining of Ctx(Ile^{21})-Ha AMP (MW = 2289.72 g mol^{-1}), shown in Figure 1.

Ctx(Ile^{21})-Ha AMP was microencapsulated with sodium alginate and coated with HPMCP (Figure 2). The final products (ERCtx) used for in vivo evaluation are represented by PEP1 and PEP2. The microencapsulation development and characterization are described according to Roque-Borda et al. [19].

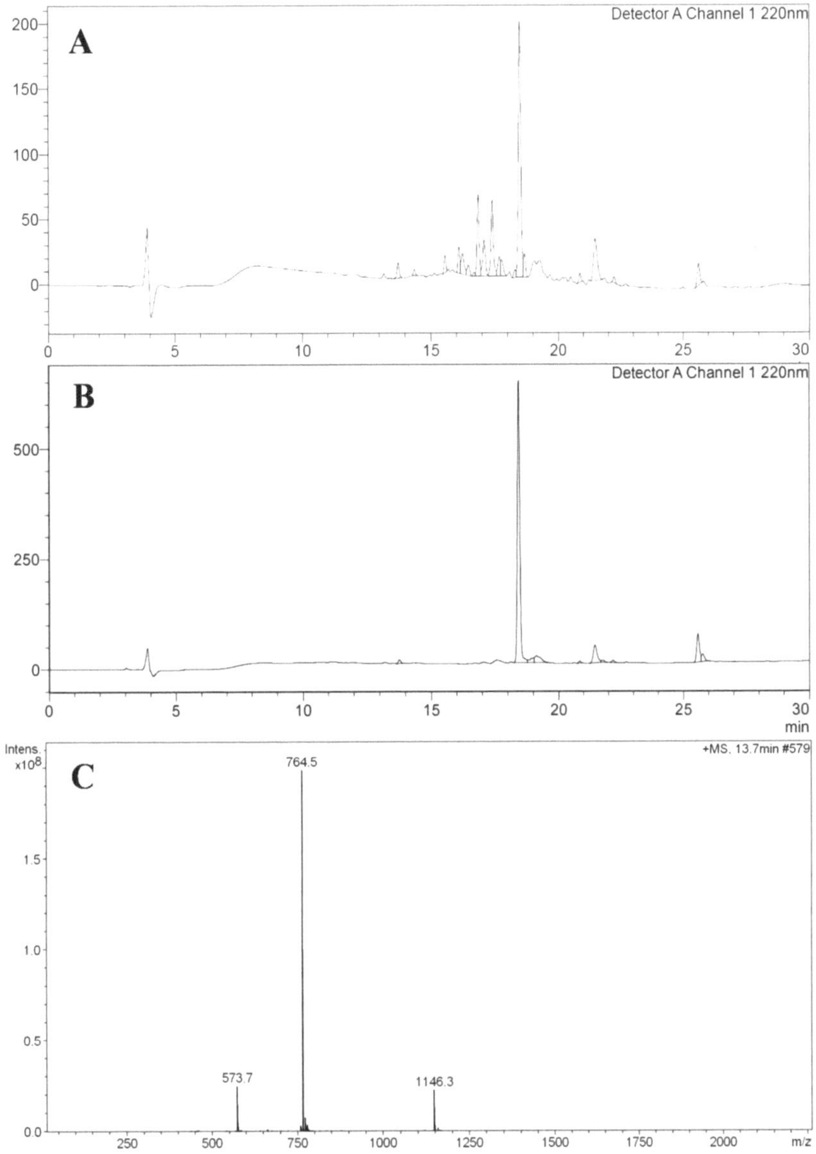

Figure 1. (**A**): Chromatographic profile of crude Ctx(Ile^{21})-Ha peptide by HPLC at 220 nm. (**B**): Chromatographic profile of purified Ctx(Ile^{21})-Ha peptide by HPLC at 220 nm. (**C**): Mass spectra of Ctx(Ile^{21})-Ha peptide, confirming the correct obtaining.

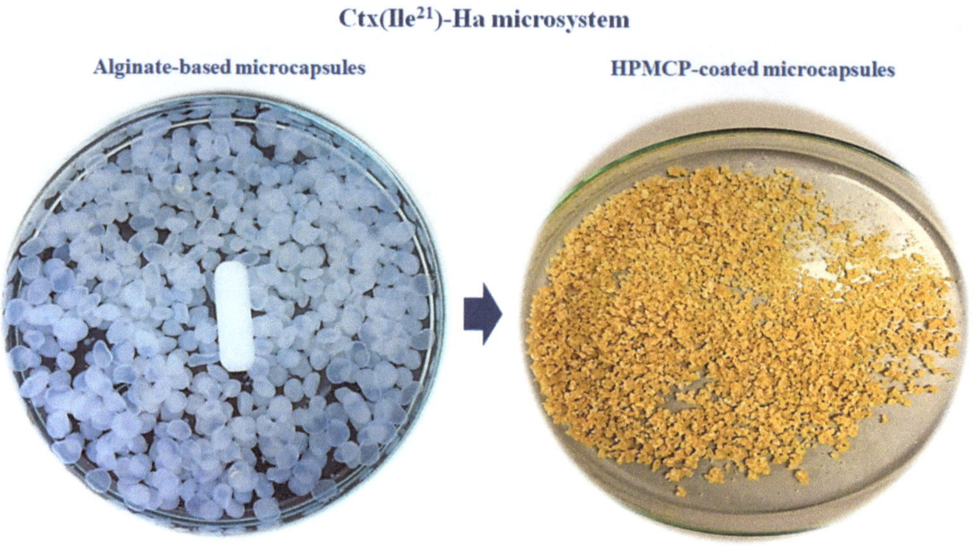

Figure 2. Microcapsules obtained after ionic gelation and fluidized bed.

3.2. *In Vivo Results*

The degree of invasiveness present in this study, together with the ethical requirements in the use of animals in experiments, added to the preservation of the quality of handling, led to the use of 45 animals per treatment, making a total of 135 animals. All the chicks were challenged with *Salmonella* Enteritidis from the first day of life, and the PEP treatment groups received a different dose of AMP (Section 2.4). Weighing difference and mortality rate were evaluated using rigorous statistical analysis described in the Materials and Methods section.

3.2.1. Post-Inoculation Treatment Study

The mortality results showed the significant ($\alpha = 0.05$) influence of the application of coated-microparticles loaded with Ctx(Ile^{21})-Ha AMP in the treatment on the registered mortality percentages (p =0.03), by using Qui-square test, with two degrees of freedom (df = 2). Therefore, mortality percentages differ significantly between treatments. In the control treatment (CTRL), the estimated risk of death for a chicken (R_{CTRL}) corresponds to the probability estimation of chick death, given the non-ingestion of the microparticles with antimicrobial peptide Ctx(Ile^{21})-Ha; that is, $R_{CTRL} = 13/45 = 28.89\%$. In parallel, risk of death for a hen treated with PEP1, which is the estimate of the probability of death of the chick given the ingestion of 20 mg of Ctx(Ile^{21})-Ha microencapsulated per kg of poultry feed, is $R_{PEP1} = 4/45 = 8.89\%$. Finally, the risk of death for a hen treated with PEP2, which corresponds to the estimated probability of death of the chick given the ingestion of 40 mg of Ctx(Ile^{21})-Ha microencapsulated per kg of poultry feed; that is, $R_{PEP2} = 6/45 = 13.33\%$.

The mortality results were explored with the percentage distribution conditioned by each treatment, where the proportion of the results was presented as a function of the corresponding treatment to which the chicks were subjected (Figure 3). Due to the statistics illustrated in Figure 3, the risk of death was compared two by two, using estimated Relative Risk (RR) statistic that quantifies the relationship between higher mortality through the relationship between risks [23], the numerator having the highest risk and the denominator, the lowest risk.

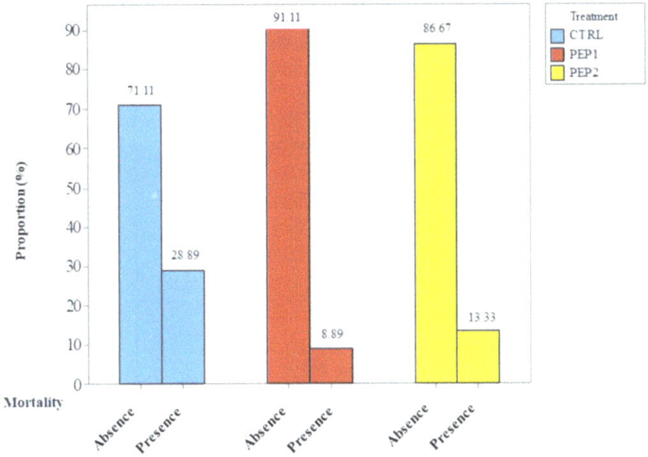

Figure 3. Percentage distribution of mortality resulted from the in vivo treatments analyzed.

In this study, PEP1 and PEP2 treatments have the function of protecting the chicks from the direct and indirect harmful effects of *S.* Enteritidis inoculation. Therefore, the control group corresponds to the exposure group and, consequently, to a higher risk. Thus, three RR estimates could be produced, but only two were of real interest for analysis.

The first was the RR of mortality among the animals in the CTRL and PEP1 treatments ($R_{CTRL\text{-}PEP1}$):

$$\hat{RR}_{CTRL-PEP1} = \frac{\hat{R}_{CTRL}}{\hat{R}_{PEP1}} \quad (1)$$

According to the results, a value of 3.25 ($p = 0.01$) was obtained. This implies that the risk of death of the hen is 3.25 times higher in the CTRL condition compared to PEP1.

The second, the estimated relative mortality risk between animals in the CTRL and PEP2 treatment ($R_{CTRL\text{-}PEP2}$):

$$\hat{RR}_{CTRL-PEP2} = \frac{\hat{R}_{CTRL}}{\hat{R}_{PEP2}} \quad (2)$$

and the following results were obtained: a value of 2.17 ($p = 0.04$) is reached, which indicates that the risk of death of the hen is 2.17 times higher in the CTRL condition compared to PEP2.

Importantly, the use of the hypothesis test (H_0 or H_1) performed was one-sided since the treatment is unlikely to increase mortality at a 5% significance level ($\alpha = 0.05$). Thus, the null hypothesis (H_0: RR = 1) is rejected in both risk tests ($p = 0.04$) in favor of the alternative hypothesis (H_1: RR > 1), which allows a 95% Confidence Interval (CI) of Relative Risks as a form of interval estimation for the RR population. This is represented by:

$$95\%\ \text{CI to}\ RR_{(CTRL-PEP1)} = [1.36, \infty) \quad (3)$$

That is, with 95% CI, it is possible to affirm that the true RR in question (the population) is at least greater than or equal to 1.36. This implies that the true mortality in a population is at least 36% higher for control group animals compared to the PEP1-treated group:

$$95\%\ \text{CI to}\ RR_{(CTRL-PEP2)} = [1.04, \infty) \quad (4)$$

Therefore, with 95% CI, it is possible to affirm that the true RR in question (the population) is at least 1.04. This implies that the true mortality in a population is at least 4% higher for the chicks in the control group, compared to the PEP2-treated group.

In this experiment there was no reduction in mortality when the peptide concentration was increased. Therefore, it is not necessary to test the statistical difference in mortality risk between these two doses. Moreover, a higher protection (lower mortality) was obtained with fewer resources (peptide mass), which is important in an industrial approach. That is, due to the results, the reduction in mortality does not improve due to the increase in concentration. However, in the best of cases, it remains the same. Furthermore, it is highlighted that there is statistical evidence that PEP1 treatment reduces total mortality, and not only due to *S.* Enteritidis infection. They can be used to establish a metric that quantifies the protection acquired by chicks, because they were also subjected to a treatment with peptides (PEP1 or PEP2). In addition, this can be due to the nature of the action of antimicrobial peptides, which is to protect the chicks against *S.* Enteritidis (Figure 4).

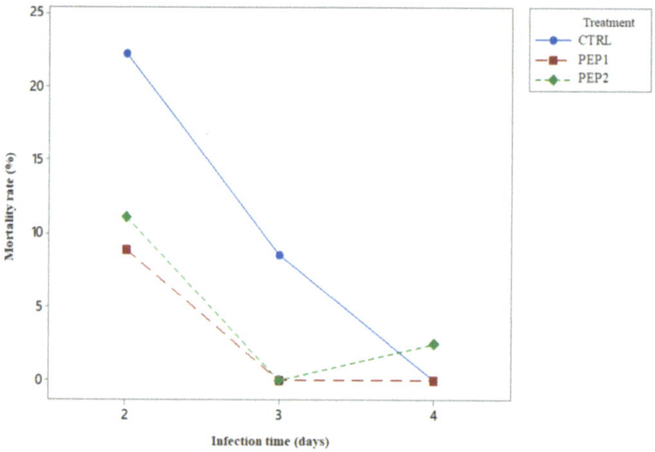

Figure 4. Mortality rate as a function of time of infection.

The Protection Factor (PF) is the statistic that quantifies the reduction in mortality risk due to the use of PEP1 or PEP2. In this case, mathematically, the PF is nothing more than the opposite of RR, shown in Equation (5). Therefore, the estimation of the Protection Factor that PEP1 treatment has on mortality, when compared with the CTRL, is given by:

$$\hat{PF}_{(CTRL-PEP1)} = 1 - \left(\hat{RR}_{(CTRL-PEP1)}\right)^{-1} \quad (5)$$

Therefore, 1 − (1/3.25) = 0.69. Thus, it is specifically estimated that treatment with PEP1 reduces the risk of death of chicks by 69% ($p < 0.01$), compared to the CTRL group. When using the one-sided interval estimation, with 95% confidence, for $\hat{PF}_{CTRL\text{-}PEP1}$:

$$CI_{95\%} \text{ to } \hat{PF}_{(CTRL-PEP1)} = [0.26, 1.00) \quad (6)$$

This implies that the reduction in mortality from the use of PEP1 is at least 26%, compared to the control group. The estimate of the protection factor is exerted by PEP2 treatment on the control group, and is given by:

$$\hat{PF}_{(CTRL-PEP2)} = 1 - \left(\hat{RR}_{(CTRL-PEP2)}\right)^{-1} \quad (7)$$

Therefore, 1 − (1/2.17) = 0.54. This result indicates that PEP2 treatment reduces the risk of mortality by 54% compared to the CTRL group ($p = 0.04$). Using the unilateral interval estimate for $\hat{PF}_{CTRL\text{-}PEP2}$, with 95% confidence:

$$CI_{95\%} \text{ to } \hat{PF}_{(CTRL-PEP2)} = [0.04, 1.00) \quad (8)$$

Consequently, the reduction in mortality from the use of PEP2 is at least 4% (more precisely, 4.05%), compared to the CTRL group.

The mortality rate after 5 dpi (days post-infection, 7th day of life) was zero for the chicks, subjected to all the treatments studied. Thus, the critical analysis period was concentrated from 2 dpi to 4 dpi per day of the experiment. With clear evidence, chicks treated with the ERCtx had a mortality rate of zero at 3 dpi (Figure 4). In relation to PEP2, there was only one death at 4 dpi, a fact that differs from the trend shown by treatments, and that may be caused by some eventuality, but it is not possible to conclude with certainty. There is a significant difference between the mortality rate of the CTRL group compared to the PEP1 and PEP2 treatments, on the second and third days of infection ($p < 0.05$). This shows that the antimicrobial peptide has the effect of reducing the risk of mortality already at the beginning of infection, when chickens ingest the microencapsulated peptide, which corresponds to the most acute phase of their mortality.

3.2.2. Using a Power Test to Analyze Results

The one-sided 95% CI showed that the reduction, in percentage points, in the mortality rate from the control group to the PEP1 treatment group would have the lower limit (LL = 0.07 = 7%). This means that the existing population reduction would be at least 7%, which is highly satisfactory. For the reduction from CTRL to PEP2, it would be with LL = 0.02 = 2%, which is less than satisfactory. For this reason, it is not necessary to increase the sample size to demonstrate the efficacy of the Ctx(Ile^{21})-Ha antimicrobial peptide, when considering the performance of PEP1 treatment in reducing the mortality rate.

When assessing the sufficiency of the sample size, analysis with the Power Test can be included, which corresponds to the sensitivity of the test to reject the null hypothesis unequivocally, which can further improve test performance [24]. For this reason, a simulation was developed for different mortality rates lower than those obtained in the control treatment, according to the alternative hypothesis. The simulation for the sample size calculations was based on the estimates obtained, with a significance level of 5% and a power test of 80%, considered by Cohen [25] as acceptable. In Figure 5, the minimum number of sample units per treatment (for example, number of chicks used) is shown for the test to detect the reduction in mortality for proportions of 25 to 5%.

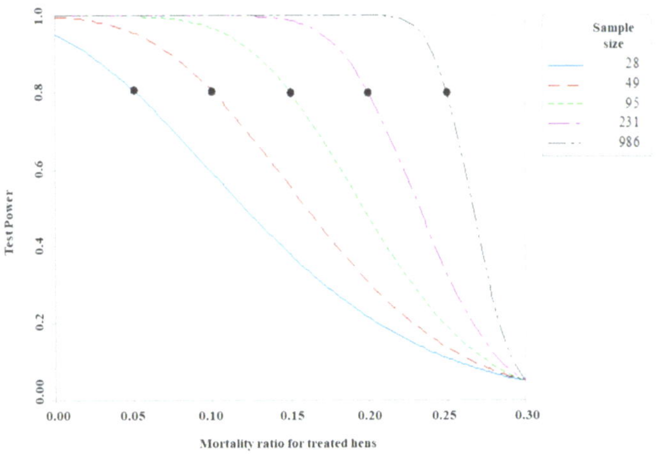

Figure 5. Calculation of the theoretical sample size to demonstrate the test power obtained in this experiment.

According to Figure 5, it is evident that the more the mortality proportion is reduced, the smaller the sample size necessary to detect the decrease in mortality, with a power of 80% and a significance of 5%. Mortality rates between 5 and 10% are known to require between 28 and 49 chicks per treatment, respectively. This result affirms that the 45 chicks used per treatment in this experiment would be sufficient to detect a reduction in mortality in the control treatment of the order of 20 percentage points or more, which occurs in the treatment with the lowest dose of peptide (PEP1). In another situation, if it is considered only for comparison (CTRL for PEP2), then a significance level greater than 5% would be adopted, or a power less than 80%, which could compromise the sensitivity of the test, or in general, test another four animals for each treatment to complete 49 animals per treatment, which would be unnecessary at this time, given the results found.

3.2.3. Cecal Content

The data for the *S.* Enteritidis count in CFU mL^{-1} required transformation to a natural logarithm (Ln), to adapt the recommended model in ANOVA. The F test for treatment purposes showed statistical evidence ($p < 0.02$) that there is a difference between treatments. Likewise, the time effect of infection on the Ln count was strongly significant ($p = 0.00$), especially on the second day of infection (5 days of life). In addition to the main effects, the interaction effect was also investigated ($p = 0.24$).

This result shows that there is no evidence of an interaction between treatment and age; that is, the treatment showing the best performance is still PEP1, especially on the second day of infection, and after that this treatment alone, does not differ significantly from the others, as shown in Figure 6.

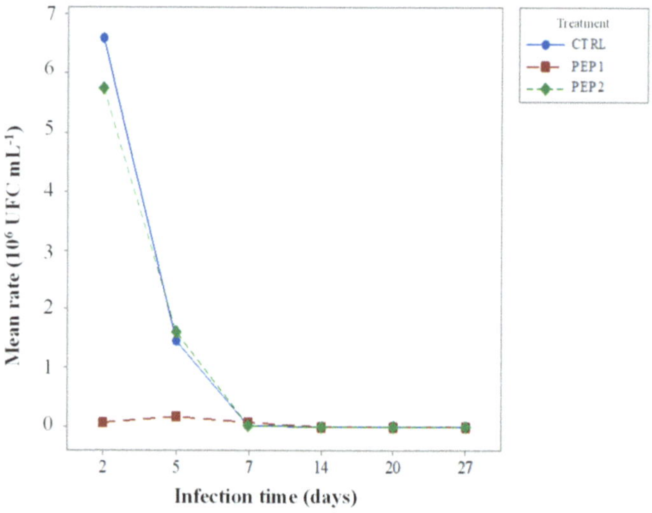

Figure 6. Mean count rate of *S.* Enteritidis, which is dependent on the treatments and time of infection.

After ANOVA, a comparison test of the control treatment (CTRL) was performed against the other treatments (PEP1 or PEP2) using Dunnett's test, which, in turn, showed statistical significance only between CTRL and PEP1 ($p < 0.05$).

3.2.4. Chick Cloacal Swab

Results of the follow-up of the infection with the swab method of the *S.* Enteritidis inoculum (Figure 7) at a concentration of 10^9 CFU mL^{-1}, were subjected to the Chi-square test ($p > 0.05$), where the *p*-value found was 0.88. This result indicates that there is no evidence that the proportion of presence or absence is different between treatments. Therefore, based on this sample, it cannot be said that the treatment influences the absence or presence of the inoculum.

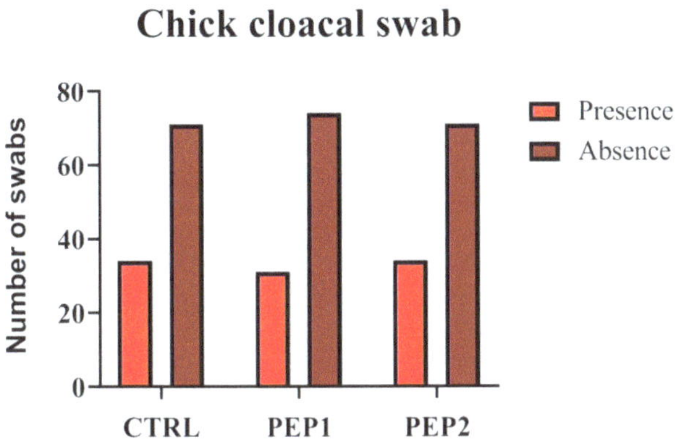

Figure 7. Evaluation of the effect of antimicrobial peptide on *Salmonella* Enteritidis fecal excretion during 28 days.

3.2.5. Weighing of the Chicks

From the inferential perspective, the F-test for treatment purposes showed moderate evidence ($p = 0.07$) that there is a difference between treatments. The effect of age on weight, on the other hand, was strongly significant ($p = 0.00$) due to the intrinsic development of the body mass of the chicks, especially in the first weeks of life. In addition to these main effects, the presence of an interaction effect was also investigated ($p = 0.74$). This result shows that there is no evidence of interaction between treatment and age; that is, the effect of the treatments does not depend on age. These results could be illustrated using a boxplot (Figure 8).

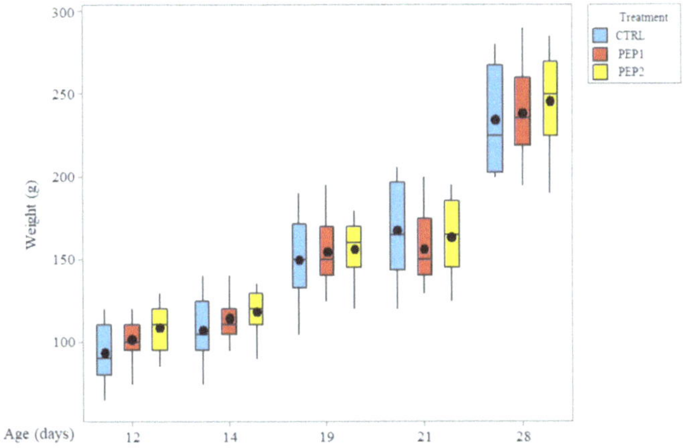

Figure 8. Boxplot of weight distribution according to the treatments and infection time to which the chicks were subjected.

4. Discussion

Due to the absence of similar studies for parameter estimations necessary for the calculations, the minimum number of chicks required to demonstrate the efficacy of the treatment in reducing mortality was not determined. This is in agreement with Montgomery and Runger [20], when they report on the minimum conditions to use the approximation of the binomial by normal distribution, which is necessary when calculating the sample size that involves proportional estimation. The approximation conditions are: $np > 5$ and $np(1 - p) > 5$, where "n" is the sample size, "p" is the proportion of the event of interest:

in this case, the death of the chicks. These same authors note that, in general, a better approximation is given for large samples ($n > 40$).

It is known that the mortality rate caused by S. Enteritidis is low [26]. However, infection with this bacterium weakens the immune system and causes collateral damage that affects nutrient absorption [27]. Consequently, other bacteria can act as opportunists, colonizing the intestine and causing poultry death. Systemic poultry infection would be linked to the influence of the flagella in some *Salmonella* sp. serovars [26]. Thus, when it comes to newborn chickens (up to 5 dpi), some studies suggest the use of immune stimulators to reduce the mortality rate [27]. Another study affirms that the BT peptide was able to promote mRNA transcription for Toll-like receptors (TLR), responsible for producing a pro-inflammatory response with cytokines and, consequently, activating the immune response. They also highlighted that the use of AMPs in the first four days of life is important, and that its best application would be orally [14].

A recent study indicates that AMPs have the same bacteriostatic potential compared to conventional antibiotics, and they also increased the content of white blood cells, making them an excellent replacement alternative for bio-sustainable poultry production, even better than other natural components [28]. In addition, due to its rapid way of acting against bacteria, the risk of acquiring or generating bacterial resistance is minimal, since the main target of lytic AMPs are the plasmatic membranes [19].

A study with essential oils in a combination of *Syzygium aromaticum* and *Cinnamomum zeylanicum* showed antimicrobial activities against S. Enteritidis and *S. typhimurium* (0.322–0.644 mg mL^{-1} and 0.644–1.289 mg mL^{-1}, respectively). However, these MIC values were very low compared (9.32 and 37.30 μg L^{-1}, respectively) to those reached by the Ctx(Ile^{21})-Ha antimicrobial peptide. It is worth mentioning that in vitro studies revealed that the microencapsulated Ctx(Ile^{21})-Ha peptide presented antimicrobial activity with pathogens from the poultry sector such as *Salmonella* Enteritidis, *Salmonella* Typhimurium and *Escherichia coli* [19].

MccJ25 is a highly studied cyclic recombinant AMP, presenting a broad bactericidal spectrum, mainly against *Salmonella* sp. [29] This AMP showed that its function is not only to eliminate the bacteria and improve the fecal microbiota, but also to influence intestinal morphology by improving texture and reducing inflammation after infection [30]. Moreover, bacteriocins are an AMP group studied for use in the poultry and swine industry. They are produced by some bacteria (the majority by Gram-positive) and present interesting effects by reducing the content of pathogenic bacteria, such as *Salmonella* sp. and *Campylobacter jejuni* [31]. Other bacteriocins were studied to reduce *Salmonella* in broilers using a dose of 2.5 g kg^{-1}, exhibiting an increase in the weight of the chickens and a slight bacterial decrease [32]. Unlike our results, which could be due to the minimum dose used in this experiment, which is thousands of times less than the reference, our work used mg (miligrams) of peptide instead of g (grams), used by the reference mentioned. However, other research indicates that the application of swine intestine [33] as a food supplement influences positively broilers' weight, as well as an increased villus height [34]. As an explanation, the hypothesis is if Ctx(Ile^{21})-Ha peptide concentration is incremented, it will be possible to visualize a more pronounced increase in weight in chicks. However, for a pilot in vivo experiment, the Ctx(Ile^{21})-Ha peptide microcapsules showed very promising and interesting results.

Studies based on previous AMP-encapsulates, such as bacteriocins, were protected using polyvinylpyrrolidone as an encapsulating material and showed promising results due to decrease content of *C. jejuni*. However, the AMP dose employed was very high compared with our encapsulated products (500 mg of AMP per kg^{-1} of poultry feed) [35]. Our product is encapsulated based on sodium alginate, which is a cheap and more biocompatible polymer [36]. Sodium alginate encapsulations loaded with specific phages (f3αSE) for S. Enteritidis have been made, achieving up to 80% protection of viability of this product at a gastric pH [37]. This confirms and corroborates that our developed microcapsules can satisfactorily contain and protect the Ctx(Ile^{21})-Ha AMP, as they also have an additional protective layer with HPMCP. This polymer is degraded only at intestinal pH used as a drug targeting, and which also protects microparticles and AMP from mechanical processes that could be subjected to in manufacturing or by the gizzard [11,19].

Consequently, this study showed a decrease in mortality rate in first days of life, which certifies the success of the encapsulated and coated antimicrobial peptide. Values of anti-*S.* Enteritidis activity in vivo did not make a significant difference. However, there is an interesting result in first days of life, decreasing the total count. This could be due to the relationship between the amount of microcapsule ingested and the total volume of the intestine, and that each time the chicks grew, this relationship would be more different. Therefore, it is suggested that further experiments employing higher doses can be performed to achieve a total bacterial decrease.

5. Conclusions

The in vivo analyses allow us to conclude that the antimicrobial peptide Ctx(Ile^{21})-Ha presented positive, significant and promising results in relation to the reduction in younger chicken's mortality and the bacterial count, mainly for PEP1 treatment, where there is a 69% reduction in the risk of death. Regarding the weight of the chickens, in two doses of antimicrobial peptide used, there was a significant difference between treatments and this result shows that there is no evidence of interaction between treatment and age; that is, the effect of the treatments does not depend on age. Finally, it is concluded that there is a potential effect of the microencapsulated-coated antimicrobial peptide Ctx(Ile^{21})-Ha in poultry, which enables the application of the peptide by using a very low mass compared to other studies in the literature.

6. Patents

The present methodology and application developed was deposited in the National Institute of Intellectual Property (INPI BR1020200220489), which is protected throughout the Brazilian territory.

Author Contributions: Conceptualization, E.F.V.; methodology, P.A.B.M.-L., E.A.L.G., N.M.S. and M.C.; validation, E.A.L.G. and N.M.S.; formal analysis, D.D.S.; investigation, L.P.P., A.B.M., E.A.L.G. and N.M.S.; resources, E.F.V.; data curation, E.F.V. and P.A.B.M.-L.; writing—original draft preparation, C.A.R.-B.; writing—review and editing, C.A.R.-B., E.F.V. and P.A.B.M.-L.; supervision, E.F.V., P.A.B.M.-L. and M.C.; funding acquisition, E.F.V. All authors have read and agreed to the published version of the manuscript.

Funding: This research was funded by São Paulo Research Foundation/FAPESP (Process number 2016/00446-7), master (Process number 2018/25707-3) and undergraduate scholarships (Process number 2017/21822-0).

Institutional Review Board Statement: Animal experiments were approved by the local Animal Ethics Committee (CEUA) from São Paulo State University (Unesp), School of Sciences and Engineering, Tupã, Brazil (Number process 06/2018).

Informed Consent Statement: Not applicable.

Data Availability Statement: Not applicable.

Acknowledgments: We thank the technical assistants of Laboratory of Chemistry and Biochemistry from São Paulo State University (Unesp), School of Sciences and Engineering, Tupã; the University of Araraquara, which kindly made available the use of the fluidized-bed equipment; the Shin-Etsu company for gently donating the HPMCP coating for the experiments; and finally, the research group "Peptides: Synthesis, Optimization and Applied Studies - PeSEAp" for continuous support.

Conflicts of Interest: The authors declare no conflict of interest.

References

1. Renu, S.; Han, Y.; Dhakal, S.; Lakshmanappa, Y.S.; Ghimire, S.; Feliciano-Ruiz, N.; Senapati, S.; Narasimhan, B.; Selvaraj, R.; Renukaradhya, G.J. Chitosan-adjuvanted Salmonella subunit nanoparticle vaccine for poultry delivered through drinking water and feed. *Carbohydr. Polym.* **2020**, *243*, 116434. [CrossRef] [PubMed]
2. Gaggìa, F.; Mattarelli, P.; Biavati, B. Probiotics and prebiotics in animal feeding for safe food production. *Int. J. Food Microbiol.* **2010**, *141*, S15–S28. [CrossRef]
3. Tacconelli, E.; Carrara, E.; Savoldi, A.; Harbarth, S.; Mendelson, M.; Monnet, D.L.; Pulcini, C.; Kahlmeter, G.; Kluytmans, J.; Carmeli, Y.; et al. Discovery, research, and development of new antibiotics: The WHO priority list of antibiotic-resistant bacteria and tuberculosis. *Lancet Infect. Dis.* **2018**, *18*, 318–327. [CrossRef]
4. World Health Organization. *Global Priority List of Antibiotic-Resistant Bacteria to Guide Research, Discovery, and Development of New Antibiotics*; World Health Organization: Geneva, Switzerland, 2017.
5. Ahmed, A.; Siman-Tov, G.; Hall, G.; Bhalla, N.; Narayanan, A. Human Antimicrobial Peptides as Therapeutics for Viral Infections. *Viruses* **2019**, *11*, 704. [CrossRef] [PubMed]
6. Lin, Z.; Wu, T.; Wang, W.; Li, B.; Wang, M.; Chen, L.; Xia, H.; Zhang, T. Biofunctions of antimicrobial peptide-conjugated alginate/hyaluronic acid/collagen wound dressings promote wound healing of a mixed-bacteria-infected wound. *Int. J. Biol. Macromol.* **2019**, *140*, 330–342. [CrossRef]
7. Ferreira Cespedes, G.; Nicolas Lorenzon, E.; Festozo Vicente, E.; Jose Soares Mendes-Giannini, M.; Fontes, W.; de Souza Castro, M.; Maffud Cilli, E. Mechanism of Action and Relationship Between Structure and Biological Activity of Ctx-Ha: A New Ceratotoxin-like Peptide from Hypsiboas albopunctatus. *Protein Pept. Lett.* **2012**, *19*, 596–603. [CrossRef]
8. Vicente, E.F.; Basso, L.G.M.; Cespedes, G.F.; Lorenzón, E.N.; Castro, M.S.; Mendes-Giannini, M.J.S.; Costa-Filho, A.J.; Cilli, E.M. Dynamics and Conformational Studies of TOAC Spin Labeled Analogues of Ctx(Ile21)-Ha Peptide from Hypsiboas albopunctatus. *PLoS ONE* **2013**, *8*, e60818. [CrossRef]
9. Ghibaudo, G.; Santospirito, D.; Sala, A.; Flisi, S.; Taddei, S.; Cavirani, S.; Cabassi, C.S. In vitro antimicrobial activity of a gel containing antimicrobial peptide AMP_{2041}, chlorhexidine digluconate and Tris-EDTA on clinical isolates of *Pseudomonas aeruginosa* from canine otitis. *Vet. Dermatol.* **2016**, *27*, 391. [CrossRef]
10. Malekkhaiat Häffner, S.; Malmsten, M. Interplay between amphiphilic peptides and nanoparticles for selective membrane destabilization and antimicrobial effects. *Curr. Opin. Colloid Interface Sci.* **2019**, *44*, 59–71. [CrossRef]
11. Roque Borda, C.A.; Saraiva de Mesquita Souza, M.; Monte, F.M.D.; Rodrigues Alves, L.B.; de Almeida, A.M.; Santiago Ferreira, T.; Spina de Lima, T.; Pereira Benevides, V.; Memrava Cabrera, J.; Meneguin, A.B.; et al. Application of HPMCAS-coated Ctx(Ile21)-Ha peptide microparticles as a potential use to prevent systemic infection caused by Salmonella Enteritidis in poultry. *bioRxiv* **2021**. [CrossRef]
12. Roque Borda, C.A.; Leite Silva, H.R.; Silveira, F.R.; Bustos Mac-Lean, P.A.; Vicente, E.F. Peptídeos antimicrobianos na produção animal: Uma alternativa biosustentável. In *Tecnologias Sustentáveis e Agronegócio*; Ferrari Putti, F., Casemiro da Silva, A.L., Almeida Gabriel Filho, L.R., Eds.; Editora ANAP: Tupã, São Paulo, Brazil, 2020; pp. 131–166. ISBN 9786586753233.
13. Silveira, R.F.; Roque Borda, C.A.; Vicente, E.F. Antimicrobial peptides as a feed additive alternative to animal production, food safety and public health implications: An overview. *Anim. Nutr.* **2021**, *7*, 603.
14. Kogut, M.H.; Genovese, K.J.; He, H.; Swaggerty, C.L.; Jiang, Y. Modulation of chicken intestinal immune gene expression by small cationic peptides as feed additives during the first week posthatch. *Clin. Vaccine Immunol.* **2013**, *20*, 1440–1448. [CrossRef] [PubMed]
15. Plazola-Jacinto, C.P.; Pérez-Pérez, V.; Pereyra-Castro, S.C.; Alamilla-Beltrán, L.; Ortiz-Moreno, A. Microencapsulation of biocompounds from avocado leaves oily extracts. *Rev. Mex. Ing. Quim.* **2019**, *18*, 1261–1276. [CrossRef]
16. Harimurti, S.; Ariyadi, B.; Wihandoyo; Akhirini, N.; Pradipta, M.S.I. Growth of probiotics for poultry in glucose yeast pepton media, production of biomass, viability and stability after encapsulation with spray drying. In Proceedings of the IOP Conference Series: Earth and Environmental Science, Graz, Austria, 11–14 September 2019; Institute of Physics Publishing: Bristol, UK, 2019; Volume 387, p. 12130.
17. Son, Y.R.; Chung, J.H.; Ko, S.; Shim, S.M. Combinational enhancing effects of formulation and encapsulation on digestive stability and intestinal transport of green tea catechins. *J. Microencapsul.* **2016**, *33*, 183–190. [CrossRef] [PubMed]
18. Momoh, M.A.; Akpa, P.A.; Ugwu, K.C.; Kenechukwu, F.C.; Kenneth, O.C. Pharmacodynamics and pharmacokinetics behaviour of insulin from PEGylated-mucin microparticles coated with pH sensitive polymer: Preparation and characterization. *Mater. Today Commun.* **2020**, *25*, 101539. [CrossRef]
19. Roque-Borda, C.A.; Silva, H.R.L.; Crusca Junior, E.; Serafim, J.A.; Meneguin, A.B.; Chorilli, M.; Macedo, W.C.; Teixeira, S.R.; Guastalli, E.A.L.; Soares, N.M.; et al. Alginate-based microparticles coated with HPMCP/AS cellulose-derivatives enable the Ctx(Ile21)-Ha antimicrobial peptide application as a feed additive. *Int. J. Biol. Macromol.* **2021**, *183*, 1236–1247. [CrossRef] [PubMed]
20. Montgomery, D.; Runger, G. *Probabilidad y Estadística Aplicadas a la Ingeniería*, 2nd ed.; Limusa SA: Mexico City, Mexico, 2012; Volume 817.
21. Berchieri, A.J.; Murphy, C.K.; Marston, K.; Barrow, P.A. Observations on the persistence and vertical transmission of Salmonella enterica serovars Pullorum and Gallinarum in chickens: Effect of bacterial and host genetic background. *Avian Pathol.* **2001**, *30*, 221–231. [CrossRef]

22. Freitas Neto, O.C.; Arroyave, W.; Alessi, A.C.; Fagliari, J.J.; Berchieri, A. Infection of commercial laying hens with Salmonella gallinarum: Clinical, anatomopathological and haematological studies. *Rev. Bras. Cienc. Avic.* **2007**, *9*, 133–141. [CrossRef]
23. González, R.J.; Sampedro, F.; Feirtag, J.M.; Sánchez-Plata, M.X.; Hedberg, C.W. Prioritization of chicken meat processing interventions on the basis of reducing the Salmonella residual relative risk. *J. Food Prot.* **2019**, *82*, 1575–1582. [CrossRef]
24. Roush, W.B.; Tozer, P.R. The power of tests for bioequivalence in feed experiments with poultry. *J. Anim. Sci.* **2004**, *82*, E110–E118. [CrossRef]
25. Cohen, J. *Statistical Power Analysis for the Behavioral Sciences*, 2nd ed.; Lawrence Erlbaum Associates Inc.: Hillsdale, MI, USA, 1988; Volume 13.
26. De Oliveira Barbosa, F.; de Freitas Neto, O.C.; Batista, D.F.A.; de Almeida, A.M.; da Silva Rubio, M.; Alves, L.B.R.; de Oliveira Vasconcelos, R.; Barrow, P.A.; Berchieri Junior, A. Contribution of flagella and motility to gut colonisation and pathogenicity of Salmonella Enteritidis in the chicken. *Braz. J. Microbiol.* **2017**, *48*, 754–759. [CrossRef] [PubMed]
27. He, H.; Lowry, V.K.; Swaggerty, C.L.; Ferro, P.J.; Kogut, M.H. In vitro activation of chicken leukocytes and in vivo protection against *Salmonella enteritidis* organ invasion and peritoneal *S. enteritidis* infection-induced mortality in neonatal chickens by immunostimulatory CpG oligodeoxynucleotide. *FEMS Immunol. Med. Microbiol.* **2005**, *43*, 81–89. [CrossRef]
28. Xu, B.; Fu, J.; Zhu, L.; Li, Z.; Jin, M.; Wang, Y. Overall assessment of antibiotic substitutes for pigs: A set of meta-analyses. *J. Anim. Sci. Biotechnol.* **2021**, *12*, 3. [CrossRef] [PubMed]
29. Vincent, P.A.; Delgado, M.A.; Farías, R.N.; Salomón, R.A. Inhibition of Salmonella enterica serovars by microcin J25. *FEMS Microbiol. Lett.* **2004**, *236*, 103–107. [CrossRef] [PubMed]
30. Wang, G.; Song, Q.; Huang, S.; Wang, Y.; Cai, S.; Yu, H.; Ding, X.; Zeng, X.; Zhang, J. Effect of Antimicrobial Peptide Microcin J25 on Growth Performance, Immune Regulation, and Intestinal Microbiota in Broiler Chickens Challenged with Escherichia coli and Salmonella. *Animals* **2020**, *10*, 345. [CrossRef] [PubMed]
31. Ben Lagha, A.; Haas, B.; Gottschalk, M.; Grenier, D. Antimicrobial potential of bacteriocins in poultry and swine production. *Vet. Res.* **2017**, *48*, 22. [CrossRef] [PubMed]
32. Wang, H.-T.; Yu, C.; Hsieh, Y.-H.; Chen, S.-W.; Chen, B.-J.; Chen, C.-Y. Effects of albusin B (a bacteriocin) of Ruminococcus albus 7 expressed by yeast on growth performance and intestinal absorption of broiler chickens-its potential role as an alternative to feed antibiotics. *J. Sci. Food Agric.* **2011**, *91*, 2338–2343. [CrossRef]
33. Wang, D.; Ma, W.; She, R.; Sun, Q.; Liu, Y.; Hu, Y.; Liu, L.; Yang, Y.; Peng, K. Effects of swine gut antimicrobial peptides on the intestinal mucosal immunity in specific-pathogen-free chickens. *Poult. Sci.* **2009**, *88*, 967–974. [CrossRef]
34. Liu, T.; She, R.; Wang, K.; Bao, H.; Zhang, Y.; Luo, D.; Hu, Y.; Ding, Y.; Wang, D.; Peng, K. Effects of rabbit sacculus rotundus antimicrobial peptides on the intestinal mucosal immunity in chickens. *Poult. Sci.* **2008**, *87*, 250–254. [CrossRef]
35. Stern, N.J.; Svetoch, E.A.; Eruslanov, B.V.; Kovalev, Y.N.; Volodina, L.I.; Perelygin, V.V.; Mitsevich, E.V.; Mitsevich, I.P.; Levchuk, V.P. Paenibacillus polymyxa purified bacteriocin to control Campylobacter jejuni in chickens. *J. Food Prot.* **2005**, *68*, 1450–1453. [CrossRef]
36. Lee, K.Y.; Mooney, D.J. Alginate: Properties and biomedical applications. *Prog. Polym. Sci.* **2012**, *37*, 106–126. [CrossRef] [PubMed]
37. Soto, M.J.; Retamales, J.; Palza, H.; Bastías, R. Encapsulation of specific Salmonella Enteritidis phage f3αSE on alginate-spheres as a method for protection and dosification. *Electron. J. Biotechnol.* **2018**, *31*, 57–60. [CrossRef]

antibiotics

Article

Natural Agents against Bovine Mastitis Pathogens

Zorana Kovačević [1,*], Miodrag Radinović [1], Ivana Čabarkapa [2], Nebojša Kladar [3] and Biljana Božin [3]

[1] Department of Veterinary Medicine, Faculty of Agriculture, University of Novi Sad, Trg Dositeja Obradovica 8, 21000 Novi Sad, Serbia; miodrag.radinovic@polj.uns.ac.rs
[2] Institute of Food Technology, University of Novi Sad, Bulevar cara Lazara 1, 21000 Novi Sad, Serbia; ivana.cabarkapa@fins.uns.ac.rs
[3] Center for Medical and Pharmaceutical Investigations and Quality Control/Department of Pharmacy, Faculty of Medicine, University of Novi Sad, Hajduk Veljkova 3, 21000 Novi Sad, Serbia; nebojsa.kladar@mf.uns.ac.rs (N.K.); biljana.bozin@mf.uns.ac.rs (B.B.)
* Correspondence: zorana.kovacevic@polj.edu.rs

Abstract: Bovine mastitis is the most widespread and economically important disease worldwide. The present study aimed to determine bioactive compounds in two essential oils (EOs) from wild *(Thymus serpyllum)* and common thyme *(Thymus vulgaris)* and to assess the antioxidant potential as well as antibacterial efficacy of the EOs against mastitis-associated bacteria. The study also included antibiotic susceptibility tests. The strains were previously isolated from lactating animals with clinical and subclinical mastitis. The antioxidant potential of the commercial EOs of wild and common thyme was evaluated by five in vitro assays. The antibacterial activity was performed using the microdilution technique, while antibiotic susceptibility testing was performed by the Kirby–Bauer disc diffusion method. The dominant compound in wild thyme was thymol (45.22%), followed by *p*-cymene (23.83%) and γ-terpinene (3.12%), while in common thyme, it was thymol (54.17%), followed by γ-terpinene (22.18%) and *p*-cymene (16.66%). Among the fourteen mastitis-associated bacteria, strain IX *Streptococcus* spp. (β-hemolytic) was the most sensitive to the tested EOs (minimum inhibitory concentration (MIC)/minimal bactericidal concentration (MBC) were 0.78/1.56 and 0.39/0.78 mg/mL for *T. serpyllum* (TS) and *T. vulgaris (TV)*, respectively). Regarding *Streptococcus* spp. β heamoliticus, MICs for *TS* ranged from 0.78 to 1.56 mg/mL, while for the same oil, MBCs ranged from 1.56 to 12.5 mg/mL. In the case of *T. vulgaris,* MICs ranged from 0.39 to 3.125 mg/ mL, while MBCs ranged from 3.125 to 6.25 mg/mL. TV is more active against *E. coli, E. sakazakii,* and *Streptococcus* spp., while it is less effective against *Staphylococcus* spp. than TS. The study revealed that the tested EOs possess remarkable antioxidative and antibacterial activities and could be used in the development of pharmaceutical formulation as an alternative to conventional mastitis therapy.

Keywords: antibacterial activity; essential oil; mastitis causing bacteria; antioxidant; thymol; antibiotics

Citation: Kovačević, Z.; Radinović, M.; Čabarkapa, I.; Kladar, N.; Božin, B. Natural Agents against Bovine Mastitis Pathogens. *Antibiotics* **2021**, *10*, 205. https://doi.org/10.3390/antibiotics10020205

Academic Editor: William N. Setzer

Received: 2 January 2021
Accepted: 13 February 2021
Published: 19 February 2021

1. Introduction

The economic rise of the dairy market all over the world with the importance of delivering healthy and safety dairy products highlights the importance of managing milk production in a secure and sustainable manner [1–3]. In Serbia, milk production is organized in two different systems; small household farms with ten to twenty animals and large farms counting several hundred to several thousand cows [4].

The most common problems influencing animals' health in both production methods are those related to the health status of the mammary gland [5]. Actually, the occurrence of mastitis is highly frequent and, according to the type of clinical manifestation, this disease has clinical and subclinical classifications that occur simultaneously [6,7]. The etiology of mastitis is complex, and both mechanical and chemical factors that can be attributed to omissions in the way of housing and the procedure of milking cows certainly could contribute to the development of this disease [8]. This problem is more represented on large farms where little human labor is employed. Besides the etiology of mastitis, microbiological factors are more important, dominant bacterial causes [5]. While intramammary administration implies application of antibiotics directly in mammary gland through teat channel in order to achieve their effect locally in the gland, parenteral administration is application where the digestive tract is bypassed (e.g., intramuscularly, subcutaneously, intravenously) in order to achieve systemic effect including mammary gland tissue.

In Serbia, the most common causative agents of mastitis are *Staphylococcus aureus* and *Streptococcus agalactiae*, and recently *E. coli*, while *Klebsiella* spp., coagulase-negative staphylococci and *Streptococcus uberis* are becoming more and more common [5].

The prevalence of bovine mastitis resulted in the extensive use of antibiotics, intramammary and parenterally [9]. Erskine, et al. [10] revealed that 90% of antibiotic residues in milk are a consequence of mastitis therapy. Hence, the use of antibiotics in the treatment of mastitis has some negative consequences, such as entry of antibiotic residues into the human food chain [11], with the possibility of antibiotic-resistant bacteria strains transmission [12]. Additionally, as a negative consequence, increasing resistance of microorganisms to antibiotics causes the degree of intramammary infections cure to be at a very low level. Moreover, the degree of cure in the case of *Staphylococcus aureus* is 20 to 75% [13].

Control of udder health is important for the dairy production chain in light of food safety issues, with control of udder pathogens being the most important in the reduction of foodborne illness and giving healthy dairy food [14,15]. Besides, development and spread of resistance to antibiotics as a consequence of mastitis treatment represent a public health threat to consumers as a global problem, influencing both human and animal health. Faced with the continued growth of antibiotic-resistant pathogens, there is a need for finding novel antimicrobial compounds [16].

Considering the facts mentioned above, many studies tend to develop alternative treatments with bioactive plant-derived products (PDPs), such as plant extracts, essential oils (EOs), hydrolates, oleoresins, and so on [17,18]. Many attempts have been made to test the potential role of EOs and their active compounds to combat antibiotic resistance in bacteria [19].

Furthermore, although many aromatic plants and essential oils are tested, especially for antioxidant and antimicrobial activity, plants belonging to the genus *Thymus*, among others, are of special interest regarding the presence of notable amounts of thymol and carvacrol, being strong antioxidant and antimicrobial agents [20–23].

Moreover, these studies highlighted a high scientific interest whereby EOs warrant special attention as they are recognized as safe. Besides, EOs do not increase antibiotic resistance during long-term usage, which represents their main advantage [24]. Additionally, synergism between plant metabolites and antibiotics has been described by Hemaiswarya, et al. [25], suggesting the use of EOs as in combination with antibiotics. Furthermore, EOs were characterized by low mammalian toxicity, low environmental effects, and wide public acceptance.

However, it is well known that several chemotypes of *Thymus serpyllum* have been described until now [26–28]; as differences in chemical composition have a notable influence on investigated biological activities, new data are of great importance. Besides, it is well known that EOs' chemical composition, contributing to their medicinal value and being responsible for the biological properties, highly depends on many factors such as geographical and climatic conditions, harvesting, isolation techniques, as well as storage [29,30].

In line with those mentioned above, this study aimed to evaluate the effectiveness of EOs of common (*Thymus vulgaris* L.) and wild thyme (*Thymus serpyllum* L.) against mastitis-associated pathogens in Serbia.

2. Results

2.1. *Bacteriological Testing of Milk Samples*

Bacteriological testing was performed on a total of 31 milk samples, while pathogens were isolated in 21 (67.74%) samples. The isolated pathogens were the most common mastitis pathogens, including *Streptococcus* spp. β heamoliticus (Strep_bh), *E. coli* (E_c), *Enterobacter sakazakii* (E_s), *Klebsiella oxytoca* (K_o), *Staphylococcus aureus* (Staph_a), *Staphylococcus* spp. coagulase negative (Staph_cn), *Streptococcus dysgalactiae* (Strep_d), *Streptococcus* spp. (Strep), and *Streptococcus uberis* (Strep_u).

The most common among the pathogens was *E. coli*, which was identified in six samples (19.35%), followed by five (16.13%) samples with *Streptococcus* spp., while *Staphylococcus* spp. coagulase negative, *Streptococcus uberis*, *Streptococcus dysgalactiae*, *Klebsiella oxytoca*, and *Enterobacter sakazakii* were found in one sample each (3.23%) (Figure 1).

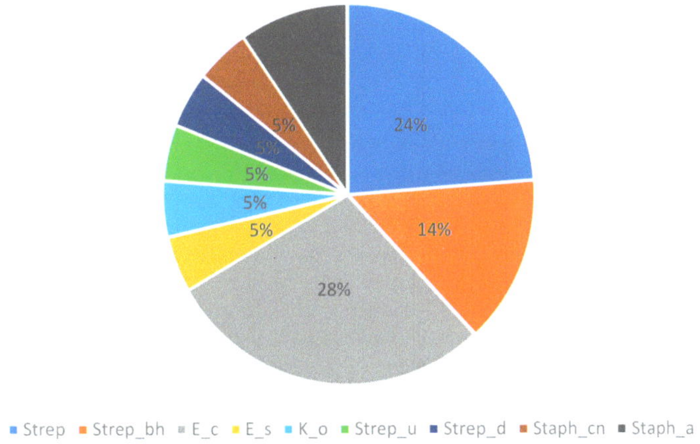

Figure 1. The proportion (%) of the evaluated bacterial strains in the collected samples.

2.2. *Antibiotic Susceptibility Testing of Mastitis-Associated Bacteria*

Antibiotic susceptibility patterns for the analyzed 16 mastitis-associated bacteria are shown in Table 1. Antibiotics included in the testing are amoxycillin (AMX), ampicillin (AMP), ceftriaxone (CRO), enrofloxacin (ENR), erythromycin (ERY), lincomycin (LIN), neomycin (NEO), penicillin (PEN), streptomycin (STR), tetracycline (TET), amoxicillin/clavulanic acid (AMC), novobiocin (NB), trimethoprim/sulfamethoxazole (SXT), and cloxacillin (CLO). In Serbia, the most used antibiotics in mastitis therapy are penicillin, streptomycin, gentamicin, tetracycline, cephalexin, sulfonamides, and enrofloxacin [31].

Table 1. Antibiotic susceptibility patterns for the mastitis-associated bacteria (S—sensitive, I—intermediate, R—resistant). AMX, moxycillin; AMP, ampicillin; CRO, ceftriaxone; ENR, enrofloxacin; ERY, erythromycin; LIN, lincomycin; NEO, neomycin; PEN, penicillin; STR, streptomycin; TET, tetracycline; AMC, amoxicillin/clavulanic acid; NB, novobiocin; SXT, trimethoprim/sulfamethoxazole; CLO, cloxacillin.

Bacterial Strains Culture	AMX	AMP	CRO	ENR	ERY	GEN	LIN	NEO	PEN	STR	TET	AMC	NB	SXT	CLO
Streptococcus spp. β heamoliticus	S	S	S	S	S	R	S	R	R	S	S	S	S	R	R
Staphylococcus spp.	R	R	R	R	R	I	R	R	R	S	R	R	R	R	R
Staphylococcus spp.	R	R	R	R	R	I	R	R	R	S	R	R	R	R	R
Staphylococcus spp. coagulase negative	S	S	I	S	S	S	S	S	R	S	S	S	S	S	R
Staphylococcus spp.	R	R	R	R	I	S	R	R	R	S	R	R	R	R	R
Streptococcus spp. β heamoliticus	I	R	S	S	R	S	R	S	R	S	I	S	I	S	R
E. coli	R	R	R	S	R	S	R	S	R	S	R	R	R	S	R
E. coli	R	R	R	S	R	S	R	S	R	S	I	R	R	S	R
Streptococcus spp. β heamoliticus	R	R	S	S	R	S	R	S	R	S	R	S	R	R	R
Klebsiella oxytoca	R	R	S	S	R	S	R	S	R	S	R	R	R	S	R

Table 1. *Cont.*

Bacterial Strains Culture	AMX	AMP	CRO	ENR	ERY	GEN	LIN	NEO	PEN	STR	TET	AMC	NB	SXT	CLO
E. coli	R	R	R	S	R	S	R	S	R	S	I	R	R	S	R
Staphylococcus spp.	R	R	I	S	R	S	I	R	R	S	R	S	R	R	R
E. coli	R	R	R	S	R	S	R	S	R	S	R	R	R	S	R
Enterobacter sakazakii	R	R	R	S	R	S	R	S	R	S	S	R	R	S	R
Staphylococcus aureus	I	R	S	S	S	S	S	S	R	S	S	S	S	S	R
E. coli	I	R	S	S	R	S	R	S	R	S	I	S	R	S	R
Streptococcus uberis	S	S	I	S	I	S	R	R	R	S	S	S	R	R	R
E. coli	I	R	S	S	R	S	R	S	R	S	S	S	R	S	R
Staphylococcus aureus	I	R	S	S	S	S	S	S	R	S	S	S	S	S	R
Streptococcus dysgalactiae	S	R	R	S	I	I	R	R	R	S	R	S	I	R	R
Staphylococcus spp.	S	S	S	S	S	S	R	R	R	R	R	S	R	R	R

Application of correspondence analysis (CA) on a dataset describing bactericidal potential of different antibiotics on bacteria isolated from the milk samples shows associations of different bacteria and the evaluated antibiotics in terms of bacteria resistance (R) or sensitivity (S). It must be stated that the results obtained for penicillin (PEN) and cloxacillin (CLO) were not included in statistical processing because of their uniformity. It was observed that the first three correspondent axes (CA1, CA2, and CA3) describe around 50% of the samples' variability (percentage of inertia for CA1, CA2, and CA3 was 22.14%, 17.83%, and 9.31%, respectively). The position of the evaluated bacteria cultures and antibiotics in the space defined by the first three correspondent axes (Figure 2) shows close association of *E. coli* (E_c), *Klebsiella oxytoca* (K_o) and *Enterobacter sakazakii* (E_s) in the negative part of CA1 and the positive part of CA2 as a result of resistance to erythromycin (ERY), amoxycillin (AMX), and amoxicillin/clavulanic acid (AMC), and sensitivity to neomycin (NEO) and trimethoprim/sulfamethoxazole (SXT). Furthermore, *Streptococcus* spp. (Strep) are localized in the negative part of CA1 and the negative part of CA2, which is closely related to resistance to SXT, NEO, enrofloxacin (ENR), tetracycline (TET), lincomycin (LIN), and ceftriaxone (CRO). *Streptococcus* spp. β-heamoliticus (Strep_bh) are sensitive to AMC, CRO, and ENR. *Staphylococcus aureus* are resistant to ampicillin (AMP), penicillin (PEN), and cloxacillin (CLO).

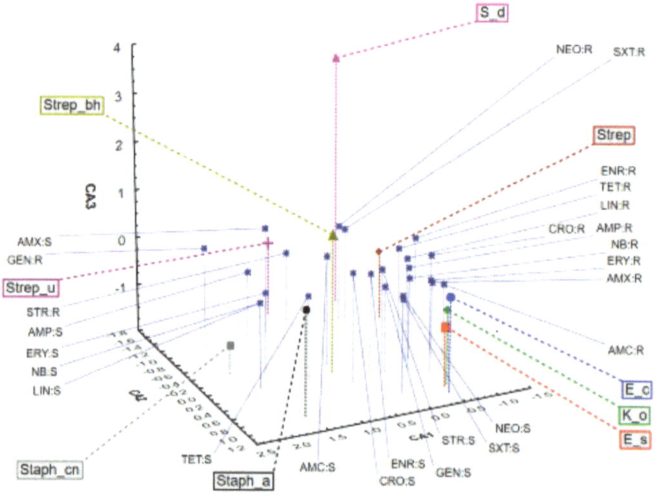

Figure 2. Position of the evaluated bacterial cultures and their sensitivity (S) or resistance (R) to antibiotics treatment in the space defined by the first three correspondent axes.

2.3. EOs' Chemical Composition Analysis

Detailed chemical compositions of the tested wild (*T. serpyllum*) and common thyme (*T. vulgaris*) EOs are listed in Table 2. In the wild thyme EO, there are 19 identified compounds (accounting for 99.29% of total volatile compounds) and, in the common thyme EO, there are 25 compounds (accounting for 99.20% of total volatile compounds). In general, the compounds in both EOs are classified as monoterpenes, with predominance of aromatic oxygenated monoterpenes (51.49% in *T. vulgaris* and 54.98% in *T. serpyllum*). The dominant compounds in *T. serpyllum* EO are thymol (54.17%), γ-terpinene (22.18%), and *p*-cymene (16.66%). In *T. vulgaris* EO, the dominant compounds are thymol (45.22%) and *p*-cymene (23.83%), while the content of γ-terpinene is notably lower (3.12%). *Trans*-β-caryophyllene, a sesquiterpene hydrocarbon, is the third main compound (4.04%) in *T. vulgaris* EO.

Table 2. Chemical composition of *T. serpyllum* and *T. vulgaris* essential oils (EOs) (%).

Peak No.	Compounds	RI [a]	*T. vulgaris*	*T. serpyllum*
	Monoterpene Hydrocarbons		**10.84**	**25.4**
1.	α-Pinene	937	1.51	0.18
2.	Camphene	952	1.67	0.19
3.	β-Pinene	978	0.21	2.15
4.	β-Myrcene	991	1.64	0.28
5.	α-Phellandrene	1005	0.11	0.08
6.	α-Terpinene	1017	0.87	0.13
8.	Limonene	1030	1.71	0.21
12.	γ-Terpinene	1060	3.12	22.18
	Aromatic Monoterpene Hydrocarbons		**23.83**	**16.66**
7.	p-Cymene	1025	23.83	16.66
	Oxygenated Monoterpenes		**7.19**	**2.05**
9.	1,8-Cineole	1032	0.93	0.16
10.	Linalool	1099	2.55	0
11.	Camphor	1145	0.33	0.77
13.	endo-Borneol	1167	1.68	0
14.	Terpinen-4-ol	1177	1.42	0.07
15.	Isomenthol	1183	0	0.84
16.	α-Terpineol	1189	0.23	0.03
19.	Bornyl acetate	1285	0.05	0.07
26.	trans-β-Ionone	1486	0	0.11
	Aromatic Oxygenated Monoterpenes		**51.49**	**54.98**
17.	Isothymol methyl ether	1230	0.92	0
18.	Thymol methyl ether	1235	1.49	0
20.	Thymol	1291	45.22	54.17
21.	Carvacrol	1299	3.86	0.81
	Sesquiterpene Hydrocarbons		**4.91**	**0.2**
22.	α-Cubebene	1351	0.08	0
23.	β-Cubenene	1388	0.03	0
24.	trans-β-Caryophyllene	1419	4.04	0.12
25.	Humulene	1454	0.41	0.08
27.	δ-Cadinene	1524	0.35	0
	Oxygenated Sesquiterpenes		**0.94**	**0**
28.	Caryophyllene oxide	1581	0.94	0
	Total of identified compounds (%)		**99.2**	**99.29**

[a] Retention indices (RI) relative to C9–C24 n-alkanes on the HP 5MS column.

2.4. EOs' Antioxidant Potential Evaluation

The antioxidant potential of the tested EOs (*T. vulgaris* and *T. serpyllum*) and the positive control substances were evaluated in a series of in vitro tests (Table 3). All results, except those obtained in the ferric reduction antioxidant potential (FRAP) test, are presented as the inhibitory concentration (IC_{50}) values, representing the concentrations of the EOs and positive controls that caused 50% of neutralization, determined by linear regression analysis.

Table 3. Antioxidant potential of the investigated essential oils of *T. serpyllum* and *T. vulgaris* and positive control substances (**AA**—ascorbic acid; **PG**—propyl gallate; **BHT**—*tert*-butylated hydroxytoluene). FRAP, ferric reduction antioxidant potential; DPPH, 2,2-diphenyl-1-picrylhydrazyl; OH, hydroxyl; LP, lipid peroxidation.

Samples	**Assay**			
	DPPH IC_{50}	**OH IC_{50} (μg / mL)**	**LP IC_{50}**	**FRAP (mg AAE [a] /mL EO)**
	$\bar{X}$ [b] ± SD [c]	$\bar{X}$ ± SD	$\bar{X}$ ± SD	$\bar{X}$ ± SD
T. vulgaris	14 ± 0.85	230 ± 1.19	19 ± 1.02	34.95 ± 3.50
T. serpyllum	16 ± 0.93	170 ± 2.02	17 ± 0.92	29.00 ± 2.90
AA	/	2003 ± 0.39	/	/
PG	0.71 ± 0.04	9.07 ± 0.59	/	/
BHT	/	0.03 ± 0.01	7.29 ± 0.56	/

[a] ascorbic acid equivalents; [b] mean value; [c] standard deviation.

DPPH assay was employed to determine the ability of the tested EOs of common and wild thyme, as well as propyl gallate (PG), to act as donors of hydrogen atoms or electrons in the transformation of $DPPH^{\bullet}$ into its reduced form DPPH-H reaction [32]. Although PG (propyl gallate) (0.71 μg/mL) exhibited very potent free radical scavenging capacity, both EOs were able to reduce the $DPPH^{\bullet}$ into DPPH-H, reaching 50% of reduction (IC_{50} = 16 for *T. serpyllum* and 14 μL/mL for *T. vulgaris*). The free radical scavenging capacity (RSC) of EOs for hydroxyl (OH) radicals was evaluated by measuring the degradation of 2-deoxyribose with OH radicals, generated in the Fenton reaction [32]. Both EOs showed a lower RSC (IC_{50} = 170 for *T. serpyllum* and 230 μg/mL for *T. vulgaris*, respectively) compared with the PG (propyl gallate) (9.07 μg/mL) and *tert*-butylated hydroxytoluene (BHT) (0.03 μg/mL) IC_{50} values, used as standard synthetic antioxidants. However, both of them exhibited protective effects on 2-deoxy-D-ribose degradation, although they were lower compared with ascorbic acid (AA) (2.03 μg/mL). Regarding the neutralization of NO, neither EO reached 50% of reduction. The testing of the ability of the examined EOs to protect the integrity of biological membranes containing lipids was evaluated through determination of lipid peroxidation (LP) inhibition potential, pointing to protective effects of the tested EOs (IC_{50} = 170 for *T. serpyllum* and 190 μg/mL for *T. vulgaris*), but notably lower from those exhibited by BHT (7.29 μg/mL).

The FRAP test showed a notable antioxidant activity for both EOs (29 mg AAE/mL for *T. serpyllum* EO and 34.95 mg AAE/mL for *T. vulgaris* EO).

Comprehensive evaluation of the antioxidant potential in several test-systems showed no significant differences between the examined EOs samples (F (4,1) = 58.82, Wilks = 0.004, p = 0.0974).

2.5. EOs Effectiveness against Mastitis-Associated Bacteria

EOs effectiveness against mastitis-associated bacteria was expressed as minimum inhibitory concentrations (MICs) and minimal bactericidal concentrations (MBCs) (Table 4). Among the fourteen mastitis-associated bacteria, strain IX *Streptococcus* spp. (β-hemolytic) showed the most sensitivity to the tested EOs (MIC/MBC were 0.78/1.56 and 0.39/0.78 mg/mL for *T. serpyllum* and *T. vulgaris*, respectively). Regarding *Streptococcus* spp. β heamoliticus, MICs for *T. serpyllum* ranged from 0.78 to 1.56 mg/mL, while for the same oil, MBCs ranged from 1.56 to 12.5 mg/mL. In the case of *T. vulgaris,* MICs ranged from 0.39 to 3.125 mg/mL, while MBCs ranged from 3.125 to 6.25 mg/mL. TV is more active against *E. coli, E. sakazakii,* and *Streptococcus* spp., while it is less effective against *Staphylococcus* spp. than TS.

Table 4. Minimum inhibitory concentrations (MICs) and minimal bactericidal concentrations (MBCs) of *T. serpyllum* and *T. vulgaris* EOs against mastitis-associated pathogens.

Sample	TV * (MIC) (mg/mL)	TV * (MBC) (mg/mL)	TS ** (MIC) (mg/mL)	TS ** (MBC) (mg/mL)
4 *E. coli*	3.125	6.25	6.25	12.5
Enterobacter sakazakii	3.125	6.25	6.25	12.5
Streptococcus spp. β heamoliticus	0.39	0.78	1.56	3.125
Streptococcus spp. β heamoliticus	0.78	1.56	1.56	3.125
Streptococcus spp. β heamoliticus	0.39	0.78	0.78	1.56
Streptococcus spp.	1.56	3.125	3.125	6.25
Streptococcus spp.	0.78	1.56	3.125	6.25
Streptococcus spp.	1.56	6.25	3.125	6.25
Staphylococcus spp.	6.25	12.5	3.125	6.25
Staphylococcus spp. coagulase negative	6.25	12.5	3.125	6.25
Klebsiella oxytoca	1.56	6.25	3.125	6.25

* T. serpyllum (TS) EO. ** T. vulgaris (TV) EO.

2.6. Interpretations of MBC, MIC, Thymus vulgaris, *and* Thymus serpyllum *EOs in Relation to the Chemical Composition of the EOs*

Application of principal components analysis (PCA) on the results describing the MIC and MBC of the tested EOs in relation to the most abundant secondary metabolites showed that the first two principal components (PCs) describe more than 95% of the dataset variability, while the principal components axis 1 (PCA1) describes more than 90% of the samples' variability. It can be observed that most of the variability is explained by the results describing the antibacterial potential in the case of *Streptococcus* spp., *Enterobacter sakazakii, Klebsiella oxytoca,* and *Staphylococcus* spp., as well as by the chemical composition in terms of carvacrol, trans-β-caryophyllene, and γ-terpinene content. Positioning of *Thymus vulgaris* EO samples in the negative part of PCA1 suggests that these samples, in relation to *Thymus serpyllum* EO, are characterized by the presence of significant amounts of carvacrol, trans-β-caryophyllene, and p-cymene. Furthermore, the thyme EO showed stronger antibacterial potential against *Streptococcus* spp. (β-hemolytic), *Streptococcus* spp. *Enterobacter sakazakii, E. coli,* and *Klebsiella oxytoca* in comparison with the wild thyme EO. On the other hand, *Thymus serpyllum* EO samples grouped in the positive part of PCA1 (as a result of higher amounts of thymol and γ-terpinen), and thus showed stronger antibacterial activity against *Staphylococcus* spp. (coagulase-negative) and *Staphylococcus* spp. (Figure 3).

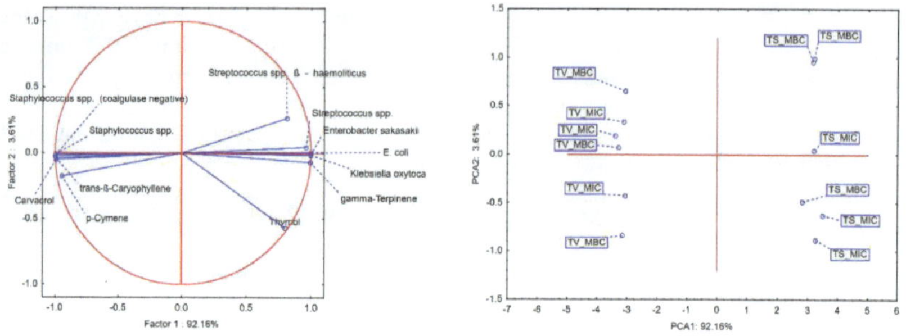

(a) (b)

Figure 3. Results of principal components analysis (PCA): (**a**) loadings of the first two principal components; (**b**) position of the examined samples in the space defined by the first two principal components. TS, *T. serpyllum*; TV, *T. vulgaris*; MIC, minimum inhibitory concentration; MBC, minimal bactericidal concentration.

3. Discussion

Considering the importance of the issue of antimicrobial resistance (AMR), scientists are trying to find an alternative to antibiotics in mastitis therapy [33–35]. Recently, phytotherapy has been finding a place in the vast drug market owing to its capacity to prevent the development and spread of AMR. Phytotherapy in this way also reduces the economic losses in the dairy industry caused by rejection of milk due to antibiotic withdrawal time [36,37].

In order to develop an EO-based pharmaceutical formulation, it is necessary to perform chemical composition analysis and testing of EOs against the most common mastitis pathogens.

Analysis of EOs' chemical composition in this study revealed that both tested essential oils are in accordance with the requirements prescribed by Ph. Eur. 10 (2020) [38] for thymol type of thyme EOs, with thymol ranging from 37 to 55% and carvacrol from 0.5 to 5.5%. According to the pharmacopoeia, the official biological source of *Thymus vulgaris* EO is only the flowering aerial parts of *Thymus vulgaris*, *T. zygis*, or a mixture of both species, while *T. serpyllum* is the biological source of *Serpylli herba*. However, the content of thymol in the wild thyme EO is higher (54.17%) than in the common thyme EO (45.22%). Unlike thymol, the content of carvacrol is reversed (3.86% in common thyme and 0.81% in wild thyme). There is a notable difference between the tested EOs in the content of *p*-cymene in common thyme (23.83%) and wild thyme (16.66%), but both EOs meet the quality criteria prescribed by the pharmacopoeia (14–28%). On the other hand, the content of γ-terpinene (3.12% for common thyme and 22.18% for wild thyme) does not comply with the pharmacopoeia requirements (4–12%). According to the prescribed content of linalool (1.5–6.5%) and terpinen-4-ol (0.1–2.5%) established by the pharmacopoeia, *T. vulgaris* EO meets the requirements related to the chemical composition for thymol type EO (2.55% for linalool and 1.42% for terpinen-4-ol). The results for *T. vulgaris* EO composition are also in line with previously published data [20,21,39]. However, because, in the wild thyme EO, several chemotypes are described [26–28], this oil could be defined as a thymol chemotype.

However, the chemical composition of *T. vulgaris* EO of commercial origin [40,41], and from different regions [36–38] showed different thymol chemotypes, with the thymol being the more abundant compound.

It is well known that plants possess significant antioxidant potential, mainly attributed to the presence of different aromatic, phenolic, and flavonoid compounds [42]. Nowadays, the trends in food and cosmetic industry suggest the use of natural products, especially as a replacement for synthetic antioxidants [43]. Although EOs in all of the tested systems exhibited weaker free radical scavenging effects, it must be emphasized that the comparison of the antioxidant potential in the present study was performed between pure compounds and EOs, which are mixtures of different secondary metabolites, meaning that some of them do not possess potential for scavenging reactive oxygen species (ROS) and preventing biological membrane degradation. Regarding their toxicity, synthetic antioxidants are abused in some food and cosmetic products, especially *tert*-butylated hydroxytoluene (BHT) [44].

Regarding that fact, the EOs tested in our study showed notable antioxidant potential, similar to the results of other authors [20,21,27,28,32,45], although the general comparison of the results obtained in different labs is sometimes difficult because of different experimental conditions and presentation of the results, different methods of antioxidant potential evaluation, and so on. In addition, in the case of various *Thymus* species EOs, the chemical composition plays a significant role in antioxidant effects as thymol and carvacrol are the main compounds responsible for RSC and inhibition of peroxidation of different lipids and biological membranes [20,21]. Both thymol and carvacrol demonstrate the ability to achieve a resonantly stable radical structure after donation of hydrogen atom or electrons to ROS, thus neutralizing the cascade of free radical reactions [42]. Hence, different chemotypes, especially of different species of wild thyme (*T. serpyllum*, *T. marschallianus*, *T. jankae*, *T. longicaulis*, *T. lonidens*, *T. pannonicus*, and so on), can show significantly weaker antioxidant effects [27]. As different plant-derived products have less toxicity and side effects compared with synthetic antioxidants, they can play an important role in the prevention of various diseases and syndromes where reactive oxygen species are involved [42]. They have also found their place as natural preservatives in the pharmaceutical, food, and cosmetic industry [43]. ROS production is linked with the inflammatory process and is provided by netrophils in milk [46].

The results obtained in this study indicated that the common thyme EO showed stronger antibacterial potential against *Streptococcus* spp. (β-hemolytic), *Streptococcus* spp. *Enterobacter sakazakii*, *E. coli*, and *Klebsiella oxytoca* in comparison with the wild thyme EO. On the other hand, wild thyme EO samples grouped in the positive part of PCA1 (as a result of higher amounts of thymol and γ-terpinen), and thus showed stronger antibacterial activity against *Staphylococcus* spp. (coagulase-negative) and *Staphylococcus* spp. (Figure 3). The significant antimicrobial activity of *T. vulgaris* EO against *Staphylococcus* spp. isolated from bovine mastitis has been previously confirmed [47,48]. These studies reported phenolic compounds such as carvacrol and thymol as major constituents of the tested EO are responsible for their antimicrobial activities.

Phenolic compounds (carvacrol and thymol) account for 54.98% of the total oil in *T. serpyllum* EO and 49.08% in *T. vulgaris* EO. The antibacterial effect of the EOs tested in our study probably depends on these compounds, and a number of studies revealed that phenolic compounds, such as carvacrol and thymol, possess antibacterial activity [21,49–51]. Furthermore, the main constituents of the EOs tested in our study are monoterpenes (thymol, carvacrol, p-cymene, and γ-terpinene), which showed a remarkable inhibitory effect against different pathogens such as *Staphylococcus aureus*, *Escherichia coli* O157:H7, *Salmonella Infantis*, *Bacillus cereus*, and *Clostridium perfringes* [21,50,52]. From the chemical point of view, carvacrol and thymol represent structural isomers and possess differently located phenolic hydroxyl on the phenolic ring [53]. Some studies indicated that the hydroxyl group has a part in increasing their hydrophilic ability, helping them to dissolve in the microbial membrane and impair them [54–57].

Compared with carvacrol, thymol also possesses similar antibacterial activity, even though its hydroxyl group is located in a different position [58]. The thymol primary mode of antibacterial action is partly understood and it is probably similar to carvacrol. This mode of action results in structural and functional alterations in the cytoplasmic membrane that can damage the outer and inner membranes and interact with membrane proteins, as well as intracellular targets [59]. In contact with the cell membrane, thymol can modify membrane permeability, leading to the release of K^+ ions and ATP [54,60,61]. Some studies revealed that thymol integrates within the polar head-groups of the lipid bilayer, causing alterations of the cell membrane [54,60,62]. In contrast to the efficiency of monoterpenes with added oxygen molecules (carvacrol and thymol), monoterpene hydrocarbons p-cymene and γ-terpinene used separately do not demonstrate remarkable inhibitory effects against bacteria growth [50,63].

However, several studies indicated that *p*-cymene can enhance the inhibitory effects of carvacrol when these two compounds are used together [58,64,65]. It was also shown that *p*-cymene, owing to its hydrophobic nature, greatly contributes to the cytoplasmic membrane swelling [61]. The findings obtained by Ultee, Bennik, and Moezelaar [61] indicated that *p*-cymene enabled carvacrol to be more easily transported into the cell. With respect to these findings, a slightly higher antibacterial effect of *T. vulgaris* EO obtained in this research could be accounted for by a slightly higher content of *p*-cymene.

Fratini et al., examining the efficiency of *Thymus vulgaris* L. ct. carvacrol and *T. vulgaris* L. ct. thymol), two selected mixtures of EOs, and two artificial mixtures of their main constituents (thymol, carvacrol, and p-cymene), against the bacterial strains involved in the pathogenesis of mastitis using the Kirby–Bauer method, confirmed that thymol and carvacrol as main constituents of tested EO are responsible for antibacterial activity. Moreover, the highest antibacterial effectiveness was obtained with the artificial mixture of pure constituents (carvacrol and thimol) with the addition of p-cymene [48].

This study revealed significant resistance of the most common mastitis pathogens to antimicrobials, indicating the importance of finding an alternative to antibiotic treatment in therapy of this disease. Moreover, it was shown that gram-negative pathogens (*E. coli*, *Klebsiella oxytoca* and *Enterobacter sakazakii*) are resistant to erythromycin, amoxycillin, and amoxicillin/clavulanic acid. This is in accordance with results of other studies, which determined resistance to the mentioned antimicrobials [66]. In addition, *Streptococcus* spp. isolated in this study showed resistance to trimethoprim/sulfamethoxazole, neomycin, enrofloxacin, tetracycline, lincomycin, and ceftriaxone, which is in line with the resistance determined in other studies [67].

Interestingly, although studies conducted so far highlighted the possibilities of EOs as a potential resistance-modifying agent, they provided limited evidence suggesting the spontaneous occurrence of resistance to EOs [68]. In fact, resistance of bacteria to EOs and their active components depends on their chemical composition, as well as their mechanism of action, which is specific and completely different compared with antibiotics. The antimicrobial activity of these natural substances has not been fully studied, but, owing to the proven ability of some EOs to inhibit bacterial cell wall synthesis, block transcription, β-lactamase production, biofilm formation, or efflux pump operation, they are considered to be useful in the treatment of infections caused by resistant microorganisms [68,69]. Besides, the difference between the mechanisms of resistance in EOs and antimicrobials is giving immense potential for the replacement of conventional antimicrobial therapy with phytotherapy.

4. Material and Methods

4.1. Essential Oils

In the present study, the essential oils of common (*Thymus vulgaris* L., Lamiaceae) and wild thyme (*Thymus serpyllum* L., Lamiaceae), commercially available on the Serbian market and produced by a certified manufacturer (Pharmanais d.o.o., Serbia), were evaluated in the study. Row plant material (*Thymi folium* and *Serpylli herba*) was sampled before distillation from the manufacturer and confirmed for identity. Voucher specimens (Tv-03/2020 and Ts-2/2020, respectivelly) were deposited at the Herbarium of drugs of the Pharmacognosy and phytotherapy laboratory, Department of Pharmacy, Faculty of Medicine, University of Novi Sad. According to the certificate obtained from the manufacturer for both samples, essential oils were obtained using the internal steam distillation technique (Cellkraft AB, Sweden).

4.2. Sampling Procedure

The milk samples were collected from four Holstein-Friesian dairy farms located in Serbia. The number of cows on the farms varied, ranging from twenty to three hundred. The samples were taken from lactating animals with clinical and subclinical mastitis, without other health problems. Clinical mastitis was diagnosed by clinical examination of udder, while subclinical mastitis was confirmed using somatic cell count in the milk samples.

Bacteriological testing was performed by taking aseptic milk samples from all animals (clinical and subclinical mastitis) during the morning milking. The samples were then taken in sterile tubes marked with an ID number of the cow and stored at 4 °C. Afterwards, the samples were processed at the Laboratory for Milk Hygiene at the Department of Veterinary Medicine, Faculty of Agriculture, University of Novi Sad. The samples were inoculated on 2% blood agar, using a platinum loop (0.01 mL), followed by incubation of the samples for 48 h at 37 °C. Biochemical and cultural characteristics of the grown microorganisms were taken into account during their determination. Isolation and identification of bacterial strain from milk samples was conducted using microbiological procedures for the diagnosis of udder infection published by National Mastitis Council. A loopful of milk sample was streaked on blood agar (Oxoid) and then subcultured on the following selective media: Mannitol Salt Agar, Edwards Agar, Salmonella-Shigella Agar, and MacConkey Agar. Then, plates were incubated aerobically at 37 °C for 24 h. After incubation, the plates were examined for colony morphology, pigmentation, and hemolytic characteristics at 24–48 h. Catalase test was applied for distinguishing between staphylococci and other Gram-positive cocci, mannitol fermentation test, coagulase test (either positive or negative), hemolytic pattern, and colony morphology. The isolates were confirmed by biochemical tests: oxidase activity, acid production (lactose sucrose and glucose fermentation), indole production, Voges–Proskauer, and hydrogen sulfide production. In addition, each strain was confirmed using Analytical Profile Index API-20 tests (API, bio Meraux, France). To isolate staphylococci, listed media were used: blood agar, nutrient agar, Ziehl–Neelsen, MSA, for *E. coli* isolation nutrient agar, MacConkey agar, and API 25 were used. For streptococci, Edwards agar and esculin were used. Of the phenotypic characteristics for staphylococci, the occurrence of α and β hemolysis and, for E. coli, there were pink colonies with precipitation. For streptococci determination, hydrolysis of esculin was used.

4.3. Antibiotic Susceptibility Testing of Mastitis-Associated Bacteria

The antibiotic susceptibility patterns for the 16 mastitis-associated bacteria were established in vitro, following the Kirby–Bauer disc diffusion method, on Mueller–Hinton agar (Oxoid) [70]. Antibiotic susceptibility testing was conducted using commercially available antibiotic disks (Bioanalyse) in the following concentrations: ampicillin (10 µg); streptomycin (10 µg); gentamicin (10 µg); trimethoprim/sulphamethoxazole (1.25/23.75 µg); enrofloxacin (5 µg); and ceftriaxone (30 µg). The isolates and reference strains were inoculated on nutrient broth separately and incubated aerobically at 37 °C. After overnight incubation, the bacterial suspension was vortexed and diluted to a turbidity equivalent to that of 0.5 McFarland standards. The bacterial suspension was then spread onto the surface of the Mueller–Hinton agar to make confluent growth. Antibiotic discs were immediately placed on the surface of the agar plate using forceps and incubated aerobically at 37 °C for 16 h. Inhibition zones for various isolates were measured and interpreted as sensitive, intermediate, or resistant according to the Clinical Laboratory Standards Institute (CLSI) [71,72].

4.4. EOs Chemical Composition Analysis

The qualitative and quantitative analysis of the EOs was carried out on HP-5MS capillary column (30 m × 0.25 mm; film thickness 0.25 µm) on Agilent 6890B gas chromatograph coupled with flame ionization detector (GC-FID) instrument coupled to Agilent 5977 mass spectrometry detector (MSD) (Agilent Technologies Inc, Santa Clara, CA, USA, USA). The samples were injected in split mode 1:20, at an inlet temperature of 220 °C. The oven temperature was set at 60 °C and increased at a rate of 3 °C/min up to 246 °C. Helium was the carrier gas (1 mL/min), while the temperature of the MSD transfer line was set to 230 °C.

Mass spectral data were collected in scan mode (m/z = 50–550), while the identification of compounds was performed using NIST (v14, National Institute of Standards and Technology, Gaithersburg, MD, USA) mass spectral database and comparison of relative retention indices (RT), as well as literature data [73].

4.5. EOs' Antioxidant Potential Evaluation

The antioxidant potential of the commercial EOs of wild (*Thymus serpyllum*) and common thyme (*Thymus vulgaris*) was evaluated in five in vitro assays, as single models are not recommended for evaluation because of the complex composition of different plant extracts [74]. The potential of the EOs to neutralize 2,2-diphenyl-1-picrylhydrazyl (DPPH), hydroxyl (OH) and nitroso (NO) radicals was assessed by previously described spectrophotometric methods [32]. Moreover, the ability of the examined EOs to inhibit the processes of lipid peroxidation (LP) is evaluated, using liposomes emulsion as a test model [20]. The potential of the examined EOs to reduce Fe^{3+} (ferric reduction antioxidant potential—FRAP test) was assessed by the method described by Lesjak et al. [45], as it is a model correlating with the neutralization of hypochlorite and peroxynitrite anion [75]. The results obtained in the FRAP assay were expressed as ascorbic acid equivalents (AAEs) based on the previously constructed calibration curve for ascorbic acid. For each sample, four replicates were recorded in all test-systems. Synthetic antioxidants, including ascorbic acid (AA), propyl gallate (PG), and *tert*-butylated hydroxytoluene (BHT), were tested under the same experimental conditions as positive control for antioxidant potential of the tested EOs.

4.6. EOs' Effectiveness Determination against Mastitis-Associated Bacteria

EOs' effectiveness on planktonically grown bacteria was determined according to the Clinical Laboratory Standards [76] with slight modifications. The bacterial suspensions were prepared using overnight cultures and adjusted to 0.5 Mc Farland standard turbidity (corresponding to 1×10^8 CFU/mL), using a densitometer DEN-1 (Biosan, Riga, Latvia). All tests were performed in Muller–Hinton broth (MHB) (Lab M, International Diagnostics Group Plc, Bury, Lancashire, UK). MHB supplemented with 0.5% Tween 80 (Polyoxyethylenesorbitan monooleate, HiMedia Laboratories Pvt. Ltd., Mumbai, India) was used for dissolving the EOs, as well as for their dilution to the concentration ranging from 1000 to 0.9 mg/mL. Twenty-microliter aliquots of each tested EO were added to 96-well microtiter plates. Afterward, aliquots of 160 μL of MHB were added to each well. As the final step, 20 μL of the standardized bacterial suspension was inoculated into each well. The test was performed in a total volume of 200 μL with final EOs' concentrations ranging from 100 to 0.09 mg/mL, while the final microbial concentration was 10^7 CFU/mL. The plates were incubated at 37 °C for 24 h. The same tests were performed simultaneously for growth control (MHB + test organism), negative control (MHB + solvent + test organism), and sterility control (MHB + test oil).

Following the incubation, 10 μL of the resazurin solution (0.01%) (Sigma-Aldrich, St Louis, MO, USA) was added to each well. Subsequently, the plates were further incubated at 37 °C for 6 h (in darkness). After visual examination, the plates were additionally incubated for 18 h. Change of color from blue (oxidized) to pink (reduced) indicated the growth of bacteria. On completion of the incubation, wells without the color change (blue color of resazurin remained unchanged) were scored as above the minimum inhibitory concentration (MIC) value. MIC was defined as the lowest concentration at which the color change occurred [77,78].

Referring to the results of the MIC assay, the wells showing complete absence of growth were identified and 100 μL of the solutions from each well was transferred to plate count agar plates (PCA) (Lab M, International Diagnostics Group Plc, Bury, Lancashire, UK) and incubated at 37 °C for 24 h. The minimal bactericidal concentration (MBC) was defined as the lowest concentration of the EOs at which 99.9% of the inoculated bacteria were killed.

4.7. Data Analysis

The results obtained in the study were processes by MS Office Excel v2019 (Microsoft Corporation, Redmond, WA, USA) and Statsoft Statistica v12.5 (Hamburg, Germany) software. The values were expressed as the mean values corrected by standard deviation (SD). Methods of univariate and multivariate statistical analysis (MANOVA, pincipal component analysis (PCA) and correspondence analysis (CA)) were applied for comprehensive evaluation of the relations in the obtained dataset.

5. Conclusions

This study highlighted that two thyme (*Thymus serpyllum* and *T. vulgaris*) EOs can be used in the development of pharmaceutical formulation as an alternative to conventional mastitis therapy, owing to the EOs' chemical composition, antioxidant potential, and effectiveness against mastitis-associated bacteria. Further research on dairy farms is needed to conduct clinical trials of EO-based formulation. Moreover, additional studies should explore their toxicity to mammalian cells and drug-like properties (pharmacokinetic and pharmacodynamic) to determine their potential as therapeutic agents. Finally, further studies also need to compare the economic aspects of the conventional versus herbal treatment of mastitis, as well as the combination of EOs with common antibiotics used in the treatment of mastitis.

Author Contributions: Conceptualization, Z.K., I.Č., and B.B.; Formal analysis, N.K.; Investigation, Z.K., M.R., I.Č., N.K., and B.B.; Methodology, Z.K. and B.B.; Supervision, Z.K.; Validation, I.Č. and N.K.; Writing—original draft, Z.K., M.R., I.Č., N.K., and B.B.; Writing—review & editing, Z.K., M.R., I.Č., N.K., and B.B.; Funding acquisition, Z.K. All authors have read and agreed to the published version of the manuscript.

Funding: This research was supported by the Science Fund of the Republic of Serbia, PROMIS, #GRANT No 6066966, InfoBomat.

Institutional Review Board Statement: Not applicable.

Informed Consent Statement: Not applicable.

Data Availability Statement: Data is contained within the article.

Conflicts of Interest: The authors declare no conflict of interest.

References

1. Gruet, P.; Maincent, P.; Berthelot, X.; Kaltsatos, V. Bovine mastitis and intramammary drug delivery: Review and perspectives. *Adv. Drug Deliv. Rev.* **2001**, *50*, 245–259. [CrossRef]
2. Garcia, S.N.; Osburn, B.I.; Cullor, J.S. A one health perspective on dairy production and dairy food safety. *One Health* **2019**, *7*, 100086. [CrossRef]
3. Halasa, T.; Huijps, K.; Osteras, O.; Hogeveen, H. Economic effects of bovine mastitis and mastitis management: A review. *Vet. Q.* **2007**, *29*, 18–31. [CrossRef] [PubMed]
4. Drašković, B.; Stošić, I.; Rajković, Z. Tržišna struktura i nestašice mleka u Srbiji. In *Agrarna i ruralna politika u Srbiji: Nužnost ubrzanja reformi: Tematski zbornik*; DAES Društvo agrarnih ekonomista Srbije: Beograd, Serbia, 2011; pp. 65–79.
5. Hristov, S.; Stanković, B.M.; Relić, R. Klinički i subklinički mastitis u krava. Biotechnol. *Anim. Husb.* **2005**, *21*, 29–39. [CrossRef]
6. Kim, T.; Heald, C.W. Inducing inference rules for the classification of bovine mastitis. *Comput. Electron. Agric.* **1999**, *23*, 27–42. [CrossRef]
7. Zadoks, R.; Fitzpatrick, J. Changing trends in mastitis. *Ir. Vet. J.* **2009**, *62* (Suppl. 4), S59–S70. [CrossRef] [PubMed]
8. Boboš, S.; Vidić, B. *Mlečna žlezda preživara, morfologija, patologija, terapija*; Univeryitet u Novom Sadu, Poljoprivredni fakultet: Novi Sad, Serbia, 2005; pp. 57–91.
9. Krömker, V.; Leimbach, S. Mastitis treatment— Reduction in antibiotic usage in dairy cows. *Reprod Dom Anim* **2017**, *52*, 21–29. [CrossRef]
10. Erskine, R.J.; Wagner, S.; DeGraves, F.J. Mastitis therapy and pharmacology. *Vet. Clin. North Am. Food Anim.* **2003**, *19*, 109–138. [CrossRef]
11. Gupta, R.; Kumar, S.; Khurana, R. Essential oils and mastitis in dairy animals: A review. *Haryana Vet.* **2020**, *59*, 1–9.
12. Sandegren, L. Selection of antibiotic resistance at very low antibiotic concentrations. *Upsala J. Med. Sci.* **2014**, *119*, 103–107. [CrossRef] [PubMed]

13. Dingwell, R.T.; Kelton, D.F.; Leslie, K.E. Management of the dry cow in control of peripartum disease and mastitis. *Vet. Clin. N. Am. Food Anim.* **2003**, *19*, 235–265. [CrossRef]
14. Oliver, S.P.; Jayarao, B.M.; Almeida, R.A. Foodborne pathogens in milk and the dairy farm environment: Food safety and public health implications. *Foodborne Pathog. Dis.* **2005**, *2*, 115–129. [CrossRef]
15. Fusco, V.; Chieffi, D.; Fanelli, F.; Logrieco, A.F.; Cho, G.S.; Kabisch, J.; Böhnlein, C.; Franz, C.M.A.P. Microbial quality and safety of milk and milk products in the 21st century. *Compr. Rev. Food Sci. Food Saf.* **2020**, *19*, 2013–2049. [CrossRef]
16. WHO. *Global Action Plan on Antimicrobial Resistance*; World Health Organization: Geneva, Switzerland, 2015; pp. 1–28.
17. Kokoska, L.; Kloucek, P.; Leuner, O.; Novy, P. Plant-Derived Products as Antibacterial and Antifungal Agents in Human Health Care. *Curr. Med. Chem.* **2019**, *26*, 5501–5541. [CrossRef] [PubMed]
18. O'Bryan, C.A.; Pendleton, S.J.; Crandall, P.G.; Ricke, S.C. Potential of Plant Essential Oils and Their Components in Animal Agriculture – in vitro Studies on Antibacterial Mode of Action. *Front. Vet. Sci.* **2015**, *2*. [CrossRef] [PubMed]
19. Ananda Baskaran, S.; Kazmer, G.W.; Hinckley, L.; Andrew, S.M.; Venkitanarayanan, K. Antibacterial effect of plant-derived antimicrobials on major bacterial mastitis pathogens in vitro. *Int. J. Dairy Sci.* **2009**, *92*, 1423–1429. [CrossRef] [PubMed]
20. Bozin, B.; Mimica-Dukic, N.; Simin, N.; Anackov, G. Characterization of the Volatile Composition of Essential Oils of Some Lamiaceae Spices and the Antimicrobial and Antioxidant Activities of the Entire Oils. *J. Agric. Food Chem.* **2006**, *54*, 1822–1828. [CrossRef]
21. Gavaric, N.; Mozina, S.S.; Kladar, N.; Bozin, B. Chemical Profile, Antioxidant and Antibacterial Activity of Thyme and Oregano Essential Oils, Thymol and Carvacrol and Their Possible Synergism. *J. Essent. Oil-Bear. Plants.* **2015**, *18*, 1013–1021. [CrossRef]
22. Lemos, M.F.; Lemos, M.F.; Pacheco, H.P.; Guimarães, A.C.; Fronza, M.; Endringer, D.C.; Scherer, R. Seasonal variation affects the composition and antibacterial and antioxidant activities of Thymus vulgaris. *Ind. Crops Prod.* **2017**, *95*, 543–548. [CrossRef]
23. Nikolić, M.; Glamočlija, J.; Ferreira, I.C.F.R.; Calhelha, R.C.; Fernandes, Â.; Marković, T.; Marković, D.; Giweli, A.; Soković, M. Chemical composition, antimicrobial, antioxidant and antitumor activity of Thymus serpyllum L., Thymus algeriensis Boiss. and Reut and Thymus vulgaris L. essential oils. *Ind. Crops Prod.* **2014**, *52*, 183–190. [CrossRef]
24. Langeveld, W.T.; Veldhuizen, E.J.; Burt, S.A. Synergy between essential oil components and antibiotics: A review. *Crit. Rev. Microbiol.* **2014**, *40*, 76–94. [CrossRef] [PubMed]
25. Hemaiswarya, S.; Kruthiventi, A.K.; Doble, M. Synergism between natural products and antibiotics against infectious diseases. *Phytomedicine* **2008**, *15*, 639–652. [CrossRef]
26. Malankina, E.L.; Kozlovskaya, L.N.; Kuzmenko, A.N.; Evgrafov, A.A. Determination of the Component Composition of Essential Oil of Thyme Species by the Method of Gas Chromatography. *Mosc. Univ. Chem. Bull.* **2020**, *74*, 310–314. [CrossRef]
27. Ćavar-Zeljković, S.; Maksimović, M. Chemical composition and bioactivity of essential oil from Thymus species in Balkan Peninsula. *Phytochem. Rev.* **2015**, *14*, 335–352. [CrossRef]
28. Tohidi, B.; Rahimmalek, M.; Arzani, A. Essential oil composition, total phenolic, flavonoid contents, and antioxidant activity of Thymus species collected from different regions of Iran. *Food Chem.* **2017**, *220*, 153–161. [CrossRef] [PubMed]
29. Helal, I.M.; El-Bessoumy, A.; Al-Bataineh, E.; Joseph, M.R.P.; Rajagopalan, P.; Chandramoorthy, H.C.; Ben Hadj Ahmed, S. Antimicrobial Efficiency of Essential Oils from Traditional Medicinal Plants of Asir Region, Saudi Arabia, over Drug Resistant Isolates. *Biomed. Res. Int.* **2019**, *2019*, 8928306. [CrossRef] [PubMed]
30. Acimovic, M.; Zoric, M.; Zheljazkov, V.D.; Pezo, L.; Cabarkapa, I.; Stankovic Jeremic, J.; Cvetkovic, M. Chemical Characterization and Antibacterial Activity of Essential Oil of Medicinal Plants from Eastern Serbia. *Molecules* **2020**, *25*, 5482. [CrossRef]
31. Radinović, M.; Davidov, I.; Kovačević, Z.; Stojanović, D.; Galfi, A.; Erdeljan, M. Basic Principles of Mastitis Therapy. *Vet. J. Republic Srpska.* **2019**, *19*. [CrossRef]
32. Bozin, B.; Kladar, N.; Grujic, N.; Anackov, G.; Samojlik, I.; Gavaric, N.; Conic, B.S. Impact of origin and biological source on chemical composition, anticholinesterase and antioxidant properties of some St. John's wort species (Hypericum spp., Hypericaceae) from the Central Balkans. *Molecules* **2013**, *18*, 11733–11750. [CrossRef]
33. Mushtaq, S.; Shah, A.M.; Shah, A.; Lone, S.A.; Hussain, A.; Hassan, Q.P.; Ali, M.N. Bovine mastitis: An appraisal of its alternative herbal cure. *Microb. Pathog.* **2018**, *114*, 357–361. [CrossRef]
34. Yang, W.-T.; Ke, C.-Y.; Wu, W.-T.; Lee, R.-P.; Tseng, Y.-H. Effective Treatment of Bovine Mastitis with Intramammary Infusion of *Angelica dahurica* and *Rheum officinale* Extracts. *Evid. Based Complementary Altern. Med.* **2019**, *2019*, 7242705. [CrossRef] [PubMed]
35. Lopes, T.S.; Fontoura, P.S.; Oliveira, A.; Rizzo, F.A.; Silveira, S.; Streck, A.F. Use of plant extracts and essential oils in the control of bovine mastitis. *Res. Vet. Sci.* **2020**, *131*, 186–193. [CrossRef]
36. McGaw, L. Use of Plant-Derived Extracts and Essential Oils against Multidrug-Resistant Bacteria Affecting Animal Health and Production. In *Fighting Multidrug Resistance with Herbal Extracts, Essential Oils and Their Components*; Rai, M.K., Kon, K.V., Eds.; Academic Press: San Diego, CA, USA, 2013; pp. 191–203. Available online: https://doi.org/10.1016/B978-0-12-398539-2.00013-6 (accessed on 12 December 2020).
37. Doehring, C.; Sundrum, A. The informative value of an overview on antibiotic consumption, treatment efficacy and cost of clinical mastitis at farm level. *Prev. Vet. Med.* **2019**, *165*, 63–70. [CrossRef] [PubMed]
38. EDQM. *European Pharmacopoeia 10.3*; The European Directorate for the Quality of Medicines & HealthCare, Council of Europe: Brusselles, Belgium, 2020; pp. 1648–1650.

39. Bogavac, M.; Karaman, M.; Janjusevic, L.; Sudji, J.; Radovanovic, B.; Novakovic, Z.; Simeunovic, J.; Bozin, B. Alternative treatment of vaginal infections-in vitro antimicrobial and toxic effects of Coriandrum sativum L. and Thymus vulgaris L. essential oils. *J. Appl. Microbiol.* **2015**, *119*, 697–710. [CrossRef] [PubMed]
40. Pinto, L.; Cefola, M.; Bonifacio, M.A.; Cometa, S.; Bocchino, C.; Pace, B.; De Giglio, E.; Palumbo, M.; Sada, A.; Logrieco, A.F.; et al. Effect of red thyme oil (Thymus vulgaris L.) vapours on fungal decay, quality parameters and shelf-life of oranges during cold storage. *Food Chem.* **2021**, *336*, 127590. [CrossRef] [PubMed]
41. Pinto, L.; Bonifacio, M.A.; De Giglio, E.; Cometa, S.; Logrieco, A.F.; Baruzzi, F. Unravelling the Antifungal Effect of Red Thyme Oil (Thymus vulgaris L.) Compounds in Vapor Phase. *Molecules* **2020**, *25*, 4761. [CrossRef]
42. Mimica-Dukic, N.; Bozin, B. Mentha L. species (Lamiaceae) as promising sources of bioactive secondary metabolites. *Curr. Pharm. Des.* **2008**, *14*, 3141–3150. [CrossRef]
43. Caleja, C.; Barros, L.; Antonio, A.L.; Oliveira, M.B.; Ferreira, I.C. A comparative study between natural and synthetic antioxidants: Evaluation of their performance after incorporation into biscuits. *Food Chem.* **2017**, *216*, 342–346. [CrossRef]
44. Lanigan, R.S.; Yamarik, T.A. Final report on the safety assessment of BHT(1). *Int. J. Toxicol.* **2002**, *21*, 19–94. [CrossRef]
45. Lesjak, M.M.; Beara, I.N.; Orčić, D.Z.; Anačkov, G.T.; Balog, K.J.; Francišković, M.M.; Mimica-Dukić, N.M. Juniperus sibirica Burgsdorf. as a novel source of antioxidant and anti-inflammatory agents. *Food Chem.* **2011**, *124*, 850–856. [CrossRef]
46. Molinari, P.C.C.; Blagitz, M.G.; Libera, A.M.M.P.D.; Batista, C.F.; Souza, F.N. Intracellular reactive oxygen species production and phagocytosis of Staphylococcus aureus by milk neutrophils as tool to diagnose mastitis and identify susceptible dairy cows. *Pesqui. Vet. Bras.* **2018**, *38*, 659–664. [CrossRef]
47. Dal Pozzo, M.; Santurio, D.F.; Rossatto, L.; Vargas, A.C.; Alves, S.H.; Loreto, E.S.; Viegas, J. Activity of essential oils from spices against Staphylococcus spp. isolated from bovine mastitis. *Arq. Bras. Med. Vet. Zootec.* **2011**, *63*, 1229–1232. [CrossRef]
48. Fratini, F.; Casella, S.; Leonardi, M.; Pisseri, F.; Ebani, V.V.; Pistelli, L.; Pistelli, L. Antibacterial activity of essential oils, their blends and mixtures of their main constituents against some strains supporting livestock mastitis. *Fitoterapia.* **2014**, *96*, 1–7. [CrossRef] [PubMed]
49. Burt, S. Essential oils: Their antibacterial properties and potential applications in foods-a review. *Int. J. Food Microbiol.* **2004**, *94*, 223–253. [CrossRef]
50. Burt, S.A.; Vlielander, R.; Haagsman, H.P.; Veldhuizen, E.J.A. Increase in Activity of Essential Oil Components Carvacrol and Thymol against Escherichia coli O157:H7 by Addition of Food Stabilizers. *J. Food Prot.* **2005**, *68*, 919–926. [CrossRef]
51. Veldhuizen, E.J.; Tjeerdsma-van Bokhoven, J.L.; Zweijtzer, C.; Burt, S.A.; Haagsman, H.P. Structural requirements for the antimicrobial activity of carvacrol. *J. Agric. Food. Chem.* **2006**, *54*, 1874–1879. [CrossRef]
52. Du, E.; Gan, L.; Li, Z.; Wang, W.; Liu, D.; Guo, Y. In vitro antibacterial activity of thymol and carvacrol and their effects on broiler chickens challenged with Clostridium perfringens. *J. Anim. Sci. Biotechnol.* **2015**, *6*, 58. [CrossRef]
53. Hayashi, M.A.; Bizerra, F.C.; Da Silva, P.I., Jr. Antimicrobial compounds from natural sources. *Front. Microbiol.* **2013**, *4*, 195. [CrossRef]
54. Xu, J.; Zhou, F.; Ji, B.P.; Pei, R.S.; Xu, N. The antibacterial mechanism of carvacrol and thymol against Escherichia coli. *Lett. Appl. Microbiol.* **2008**, *47*, 174–179. [CrossRef]
55. Sikkema, J.; De Bont, J.A.M.; Poolman, B. Mechanisms of membrane toxicity of hydrocarbons. *Microbiol. Rev.* **1995**, *59*, 201–222. [CrossRef]
56. Nazzaro, F.; Fratianni, F.; De Martino, L.; Coppola, R.; De Feo, V. Effect of Essential Oils on Pathogenic Bacteria. *Pharmaceuticals* **2013**, *6*, 1451–1474. [CrossRef] [PubMed]
57. Marinelli, L.; Di Stefano, A.; Cacciatore, I. Carvacrol and its derivatives as antibacterial agents. *Phytochem. Rev.* **2018**, *17*, 903–921. [CrossRef]
58. Ultee, A.; Slump, R.A.; Steging, G.; Smid, E.J. Antimicrobial activity of carvacrol toward Bacillus cereus on rice. *J. Food Prot.* **2000**, *63*, 620–624. [CrossRef]
59. Chouhan, S.; Sharma, K.; Guleria, S. Antimicrobial Activity of Some Essential Oils-Present Status and Future Perspectives. *Medicines* **2017**, *4*, 58. [CrossRef]
60. Lambert, R.J.W.; Skandamis, P.N.; Coote, P.J.; Nychas, G.J.E. A study of the minimum inhibitory concentration and mode of action of oregano essential oil, thymol and carvacrol. *J. Appl. Microbiol.* **2001**, *91*, 453–462. [CrossRef] [PubMed]
61. Ultee, A.; Bennik, M.H.; Moezelaar, R. The phenolic hydroxyl group of carvacrol is essential for action against the food-borne pathogen Bacillus cereus. *Appl. Environ. Microbiol.* **2002**, *68*, 1561–1568. [CrossRef]
62. Helander, I.K.; Alakomi, H.L.; Latva-Kala, K.; Mattila-Sandholm, T.; Pol, I.; Smid, E.J.; von Wright, A. Characterization of the action of selected essential oil components on Gram-negative bacteria. *J. Agric. Food Chem.* **1998**, *46*, 3590–3595. [CrossRef]
63. Dorman, H.J.D.; Deans, S.G. Antimicrobial agents from plants: Antibacterial activity of plant volatile oils. *J. Appl. Microbiol.* **2000**, *88*, 308–316. [CrossRef]
64. Cristani, M.; D'Arrigo, M.; Mandalari, G.; Castelli, F.; Sarpietro, M.G.; Micieli, D.; Venuti, V.; Bisignano, G.; Saija, A.; Trombetta, D. Interaction of four monoterpenes contained in essential oils with model membranes: Implications for their antibacterial activity. *J. Agric. Food Chem.* **2007**, *55*, 6300–6308. [CrossRef]
65. Marchese, A.; Arciola, C.R.; Barbieri, R.; Silva, A.S.; Nabavi, S.F.; Tsetegho Sokeng, A.J.; Izadi, M.; Jafari, N.J.; Suntar, I.; Daglia, M.; et al. Update on Monoterpenes as Antimicrobial Agents: A Particular Focus on p-Cymene. *Materials* **2017**, *10*, 947. [CrossRef]
66. Belmar-Liberato, R.; Gonzalez-Canga, A.; Tamame-Martin, P.; Escribano-Salazar, M. Amoxicillin and amoxicillin-clavulanic acid resistance in veterinary medicine—the situation in Europe: A review. *Vet. Med. (Praha)* **2011**, *56*, 473–485. [CrossRef]

67. Supre, K.; Lommelen, K.; De Meulemeester, L. Antimicrobial susceptibility and distribution of inhibition zone diameters of bovine mastitis pathogens in Flanders, Belgium. *Vet. Microbiol.* **2014**, *171*, 374–381. [CrossRef] [PubMed]
68. Yap, P.S.; Yiap, B.C.; Ping, H.C.; Lim, S.H. Essential oils, a new horizon in combating bacterial antibiotic resistance. *Open Microbiol. J.* **2014**, *8*, 6–14. [CrossRef] [PubMed]
69. Cuaron, J.A.; Dulal, S.; Song, Y.; Singh, A.K.; Montelongo, C.E.; Yu, W.; Nagarajan, V.; Jayaswal, R.K.; Wilkinson, B.J.; Gustafson, J.E. Tea tree oil-induced transcriptional alterations in Staphylococcus aureus. *Phytother. Res.* **2013**, *27*, 390–396. [CrossRef]
70. Hudzicki, J. *Kirby-Bauer Disk Diffusion Susceptibility Protocol*; American Society for Microbiology (ASM): Washington, DC, USA, 2009; Available online: https://www.asmscience.org/docserver/fulltext/education/protocol/protocol.3189.pdf?expires=1613515898&id=id&accname=guest&checksum=835F5125F08BB2AB46FF21C23963C9B7 (accessed on 1 December 2020).
71. CLSI. *Performance Standards for Antimicrobial Disk and Dilution Susceptibility Tests for Bacteria Isolated from Animals*, 3rd ed.; CLSI: Wayne, PA, USA, 2008.
72. CLSI. *Performance Standards for Antimicrobial Disk Susceptibility Tests*; Approved standard M02-A12; CLSI: Wayne, PA, USA, 2012.
73. Adams, R.P. *Identification of Essential Oil Components by Gas Chromatography/Mass Spectrometry*, 4th ed.; Allured Publishing Corporation: Carol Stream, IL, USA, 2007.
74. Nuutila, A.M.; Puupponen-Pimiä, R.; Aarni, M.; Oksman-Caldentey, K.-M. Comparison of antioxidant activities of onion and garlic extracts by inhibition of lipid peroxidation and radical scavenging activity. *Food Chem.* **2003**, *81*, 485–493. [CrossRef]
75. MacDonald-Wicks, L.K.; Wood, L.G.; Garg, M.L. Methodology for the determination of biological antioxidant capacity in vitro: A review. *J. Sci. Food Agric.* **2006**, *86*, 2046–2056. [CrossRef]
76. CLSI. *Methods for Dilution Antimicrobial Susceptibility Tests for Bacteria That Grow Aerobically*, 11th ed.; Approved Standard document M07; Clinical and Laboratory Standards Institute: Wayne, PA, USA, 2018; Available online: https://clsi.org/media/1928/m07ed11_sample.pdf (accessed on 1 December 2020).
77. Elshikh, M.; Ahmed, S.; Funston, S.; Dunlop, P.; McGaw, M.; Marchant, R.; Banat, I.M. Resazurin-based 96-well plate microdilution method for the determination of minimum inhibitory concentration of biosurfactants. *Biotechnol. Lett.* **2016**, *38*, 1015–1019. [CrossRef] [PubMed]
78. Čabarkapa, I.; Čolović, R.; Đuragić, O.; Popović, S.; Kokić, B.; Milanov, D.; Pezo, L. Anti-biofilm activities of essential oils rich in carvacrol and thymol against Salmonella Enteritidis. *Biofouling* **2019**, *35*, 361–375. [CrossRef] [PubMed]

antibiotics

Article

Antimicrobial Activity of Selected Essential Oils against Selected Pathogenic Bacteria: In Vitro Study

Nikola Puvača [1,2,*], Jovana Milenković [3], Tamara Galonja Coghill [2], Vojislava Bursić [4], Aleksandra Petrović [4], Snežana Tanasković [5], Miloš Pelić [6], Dragana Ljubojević Pelić [6] and Tatjana Miljković [7]

1 Faculty of Biomedical and Health Sciences, Jaume I University, Avinguda de Vicent Sos Baynat, s/n, 12071 Castelló de la Plana, Spain
2 Department of Engineering Management in Biotechnology, Faculty of Economics and Engineering Management in Novi Sad, University Business Academy in Novi Sad, Cvećarska 2, 21000 Novi Sad, Serbia; galonja@fimek.edu.rs
3 Faculty of Pharmacy, University of Belgrade, Vojvode Stepe 450, 11221 Belgrade, Serbia; jovana.milenkovicbg1987@gmail.com
4 Department for Phytomedicine and Environmental Protection, Faculty of Agriculture, University of Novi Sad, Trg Dositeja Obradovića 8, 21000 Novi Sad, Serbia; bursicv@polj.uns.ac.rs (V.B.); aleksandra.petrovic@polj.uns.ac.rs (A.P.)
5 Faculty of Agronomy in Čačak, University of Kragujevac, Cara Dušana 34, 32102 Čačak, Serbia; stanasko@kg.ac.rs
6 Scientific Veterinary Institute Novi Sad, Rumenački put 20, 21000 Novi Sad, Serbia; milosp@niv.ns.ac.rs (M.P.); dragana@niv.ns.ac.rs (D.L.P.)
7 Faculty of Medicine, University of Novi Sad, Hajduk Veljkova 3, 21000 Novi Sad, Serbia; tatjana.miljkovic@mf.uns.ac.rs
* Correspondence: nikola.puvaca@fimek.edu.rs; Tel.: +381-65-219-1284

Citation: Puvača, N.; Milenković, J.; Galonja Coghill, T.; Bursić, V.; Petrović, A.; Tanasković, S.; Pelić, M.; Ljubojević Pelić, D.; Miljković, T. Antimicrobial Activity of Selected Essential Oils against Selected Pathogenic Bacteria: In Vitro Study. *Antibiotics* **2021**, *10*, 546. https://doi.org/10.3390/antibiotics10050546

Academic Editor: William N. Setzer

Received: 1 April 2021
Accepted: 6 May 2021
Published: 8 May 2021

Abstract: The worldwide problem of infectious diseases has appeared in recent years, and antimicrobial agents are crucial in reducing disease emergence. Nevertheless, the development and distribution of multidrug-resistant (MDR) strains in pathogenic bacteria, such as *Escherichia coli*, *Staphylococcus aureus*, *Salmonella Typhi* and *Citrobacter koseri*, has become a major society health hazard. Essential oils could serve as a promising tool as a natural drug in fighting the problem with these bacteria. The current study aimed to investigate the antimicrobial effectiveness of tea tree (*Melaleuca alternifolia* (Maiden and Betche) Cheel), rosemary (*Rosmarinus officinalis* L.), eucalyptus (*Eucalyptus obliqua* L'Hér.), and lavender (*Lavandula angustifolia* Mill) essential oils. The antimicrobial properties of essential oils were screened against four pathogenic bacteria, *E. coli*, *S. aureus*, *S. Tyhpi*, and *C. koseri*, and two reference bacterial strains, while for the testing, the agar well diffusion method was used. Gas chromatography (GC) and gas chromatography–mass spectrometric (GC–MSD) analyses were performed on essential oils. The obtained results showed that *M. alternifolia* essential oil is the richest in terpinen-4-ol, *R. officinalis* and *E. oblique* essential oils in 1,8-cineole, and *L. angustifolia* essential oil in α-terpinyl acetate. In addition, the main bioactive compounds present in the essential oil of tea tree are rich in α-pinene (18.38%), limonene (7.55%) and γ-terpinene (14.01%). The essential oil of rosemary is rich in α-pinene (8.38%) and limonene (11.86%); eucalyptus essential oil has significant concentrations of α-pinene (12.60%), *p*-cymene (3.24%), limonene (3.87%), and γ-terpinene (7.37%), while the essential oil of lavender is rich in linalool (10.71%), linalool acetate (9.60%), α-terpinyl acetate (10.93%), and carbitol (13.05%) bioactive compounds, respectively. The obtained results from the in vitro study revealed that most of the essential oils exhibited antimicrobial properties. Among the tested essential oils, tea tree was discovered to demonstrate the strongest antimicrobial activity. The recorded MIC of *S. Typhi* was 6.2 mg/mL, 3.4 mg/mL of *C. koseri*, 3.1 mg/mL of *E. coli*, and 2.7 mg/mL of *E. coli* ATCC 25922, compared to *M. alternifolia*. Similarly, only *S. aureus* ATCC 25923 showed antimicrobial activity towards *R. officinalis* (1.4 mg/mL), *E. oblique* (2.9 mg/mL), and *L. angustifolia* (2.1 mg/mL). Based on the obtained results, it is possible to conclude that tea tree essential oil might be used as an ecological antimicrobial in treating infectious diseases caused by the tested pathogens.

Keywords: antibiotic resistance; microbes; essential oils; *E. coli*; *S. aureus*; *S. Thypi*; *C. koseri*

1. Introduction

The worldwide dispersion of resistant clinical isolates has led to the necessity to discover new antimicrobial agents [1]. Nevertheless, the earlier record of the precipitous, prevalent resistance to freshly created antimicrobial agents suggests that new families of antimicrobial agents will also have a short lifespan [2–5]. Many aromatic and medicinal plants, herbs, and spices have been proposed as a significant source of natural antimicrobials as an alternative to synthetic drugs to treat bacterial infections [6]. Medicinal plants and the essential oil extracted from them due to the high concentration of bioactive compounds have been widely used for this purpose [7–9]. It has been proven that essential oils have been used to treat urinary tract infectious diseases [10], respiratory diseases [11], intestinal disorders [12], and dermal illnesses [13].

Tea tree (*Melaleuca alternifolia* (Maiden and Betche) Cheel), rosemary (*Rosmarinus officinalis*), eucalyptus (*Eucalyptus obliqua* L'Hér.), and lavender (*Lavandula angustifolia* Mill) are aromatic and medicinal plants that belong to two different botanical families. With industrial development, especially in the past twenty years, large efforts have been made to identify and quantify these plants' phenolic components [9,14]. The essential oils of these plants are rich in thymol, carvacrol, *p*-cymene, and γ-terpinene [15]. A series of studies have shown the positive effect of essential oils and their bioactive compounds thymol and carvacrol due to several biological properties: antioxidant [16], antimicrobial [17], antiviral [18], diaphoretic [19], expectorant [20], insecticidal [21], and genotoxic [22]. Due to their typical aroma and proximate composition, tea tree, rosemary, eucalyptus, lavender, are commonly utilized in agriculture, pharmaceutical, cosmetic, and food industries, respectively.

Research on extracts of both Myrtle and Lamiaceae family plant chemicals has investigated their composition and their other beneficial properties in in vitro and in vivo experiments [23,24]. As they are secondary plant metabolites, the concentration is influenced by genetic and paragenetic factors, so the constant investigation and determination of their concentrations in plants are of high importance [25].

In recent decades, *E. coli* and *S. aureus* have accounted for the most significant number of outbreaks, cases, and deaths worldwide [1]. To decrease health hazards and economic losses due to the emergence of these pathogens, the use of natural antibacterial alternatives seems to be an appealing way to control the incidence of pathogenic bacteria [26].

Salmonella Tyhpi is most often the cause of typhoid fever, which is a profoundly severe intrusive bacterial disease of humans. *S. Tyhpi* can aggressively colonize the mucosal surface of the humane digestive tract but are generally confined in healthy people by the local immune defense mechanisms. Still, *S. Typhi* has developed the capability to propagate to deeper tissues, such as the bone marrow, spleen, and liver [27]. A distinctive characteristic of *Citrobacter koseri* is the exceedingly elevated tendency to initiate brain abscesses in neonatal meningitis. Earlier reports and studies on infant rats have documented many *Citrobacter*-filled macrophages within the ventricles and brain abscesses. It has been hypothesized that intracellular survival and replication within macrophages may be a mechanism by which *C. koseri* subverts the host response and elicits chronic infection, resulting in brain abscess formation [28].

Contemplating the considerable capability of essential oils as sources for natural antimicrobial drugs, this study aimed to investigate the antimicrobial effectiveness of tea tree, rosemary, eucalyptus, and lavender essential oils against pathogenic bacteria *E. coli*, *S. aureus*, *S. Tyhpi*, and *C. koseri* in in vitro conditions.

2. Results and Discussion

Bioactive substances are types of chemicals found in small amounts in plants and certain food (such as fruits, vegetables, nuts, oils, and whole grains). Actions in the body that are provided by bioactive compounds may promote good health [29]. They have been studied in the prevention of cancer, heart disease, and other diseases [30,31]. Different subgroups, including phenolic acids, flavonoids, tannins, coumarins, lignans, quinones, stilbenes, and curcuminoids, may be segregated by their chemical structures [32]. The results shown in Table 1 present the most dominant subgroup of the bioactive compound of each investigated essential oil.

Table 1. Identified bioactive compounds of analyzed essential oils, % ± SD.

Compound	Retention Indices	Retention Indices NIST [1]	Retention Time	Tea Tree	Rosemary	Eucalyptus	Lavender
α-Thujene	922	924	5.636	1.10 ± 0.01	0.03 ± 0.00	0.06 ± 0.00	0.05 ± 0.01
α-Pinene	930	932	5.862	18.38 ± 0.08	8.38 ± 0.02	12.60 ± 0.01	0.72 ± 0.00
Camphene	945	946	6.241	0.08 ± 0.00	0.03 ± 0.00	0.10 ± 0.00	0.25 ± 0.01
Thuja-2,4(10)-diene	950	952	6.378			0.01 ± 0.00	
Sabinene	970	969	6.932	0.35 ± 0.01			0.12 ± 0.00
β-Pinene	974	974	7.047	3.19 ± 0.01	0.38 ± 0.01	0.84 ± 0.01	0.60 ± 0.02
Myrcene	988	988	7.428	0.45 ± 0.00	0.49 ± 0.00	0.58 ± 0.01	0.56 ± 0.01
Carbitol	1003	1001	7.863				13.05 ± 0.04
α-Phellandrene	1004	1002	7.9	0.09 ± 0.00	0.68 ± 0.00	0.94 ± 0.00	
Δ3-Carene	1009	1008	8.098	0.09 ± 0.00	1.45 ± 0.03	0.05 ± 0.01	
Hexyl acetate	1011	1009	8.146				0.13 ± 0.01
1,4-Cineole	1013	1012	8.235				
α-Terpinene	1015	1014	8.311	2.35 ± 0.01	2.02 ± 0.01	0.15 ± 0.00	0.41 ± 0.00
p-Cymene	1023	1020	8.598	4.30 ± 0.01	4.30 ± 0.05	3.24 ± 0.00	0.87 ± 0.01
Limonene	1027	1024	8.758	7.55 ± 0.01	11.86 ± 0.01	3.87 ± 0.01	2.23 ± 0.02
1,8-Cineole	1033	1026	8.864	2.15 ± 0.05	64.02 ± 0.04	64.71 ± 0.04	5.55 ± 0.01
(Z)-β-ocimene	1035	1032	9.035			0.28 ± 0.00	0.06 ± 0.00
β-(E)-Ocimene	1046	1046	9.45	0.08 ± 0.00	0.11 ± 0.00	0.02 ± 0.00	
γ-Terpinene	1058	1054	9.89	14.01 ± 0.01	4.06 ± 0.00	7.37 ± 0.00	0.05 ± 0.00
p-Mentha-2,4(8)-diene	1085	1083	10.891	0.38 ± 0.01			
Terpinolene	1088	1086	10.991	3.56 ± 0.02	0.31 ± 0.00	0.35 ± 0.00	0.04 ± 0.00
Linalool	1099	1095	11.423	0.05 ± 0.00		0.10 ± 0.00	10.71 ± 0.02
trans-Sabinol	1137	1137	13.036	0.06 ± 0.00		0.14 ± 0.00	
Camphor	1143	1141	13.267	0.12 ± 0.00			3.72 ± 0.03
Isoborneol	1154	1155	13.787				1.04 ± 0.02
Borneol	1164	1165	14.24	0.14 ± 0.00			0.46 ± 0.01
Isononyl acetate	1171	1171	14.53				3.45 ± 0.01
Terpinen-4-ol	1180	1174	14.944	38.53 ± 0.04		0.95 ± 0.00	0.90 ± 0.02
α-Terpineol	1190	1186	15.34	2.16 ± 0.03		2.50 ± 0.01	2.00 ± 0.00
γ-Terpineol	1196	1199	15.606	0.21 ± 0.00			
Citronellol	1226	1223	16.923				2.50 ± 0.00
Geraniol	1254	1249	18.11				1.28 ± 0.00
Linalool acetate	1255	1254	18.194				9.60 ± 0.02
Bornyl acetate	1285	1287	19.562				0.21 ± 0.00
α-terpinyl acetate	1349	1346	22.374				10.93 ± 0.06
Neryl acetate	1364	1359	23.038				0.44 ± 0.00
Geranyl acetate	1384	1379	23.898				0.80 ± 0.02
α-Gurjunene	1409	1409	25.023			0.12 ± 0.00	
(E)-Caryophyllene	1420	1417	25.443	0.38 ± 0.01			1.80 ± 0.00
Aromadendrene	1439	1439	26.282			0.69 ± 0.01	
9-epi-Caryophyllene	1462	1464	27.225			0.17 ± 0.00	
Viridiflorene	1497	1496	28.693			0.07 ± 0.00	
Total peak area				564,685,150	117,582,225	142,637,552	98,030,240
Total of identified compounds (%)				99.76	98.12	99.91	74.53

[1]—Retention indices based on n-alkane series under identical experimental conditions and comparison was performed with the mass spectra library search NIST [33]; SD—standard deviation calculated for n (n = 3) GC–MSD analysis.

Conducted analyses show that the tea tree essential oil is richest in terpinen-4-ol, rosemary and eucalyptus essential oils in 1,8-cineole, and lavender essential oil in α-terpinyl acetate, respectively (Figure 1). Nevertheless, investigated essential oils in our research came with a declaration of origin, but the lack of regulation of the chemical composition of essential oils and the growing popularity of these oils among consumers present an urgent need for the accurate characterization of various oil types from a variety of manufacturers. Many essential oils in retail stores contain chemical substances of adulterants with potential toxicity [34]. In addition to the main bioactive compounds, the results of our research showed that the essential oil of tea tree is rich in α-pinene (18.38%), limonene (7.55%), and γ-terpinene (14.01%), respectively. Obtained results showed that rosemary essential oil was rich in α-pinene (8.38%) and limonene (11.86%); eucalyptus was rich in α-pinene (12.60%), *p*-cymene (3.24%), limonene (3.87%), and γ-terpinene (7.37%); and lavender was rich in linalool (10.71%), carbitol (13.05%), linalool acetate (9.60%), and α-terpinyl acetate (10.93%), respectively.

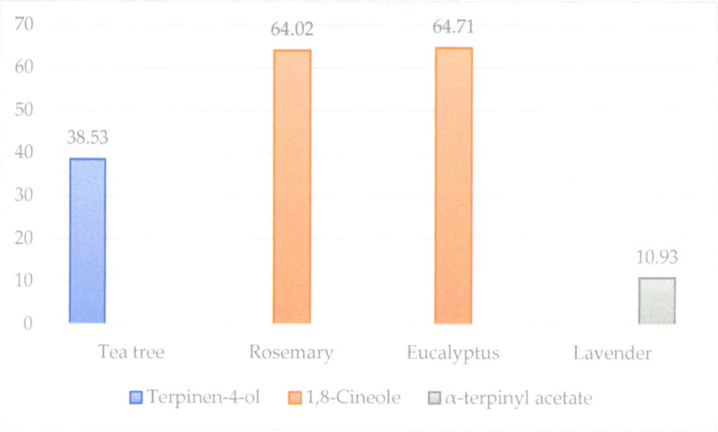

Figure 1. The highest concentrations of bioactive compounds in analyzed essential oils, %.

The two most popular essential oils on the market are tea tree and lavender oil [34]. Dubnicka et al. [34] investigated the adulteration of essential oils, which showed that six store brand essential oils, tea tree, lavender, sandalwood, rose, eucalyptus, and lemongrass, contained carbitol in concentrations from 23% to 35%, and four of the six oils contained diethyl phthalate in concentrations ranging from 0.33% to 16%. These toxicants are particularly concerning because they are known inhalation hazards, and the intended usage of these oils is for aromatherapy [34]. Based on our results and the high concentration of carbitol (13.05%) in lavender essential oil, we can assume that our lavender essential oil was not natural, which was revealed by the high concentration of carbitol as the contaminant and should be pointed out as a possible threat. Alpha-pinene presents a polyphenolic terpene organic compound [35]. It has been reported that α-pinene is a strong antioxidant agent which inhibits prostaglandin E1 and NF-κB and thus contributes to its anti-inflammatory and anticarcinogenic effects. Terpene is a part of many medical, aromatic, and spice plants [36]. Research has shown that limonene is usually found in oils obtained from citrus plants, but it has also been found in cannabis. Limonene is used to performed the percutaneous transfer of medicines in vitro and in vivo [37]. Gamma-terpinene is one of four isomeric monoterpenes. It is a naturally occurring terpenine and has been isolated from many different botanical sources [38]. It has the highest boiling point of the four known terpnine isomers (α-terpinine, β-terpinene, and δ-terpinine). It is a major component of various essential oils and has strong antioxidant activity [39,40]. It has a lemon-like or lime-like odor that is most commonly used in the food, aroma, soap, cosmetics, pharmaceuticals, tobacco, clothing and perfume industries.

Many experiments have shown the positive influence of these bioactive compounds found in essential oils, which was the topic of our research. Hendel et al. [31] in their research analyzed essential oils from the aerial parts of 15 samples of Algerian rosemary. The GC-MSD, as in our study, for the determination of phenolic compound was used. Thirty-eight components were characterized, with the highest share of α-pinene, camphene, and limonene as the main components; camphor, 1,8-cineole, and borneol as the principal oxygenated substances; caryophyllene, α-bisabolol, and humulene as the most represented sesquiterpenes. Furthermore, Hendel et al. [41] evaluated essential oils for their antimicrobial activity against *E. coli* and *S. aureus* and against ten fungal strains belonging to Aspergillus *Alternaria*, *Candida*, *Fusarium*, *Penicillium*, and *Saccharomyces* species, where the results showed moderate antimicrobial activity. Our results showed that eucalyptus essential oil is richest in eucalyptol (1,8-cineole), (Figure 1), while significant concentrations of α-pinene (12.60%), *p*-cymene (3.24%), limonene (3.87%), and γ-terpinene (7.37%) were reordered, respectively (Table 1). Eucalyptus essential oil, as well as rosemary, poses numerous beneficial properties. For example, phenolic compounds, such as camphene, α-pinene, and 2-phenyl ethanol, have high insecticidal properties of eucalyptus essential oil, so they present a potential candidate for application in integrated pest management approaches [42]. Reyes et al. [33] confirmed the fumigant and repellent action of eucalyptus essential oil against *Hypothenemus hampei*. The toxic effect of eucalyptus essential oil on the coffee berry borer is due to a synergistic effect involving 1,8-cineole, α-pinene, and *p*-cymene, according to investigations of Reyes et al. [43]. Results of our study showed that the essential oil of lavender was rich in linalool (10.71%), linalool acetate (9.60%), and α-terpinyl acetate (10.93%) bioactive compounds, respectively. Additionally, we found a significant concentration of carbitol (13.05%) in investigated lavender essential oil, which is a particular indication of essential oil adulteration. Our assumptions have also been confirmed by another study [34]. In addition to the bioactive compounds that we isolated from lavender essential oil in our research, Yadikar et al. [44] reported results that indicate isolations of seven new bioactive compounds from lavender. The same authors reported that they isolated lavandunat, lavandufurandiol, lavandufluoren, lavandupyrones A and B, and lavandudiphenyls A and B, along with five known compounds, benzoic acid, methyl propanoate, rosmarinic acid, and isosalvianolic acid C, from the ethyl acetate extract of the remaining material, which was obtained from lavender essential oil. According to the research of Sen et al. [45], in addition to the aforementioned essential oils, stated that the most produced peppermint essential oil in the Indian market also often has a high concentration of carbitol, which indicates adulteration. We also come to the same conclusion regarding the usage of lavender essential oil in our study. Donadu et al. [46] investigated the in vitro activity of lavender essential oil against drug-resistant strains of *P. aeruginosa*. Bearing in mind that lavender essential oil has been used for its anti-inflammatory, antidepressant, antiseptic, antifungal, and antimicrobial properties, the positive result in this research was expected. Donadu et al. [35] showed that lavender essential oil did not possess a cytotoxic effect when administered in very low concentration, while the same essential oil significantly reduced nitric oxide synthase activity on murine macrophages, which was also evaluated. Increased drug resistance and the absence of new antibiotics can promote the production of natural antimicrobial replacements, which is in agreement with numerous investigations of Puvača et al. [47]. Figure 2 presents the peaks of chromatography analysis of the essential oils of tea tree (a), rosemary (b), eucalyptus (c), and lavender (d) used in this research.

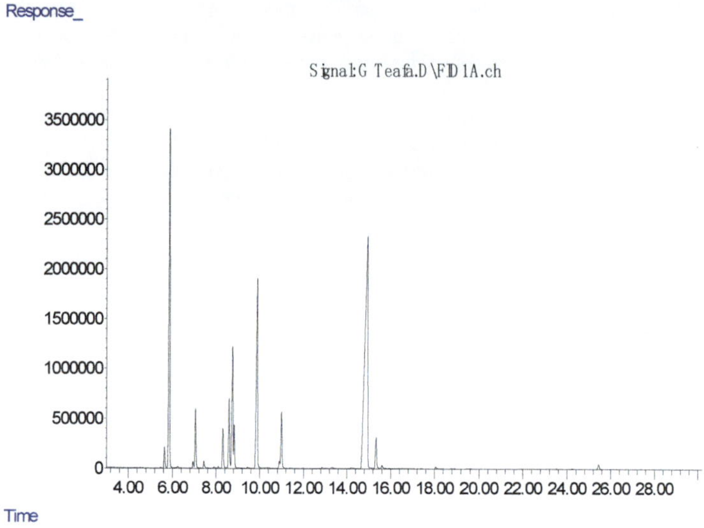

(a)

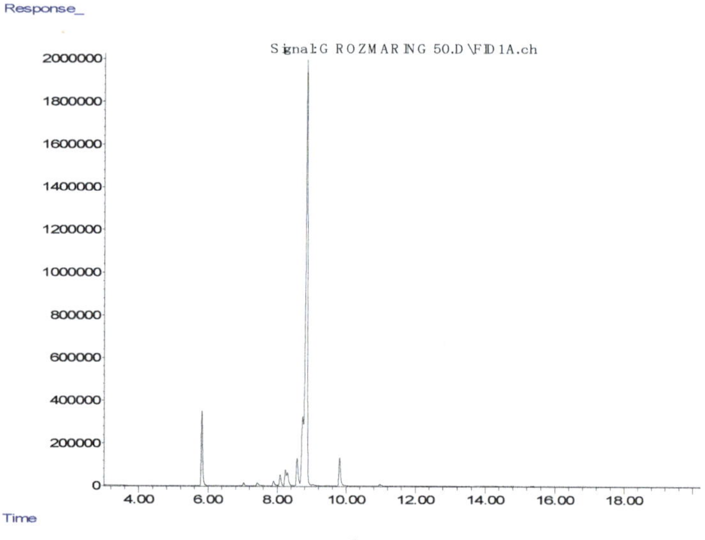

(b)

Figure 2. *Cont.*

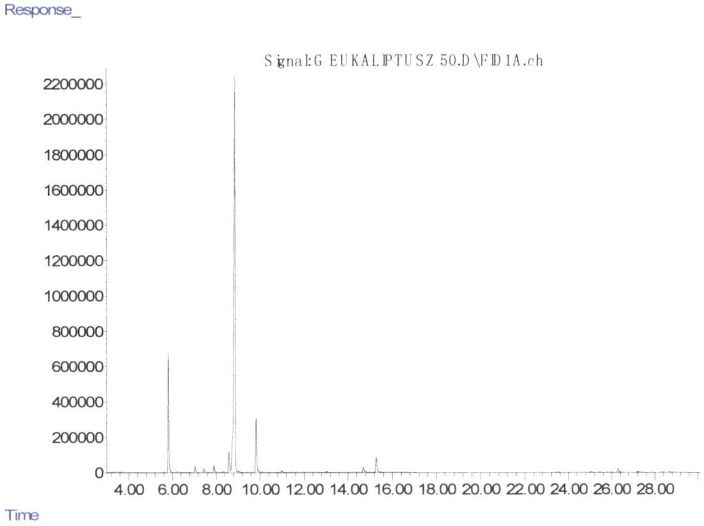

(**c**)

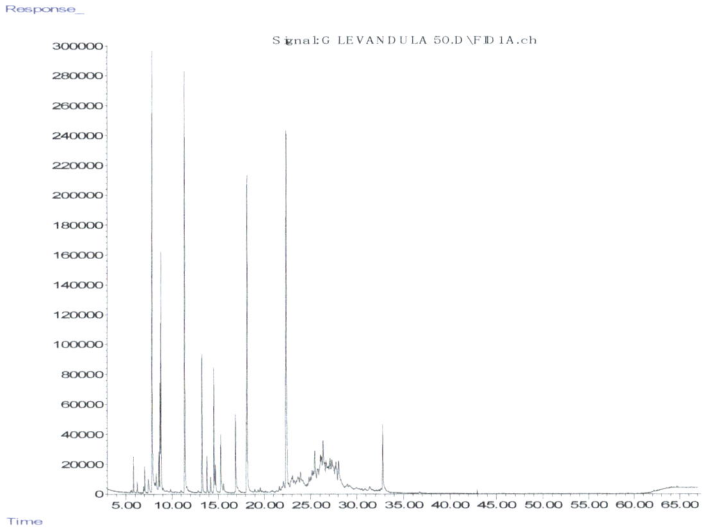

(**d**)

Figure 2. The peaks of chromatography analysis of tea tree (**a**), rosemary (**b**), eucalyptus (**c**), and lavender (**d**) essential oils.

The bioactive compounds of essential oils were tentatively identified (Table 1). All investigated essential oils in our research with their main components exhibit a broad spectrum of antimicrobial activity, which can be principally attributed to terpinen-4-ol (tea tree), 1,8-cineole (rosemary and eucalyptus), and carbitol (lavender), as active substances (Figure 1).

All worldwide countries, developed or developing, are equally affected by antibiotic resistance [48]. The development and distributions of MDR pathogens have significantly compromised the present antibacterial therapy [49]. This emergence and antibiotic resistance emergence have led to a search for new antimicrobial substances of natural origin. Essential oils are known to be rich in bioactive compounds with numerous curative properties [50]. Our research was performed to investigate four different essential oils' antimicrobial activities, with different main bioactive compounds compared to human pathogens and two reference bacterial strains.

The assessment of the antimicrobial activity in essential oils used in our study was determined by the disc diffusion method compared to *E. coli*, *S. aureus*, *S. Thypi*, and *C. koseri*. The tested pathogenic bacteria are repeatedly implicated in the occurrence of many diseases [51]. Our study showed that all essential oils that were used displayed a differing level of antimicrobial activity compared to pathogenic bacteria (Table 2).

Table 2. Zone of inhibition of essential oils used in the study (mm).

Bacteria	Tea Tree	Rosemary	Eucalyptus	Lavender
E. coli	21			
S. aureus		13	13	13
E. coli ATCC 25922	18			
S. aureus ATCC 25923		13	13	13
S. Typhi	15		15	
C. koseri	13			

The obtained results also revealed that the tea tree essential oil was the most useful among all the tested essential oils. The recorded zone of inhibition against *E. coli* was 21 mm, and against reference strain *E. coli* ATCC 25922 18 mm, 15 mm against *S. Typhi*, and 13 mm against *C. koseri*, respectively, while antimicrobial activity against *S. aureus* was not recorded. Other essential oils used in our study, rosemary, eucalyptus, and lavender, exhibited their antimicrobial activity against *S. aureus* and its reference strain with a zone of inhibition of 13 mm (Table 2), and *S. Typhi* with 15 mm, without any antimicrobial activity towards *E. coli* or its strain, or towards *C. koseri*.

The antimicrobial efficiency of essential oils was determined by measuring the minimum inhibitory concentration (MIC), as shown in Table 3. Among the tested essential oils in our study, tea tree was discovered to demonstrate strong antimicrobial activity. The recorded MIC of *S. Typhi* was 6.2 mg/mL, 3.4 mg/mL of *C. koseri*, 3.1 mg/mL of *E. coli*, and 2.7 mg/mL of *E. coli* ATCC 25922, compared to tea tree. Similarly, only *S. aureus* ATCC 25923 showed antimicrobial activity towards rosemary (1.4 mg/mL), eucalyptus (2.9 mg/mL), and lavender (2.1 mg/mL).

Table 3. Minimum inhibitory concentration (MIC); values of essential oils against bacteria (mg/mL) [1].

Bacteria	Tea Tree	Rosemary	Eucalyptus	Lavender
E. coli	3.1			
S. aureus				
E. coli ATCC 25922	2.7			
S. aureus ATCC 25923		1.4	2.9	2.1
S. Typhi	6.2			
C. koseri	3.4			

[1]—Values expressed the MIC as >the maximum concentration tested (50 mg/mL).

While tea tree essential oil showed a good antibacterial activity in nearly all bacterial isolates and strains of *E. coli* and *S. aureus*, other essential oils used in our study showed a constrained antibacterial activity contrary to the test bacterial isolates according to the obtained MIC values. Our result was similar to other findings that have reported antibacterial activity [52–56].

More stringent criteria regarding the activity were described by Saraiva [57] and Silva et al. [58], which specifically indicated that when MIC values < 100 µg/mL have been recorded, activity is described as high; when the obtained values are between 100 and 500 µg/mL, it is considered active; for those between 500 and 1000 µg/mL, activity is described as moderately active; for those between 1000 and 2000 μg/mL, activity is described as low; and those with MIC > 2000 μg/mL are described as inactive.

If taking into account the previously stated results, the effect observed in this study could be considered inactive (except for the effect of rosemary on *S. aureus*, where 1.4 mg/mL may be considered of low activity).

The in vitro antibacterial and antifungal activities of tea tree oil were investigated, and MICs for sixteen different microorganisms were determined by applying the broth dilution method. Tea tree oil showed the best overall antimicrobial effect [59]. The antimicrobial activity of tea tree essential oil has been known for a long time. Li et al. [52] investigated the dynamics and mechanism of its antimicrobial activities of tea tree essential oil in two bacterial strains. Poisoned food technique assessment showed that the MICs of tea tree essential oil for *E. coli* and *S. aureus* were 1.08 and 2.17 mg/mL, respectively. Antimicrobial dynamic curves showed that with increasing concentrations of essential oil, the rate of cell killing and the duration of the growth lag phase increased correspondingly [52]. The essential oil of tea tree exhibited a broad spectrum of antimicrobial activity. Its mode of action against the Gram-negative bacterium *E. coli* and the Gram-positive bacterium *S. aureus* was investigated using various methods. It has been reported that the exposure of these organisms to minimum inhibitory concentrations of tea tree oil inhibit respiration and increase the permeability of bacterial cytoplasmic and yeast plasma membranes [60].

The antimicrobial efficiency of essential oils was also determined by measuring the minimal bactericidal concentration (MBC), which is shown in Figure 3. Results of the MBC show that tea tree demonstrated the strongest antimicrobial activity. The recorded MBC of *S. Typhi* was 12.4 mg/mL, 6.8 mg/mL of *C. koseri*, 6.2 mg/mL of *E. coli*, and 5.4 mg/mL of *E. coli* ATCC 25922, compared to tea tree. Exceptionally, *S. aureus* ATCC 25923 showed bactericidal activity towards rosemary of 2.8 mg/mL, eucalyptus of 5.8 mg/mL, and lavender of 4.1 mg/mL.

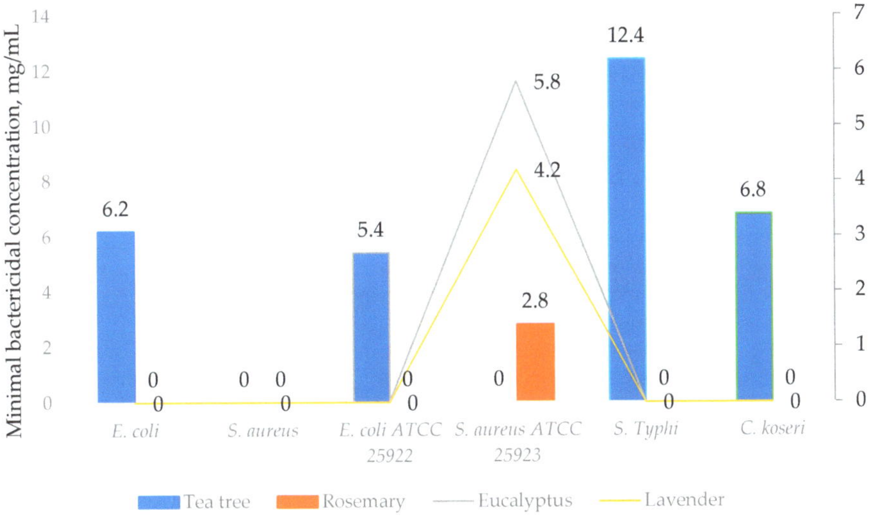

Figure 3. Minimal bactericidal concentration (MBC); values of essential oils against bacteria (mg/mL). Values expressed the MBC as >the maximum concentration tested (50 mg/mL).

Mohsen et al. [61] performed a study to evaluate the antimicrobial activity of rosemary essential oil human pathogenic bacteria. *E. coli* and *S. aureus* were selected for investigation, as well as three other bacteria. The antimicrobial activity of in vitro conditions showed that based on the disc diffusion agar method, the inhibition zone diameter of rosemary essential oil for *E. coli* was 12.10 mm. Authors concluded that rosemary essential oil is a suitable antibacterial agent and can be used as a natural alternative in the control of pathogenic microorganism growth [61].

Elaissi et al. [62] investigated the antibacterial activity of several *Eucalyptus* species and their correlation with chemical composition. The main chemical compounds were determined to be 1,8-cineole, spathulenol, α-pinene, *p*-cymene, and limonene. The most potent antibacterial activity was recorded against *S. aureus* and *E. coli*, while the correlation between the levels of active compounds in essential oil and the antibacterial activities was noticed. Similar results, which are in accordance with our findings, were demonstrated in the study of Vaghasiya and Chanda [63]. Authors investigated the antimicrobial and antifungal properties of eucalyptus essential oil and concluded that the most susceptible bacterium was *Citrobacter freundii*, while the most resistant was *Proteus vulgaris*.

Unfortunately, the antimicrobial properties of eucalyptus essential oil are very limited, but lavender essential oil and its effects in various fields have been investigated. Adaszyńska-Skwirzyńska and Szczerbińska [64] investigated the antimicrobial activity of lavender essential oil and its influence on the production performance of broiler chickens. Researchers concluded that the addition of 0.4 mL/L to the drinking water of broiler chickens had significantly improved production results, with a proven significant effect on bacterial growth inhibition. Another study was performed to verify the antimicrobial activity of lavender essential oil as the component of a preservative system in oil in water body milk [65]. The obtained results showed a reduction in bacteria in the inoculum by 3 logarithmic units within 7 days with no increase up to the 28th day. Bosnić et al. [66] investigated the antimicrobial activity of sage, rosemary, eucalyptus, melissa, lavender, and thyme essential oils against Gram-positive and Gram-negative bacteria. Based on their findings, it was concluded that the most active essential oils were eucalyptus and rosemary, with the MICs ranging from 0.097 to 0.390 mg/mL. The results of Shirugumbi Hanamanthagouda et al. [67] confirmed that lavender essential oil was inhibitory against various bacterial and fungal strains, respectively.

Although a certain number of essential oils show good antibacterial activity, some oils' narrow antibacterial activities do not provide a complete picture for the usage of essential oil against the occurrence of infectious diseases. Nevertheless, further study is necessary to investigate their efficacy in inhibiting the growth of bacteria, fungi, parasites, and viruses.

3. Material and Methods

Commercially available essential oils of tea tree, rosemary, eucalyptus, and lavender used in this research were purchased from a local distributor in Novi Sad, Serbia. According to certification, essential oils from plants were extracted using supercritical CO_2 in the conventional semi-continuous method to separate 1,8-cineole, linalool, linalyl acetate, and camphor.

Gas chromatography (GC) and gas chromatography–mass spectrometric (GC–MS) analyses were performed using an Agilent 7890A GC equipped with an inert 5975C XL EI/CI mass spectrometer detector (MSD) and flame ionization detector (FID) connected by a capillary flow technology 2-way splitter with make-up. The HP-5MS capillary column (30 m × 0.25 mm × 0.25 μm) was used. The GC oven temperature was programmed from 60 to 300 °C at a rate of 3 °C min^{-1} and held for 15 min. Helium was used as the carrier gas at 16.255 psi (constant pressure mode). An auto-injection system (Agilent 7683B Series Injector - Agilent Technologies Inc, Santa Clara, CA, USA) was employed to inject 1 μL of sample. The sample was analyzed in the splitless mode. The injector temperature was 300 °C and the detector temperature 300 °C. MS data were acquired in the EI mode with a scan range of 30–550 m/z, source temperature of 230 °C, and quadruple temperature of 150 °C; the solvent delay was 3 min.

The identification of all compounds in the analyses was matched by comparing their linear retention indices (relative to C8–C36 n-alkanes on the HP-5MSI column) and MS spectra with those of authentic standards from NIST11 databases.

Previously used structural, physical, and standard biochemistry assessments were used to pinpoint bacterial strains, followed by an antimicrobial susceptibility test by a modified Kirby Bauer disc diffusion method and the Clinical and Laboratory Standards Institute guidelines. Resistant isolates were identified as the isolates resistant to amikacin antibiotic.

A total of six human pathogenic strains were used in this study. All Gram-positive organisms were identified by conventional methods, such as Gram stain, positive catalase, tube coagulase, deoxyribonucleases (DNAse) tests. An API 20E kit was used to identify the Gram-negative organism.

The agar well diffusion method in Mueller-Hinton agar plates was used for antimicrobial testing of essential oils. Incubation of inoculated bacteria was conducted for 12 h at a temperature of 37 °C, in Nutrient broth. A Mueller-Hinton agar plate was cultured with standardized microbial culture broth. Essential oils in concentrations of 50 mg/mL were prepared in organosulfur solvent ($(CH_3)_2SO$). Four wells of 8 mm were bored in the inoculated media. Each well was filled with 50 µL of essential oils: positive control of amikacin (30 mcg) and nitrofurantoin (300 mcg) and negative control. The diffusion process lasted for about 30 min at a temperature of 22.5 °C and incubation time for 18–24 h at 37 °C. Following incubation, plates were examined to develop a clear zone around the well which corresponded to the antimicrobial activity. The zone of inhibition was detected and assessed (mm).

The broth microdilution method was used to establish the minimal inhibitory concentrations corresponding to the Clinical and Laboratory Standards Institute guidelines. Twin successive dilutions of essential oils were conducted directly in a microtiter plate containing Mueller-Hinton broth. The bacterial inoculum was added to 5 × 105 CFU/mL in each well. An antibiotic amikacin was used for the control reference. Incubation of plates was performed at temperature of 37 °C for 24 h. Resazurin was added to each well of the microtiter plate and incubated at 37 °C for 30 min. The occurrence of pink color was associated with wells which displayed bacterial growth, while the blue color was associated with those without bacterial growth. The minimal inhibitory concentrations were considered as the lowest concentration of the essential oil that completely inhibits bacterial growth.

4. Conclusions

Based on the obtained results, it can be concluded that tea tree essential oil is richest in terpinen-4-ol, rosemary, and eucalyptus essential oils in 1,8-cineole, and lavender essential oil in α-terpinyl acetate. In addition to the main bioactive compounds, the results of our research showed that the essential oil of tea tree is rich in α-pinene (18.38%), limonene (7.55%), and γ-terpinene (14.01%). The essential oil of rosemary is rich in α-pinene (8.38%) and limonene (11.86%); eucalyptus essential oil has significant concentrations of α-pinene (12.60%), *p*-cymene (3.24%), limonene (3.87%), and γ-terpinene (7.37%), while the essential oil of lavender is rich in linalool (10.71%), linalool acetate (9.60%), and α-terpinyl acetate (10.93%), respectively. It has also been found that lavender essential oil is rich in carbitol (13.05%) as a potentially toxic compound.

Our research showed tea tree essential oil's antimicrobial activity towards *E. coli*, *S. Typhi*, and *C. koseri*, while the other essential oils exhibited their antimicrobial activity towards *S. aureus*. Although results showed some potential in the in vitro activity of investigated essential oils for pathogenic bacteria, these obtained results still may not be applied in vivo. Based on our in vitro findings, further research in in vivo conditions is necessary to evaluate the antimicrobial activity of investigated essential oils fully.

Author Contributions: Conceptualization, N.P. and D.L.P.; methodology, N.P.; software, A.P.; validation, N.P., T.G.C., and M.P.; formal analysis, D.L.P.; investigation, N.P. and T.M.; resources, J.M.; data curation, V.B.; writing—original draft preparation, N.P.; writing—review and editing, D.L.P.; visualization, N.P.; supervision, S.T.; project administration, N.P.; funding acquisition, N.P. All authors have read and agreed to the published version of the manuscript.

Funding: This research was funded by the Ministry of Education, Science and Technological Development of the Republic of Serbia.

Data Availability Statement: Data is contained within the article.

Acknowledgments: This research was supported by the Ministry of Education, Science and Technological Development of the Republic of Serbia.

Conflicts of Interest: The authors declare no conflict of interest. The funders had no role in the design of the study; in the collection, analyses, or interpretation of data; in the writing of the manuscript, or in the decision to publish the results.

References

1. Puvača, N.; de Llanos Frutos, R. Antimicrobial Resistance in *Escherichia coli* Strains Isolated from Humans and Pet Animals. *Antibiotics* **2021**, *10*, 69. [CrossRef]
2. Toombs-Ruane, L.J.; Benschop, J.; French, N.P.; Biggs, P.J.; Midwinter, A.C.; Marshall, J.C.; Chan, M.; Drinković, D.; Fayaz, A.; Baker, M.G.; et al. Carriage of Extended-Spectrum-Beta-Lactamase- and AmpC Beta-Lactamase-Producing *Escherichia coli* Strains from Humans and Pets in the Same Households. *Appl. Environ. Microbiol.* **2020**, *86*. [CrossRef] [PubMed]
3. Friedrich, A.W. Control of Hospital Acquired Infections and Antimicrobial Resistance in Europe: The Way to Go. *Wien. Med. Wochenschr.* **2019**, *169*, 25–30. [CrossRef] [PubMed]
4. Ljubojević, D.; Pelić, M.; Puvača, N.; Milanov, D. Resistance to Tetracycline in *Escherichia coli* Isolates from Poultry Meat: Epidemiology, Policy and Perspective. *World's Poult. Sci. J.* **2017**, *73*, 409–417. [CrossRef]
5. Ljubojević, D.; Velhner, M.; Todorović, D.; Pajić, M.; Milanov, D. Tetracycline Resistance in *Escherichia coli* Isolates from Poultry. *Arch. Vet. Med.* **2016**, *9*, 61–81. [CrossRef]
6. Puvača, N.; Lika, E.; Tufarelli, V.; Bursić, V.; Pelić, D.L.; Nikolova, N.; Petrović, A.; Prodanović, R.; Vuković, G.; Lević, J.; et al. Influence of Different Tetracycline Antimicrobial Therapy of Mycoplasma (*Mycoplasma synoviae*) in Laying Hens Compared to Tea Tree Essential Oil on Table Egg Quality and Antibiotic Residues. *Foods* **2020**, *9*, 612. [CrossRef]
7. Cosentino, S.; Tuberoso, C.I.G.; Pisano, B.; Satta, M.; Mascia, V.; Arzedi, E.; Palmas, F. In-Vitro Antimicrobial Activity and Chemical Composition of Sardinian Thymus Essential Oils. *Lett. Appl. Microbiol.* **1999**, *29*, 130–135. [CrossRef]
8. Canter, P.H.; Thomas, H.; Ernst, E. Bringing Medicinal Plants into Cultivation: Opportunities and Challenges for Biotechnology. *Trends Biotechnol.* **2005**, *23*, 180–185. [CrossRef]
9. Joana Gil-Chávez, G.; Villa, J.A.; Fernando Ayala-Zavala, J.; Basilio Heredia, J.; Sepulveda, D.; Yahia, E.M.; González-Aguilar, G.A. Technologies for Extraction and Production of Bioactive Compounds to Be Used as Nutraceuticals and Food Ingredients: An overview. *Compr. Rev. Food Sci. Food Saf.* **2013**, *12*, 5–23. [CrossRef]
10. Ebani, V.V.; Nardoni, S.; Bertelloni, F.; Pistelli, L.; Mancianti, F. Antimicrobial Activity of Five Essential Oils against Bacteria and Fungi Responsible for Urinary Tract Infections. *Molecules* **2018**, *23*, 1668. [CrossRef]
11. Ali, B.; Al-Wabel, N.A.; Shams, S.; Ahamad, A.; Khan, S.A.; Anwar, F. Essential Oils Used in Aromatherapy: A Systemic Review. *Asian Pac. J. Trop. Biomed.* **2015**, *5*, 601–611. [CrossRef]
12. Tanveer, M.; Wagner, C.; ul Haq, M.I.; Ribeiro, N.C.; Rathinasabapathy, T.; Butt, M.S.; Shehzad, A.; Komarnytsky, S. Spicing up Gastrointestinal Health with Dietary Essential Oils. *Phytochem. Rev.* **2020**, *19*, 243–263. [CrossRef]
13. Abu-Al-Basal, M.A. Healing Potential of *Rosmarinus officinalis* L. on Full-Thickness Excision Cutaneous Wounds in Alloxan-Induced-Diabetic BALB/c Mice. *J. Ethnopharmacol.* **2010**, *131*, 443–450. [CrossRef]
14. Ignat, I.; Volf, I.; Popa, V.I. A Critical Review of Methods for Characterisation of Polyphenolic Compounds in Fruits and Vegetables. *Food Chem.* **2011**, *126*, 1821–1835. [CrossRef] [PubMed]
15. Nhu-Trang, T.-T.; Casabianca, H.; Grenier-Loustalot, M.-F. Deuterium/Hydrogen Ratio Analysis of Thymol, Carvacrol, γ-Terpinene and *p*-Cymene in Thyme, Savory and Oregano Essential Oils by Gas Chromatography–Pyrolysis–Isotope Ratio Mass Spectrometry. *J. Chromatogr. A* **2006**, *1132*, 219–227. [CrossRef]
16. Misharina, T.A.; Terenina, M.B.; Krikunova, N.I. Antioxidant Properties of Essential Oils. *Appl. Biochem. Microbiol.* **2009**, *45*, 642–647. [CrossRef]
17. Bassolé, I.H.N.; Juliani, H.R. Essential Oils in Combination and Their Antimicrobial Properties. *Molecules* **2012**, *17*, 3989–4006. [CrossRef]
18. Reichling, J.; Schnitzler, P.; Suschke, U.; Saller, R. Essential Oils of Aromatic Plants with Antibacterial, Antifungal, Antiviral, and Cytotoxic properties—An Overview. *Complement. Med. Res.* **2009**, *16*, 79–90. [CrossRef]
19. Formisano, C.; Oliviero, F.; Rigano, D.; Saab, A.M.; Senatore, F. Chemical Composition of Essential Oils and in Vitro Antioxidant Properties of Extracts and Essential Oils of Calamintha Origanifolia and Micromeria Myrtifolia, Two Lamiaceae from the Lebanon Flora. *Ind. Crops Prod.* **2014**, *62*, 405–411. [CrossRef]

20. Wannissorn, B.; Jarikasem, S.; Siriwangchai, T.; Thubthimthed, S. Antibacterial Properties of Essential Oils from Thai Medicinal Plants. *Fitoterapia* **2005**, *76*, 233–236. [CrossRef]
21. Pavela, R. Insecticidal Properties of Several Essential Oils on the House Fly (*Musca domestica* L.). *Phytother. Res.* **2008**, *22*, 274–278. [CrossRef] [PubMed]
22. Puškárová, A.; Bučková, M.; Kraková, L.; Pangallo, D.; Kozics, K. The Antibacterial and Antifungal Activity of Six Essential Oils and Their Cyto/Genotoxicity to Human HEL 12469 Cells. *Sci. Rep.* **2017**, *7*, 8211. [CrossRef]
23. Romero Rocamora, C.; Ramasamy, K.; Meng Lim, S.; Majeed, A.B.A.; Agatonovic-Kustrin, S. HPTLC Based Approach for Bioassay-Guided Evaluation of Antidiabetic and Neuroprotective Effects of Eight Essential Oils of the Lamiaceae Family Plants. *J. Pharm. Biomed. Anal.* **2020**, *178*, 112909. [CrossRef] [PubMed]
24. Usai, M.; Marchetti, M.; Culeddu, N.; Mulas, M. Chemical Composition of Myrtle (*Myrtus communis* L.) Berries Essential Oils as Observed in a Collection of Genotypes. *Molecules* **2018**, *23*, 2502. [CrossRef]
25. Jamoussi, B.; Romdhane, M.; Abderraba, A.; Hassine, B.B.; Gadri, A.E. Effect of Harvest Time on the Yield and Composition of Tunisian Myrtle Oils. *Flavour Fragr. J.* **2005**, *20*, 274–277. [CrossRef]
26. Puvača, N.; Stanaćev, V.; Glamočić, D.; Lević, J.; Perić, L.; Stanaćev, V.; Milić, D. Beneficial Effects of Phytoadditives in Broiler Nutrition. *World's Poult. Sci. J.* **2013**, *69*, 27–34. [CrossRef]
27. Parkhill, J.; Dougan, G.; James, K.D.; Thomson, N.R.; Pickard, D.; Wain, J.; Churcher, C.; Mungall, K.L.; Bentley, S.D.; Holden, M.T.G.; et al. Complete Genome Sequence of a Multiple Drug Resistant Salmonella Enterica Serovar Typhi CT18. *Nature* **2001**, *413*, 848–852. [CrossRef]
28. Townsend, S.M.; Pollack, H.A.; Gonzalez-Gomez, I.; Shimada, H.; Badger, J.L. *Citrobacter koseri* Brain Abscess in the Neonatal Rat: Survival and Replication within Human and Rat Macrophages. *Infect. Immun.* **2003**, *71*, 5871–5880. [CrossRef]
29. Weaver, C.M. Bioactive Foods and Ingredients for Health. *Adv. Nutr.* **2014**, *5*, 306S–311S. [CrossRef]
30. Singla, R.; Mishra, A.; Joshi, R.; Jha, S.; Sharma, A.R.; Upadhyay, S.; Sarma, P.; Prakash, A.; Medhi, B. Human Animal Interface of SARS-CoV-2 (COVID-19) Transmission: A Critical Appraisal of Scientific Evidence. *Vet. Res. Commun.* **2020**, *44*, 119–130. [CrossRef]
31. Kris-Etherton, P.M.; Hecker, K.D.; Bonanome, A.; Coval, S.M.; Binkoski, A.E.; Hilpert, K.F.; Griel, A.E.; Etherton, T.D. Bioactive Compounds in Foods: Their Role in the Prevention of Cardiovascular Disease and Cancer. *Am. J. Med.* **2002**, *113*, 71S–88S. [CrossRef]
32. Crozier, A.; Jaganath, I.B.; Clifford, M.N. Dietary Phenolics: Chemistry, Bioavailability and Effects on Health. *Nat. Prod. Rep.* **2009**, *26*, 1001–1043. [CrossRef]
33. Stein, S.E.; Mikaia, A.; Linstrom, P.; Mirokhin, Y.; Tchekhovskoi, D.; Yang, X.; Mallard, W.G.; Sparkman, O.D.; Sparkman, J.A. NIST 11. Standard Reference Database 1A, Mass Spectral Database. 2011. Available online: https://www.nist.gov/sites/default/files/documents/srd/NIST1a11Ver2-0Man.pdf (accessed on 8 April 2021).
34. Dubnicka, M.; Cromwell, B.; Levine, M. Investigation of the Adulteration of Essential Oils by GC-MS. *Curr. Anal. Chem.* **2020**, *16*, 965–969. [CrossRef]
35. Zhou, J.; Tang, F.; Mao, G.; Bian, R. Effect of Alpha-Pinene on Nuclear Translocation of NF-Kappa B in THP-1 Cells. *Acta Pharmacol. Sin.* **2004**, *25*, 480–484. [PubMed]
36. Gershenzon, J.; Dudareva, N. The Function of Terpene Natural Products in the Natural World. *Nat. Chem. Biol.* **2007**, *3*, 408–414. [CrossRef]
37. Ciriminna, R.; Lomeli-Rodriguez, M.; Demma Carà, P.; Lopez-Sanchez, J.A.; Pagliaro, M. Limonene: A Versatile Chemical of the Bioeconomy. *Chem. Commun.* **2014**, *50*, 15288–15296. [CrossRef]
38. Ramalho, T.; Pacheco de Oliveira, M.; Lima, A.; Bezerra-Santos, C.; Piuvezam, M. Gamma-Terpinene Modulates Acute Inflammatory Response in Mice. *Planta Med.* **2015**, *81*, 1248–1254. [CrossRef]
39. Pateiro, M.; Barba, F.J.; Domínguez, R.; Sant'Ana, A.S.; Mousavi Khaneghah, A.; Gavahian, M.; Gómez, B.; Lorenzo, J.M. Essential Oils as Natural Additives to Prevent Oxidation Reactions in Meat and Meat Products: A Review. *Food Res. Int.* **2018**, *113*, 156–166. [CrossRef]
40. Puvača, N.; Čabarkapa, I.; Petrović, A.; Bursić, V.; Prodanović, R.; Soleša, D.; Lević, J. Tea Tree (*Melaleuca alternifolia*) and Its Essential Oil: Antimicrobial, Antioxidant and Acaricidal Effects in Poultry Production. *World's Poult. Sci. J.* **2019**, *75*, 235–246. [CrossRef]
41. Hendel, N.; Napoli, E.; Sarri, M.; Saija, A.; Cristani, M.; Nostro, A.; Ginestra, G.; Ruberto, G. Essential Oil from Aerial Parts of Wild Algerian Rosemary: Screening of Chemical Composition, Antimicrobial and Antioxidant Activities. *J. Essent. Oil Bear. Plants* **2019**, *22*, 1–17. [CrossRef]
42. Pant, M.; Dubey, S.; Patanjali, P.K.; Naik, S.N.; Sharma, S. Insecticidal Activity of Eucalyptus Oil Nanoemulsion with Karanja and Jatropha Aqueous Filtrates. *Int. Biodeterior. Biodegrad.* **2014**, *91*, 119–127. [CrossRef]
43. Reyes, E.I.M.; Farias, E.S.; Silva, E.M.P.; Filomeno, C.A.; Plata, M.A.B.; Picanço, M.C.; Barbosa, L.C.A. Eucalyptus Resinifera Essential Oils Have Fumigant and Repellent Action against *Hypothenemus hampei*. *Crop Prot.* **2019**, *116*, 49–55. [CrossRef]
44. Yadikar, N.; Bobakulov, K.; Li, G.; Aisa, H.A. Seven New Phenolic Compounds from *Lavandula angustifolia*. *Phytochem. Lett.* **2018**, *23*, 149–154. [CrossRef]
45. Sen, I.; Shrivastava, D.; Aggarwal, M.; Kumar Khandal, R. Carbitol as Adulterant in Menthol; Analytical Method for Quantitative Analysis of Adulteration. *AIMS Agric. Food* **2020**, *5*, 129–136. [CrossRef]

46. Donadu, M.; Usai, D.; Pinna, A.; Porcu, T.; Mazzarello, V.; Fiamma, M.; Marchetti, M.; Cannas, S.; Delogu, G.; Zanetti, S.; et al. In Vitro Activity of Hybrid Lavender Essential Oils against Multidrug Resistant Strains of Pseudomonas Aeruginosa. *J. Infect. Dev. Ctries* **2018**, *12*. [CrossRef] [PubMed]
47. Puvača, N.; Bursić, V.; Petrović, A.; Prodanović, R.; Kharud, M.M.; Obućinski, D.; Vuković, G.; Marić, M. Influence of tea tree essential oil on the synthesis of mycotoxins: Ochratoxin A. *Maced. J. Anim. Sci.* **2019**, *9*, 25–29.
48. Jasovský, D.; Littmann, J.; Zorzet, A.; Cars, O. Antimicrobial Resistance—A Threat to the World's Sustainable Development. *Upsala J. Med Sci.* **2016**, *121*, 159–164. [CrossRef]
49. De Oliveira, D.M.P.; Forde, B.M.; Kidd, T.J.; Harris, P.N.A.; Schembri, M.A.; Beatson, S.A.; Paterson, D.L.; Walker, M.J. Antimicrobial Resistance in ESKAPE Pathogens. *Clin. Microbiol. Rev.* **2020**, *33*, e00181-19. [CrossRef]
50. Farzaneh, V.; Carvalho, I.S. A Review of the Health Benefit Potentials of Herbal Plant Infusions and Their Mechanism of Actions. *Ind. Crops Prod.* **2015**, *65*, 247–258. [CrossRef]
51. Poolman, J.T.; Anderson, A.S. *Escherichia coli* and *Staphylococcus aureus*: Leading Bacterial Pathogens of Healthcare Associated Infections and Bacteremia in Older-Age Populations. *Expert Rev. Vaccines* **2018**, *17*, 607–618. [CrossRef]
52. Li, W.-R.; Li, H.-L.; Shi, Q.-S.; Sun, T.-L.; Xie, X.-B.; Song, B.; Huang, X.-M. The Dynamics and Mechanism of the Antimicrobial Activity of Tea Tree Oil against Bacteria and Fungi. *Appl. Microbiol. Biotechnol.* **2016**, *100*, 8865–8875. [CrossRef]
53. Jiang, H.; Zheng, H. Efficacy and Adverse Reaction to Different Doses of Atorvastatin in the Treatment of Type II Diabetes Mellitus. *Biosci. Rep.* **2019**, *39*, BSR20182371. [CrossRef]
54. Jafari-Sales, A.; Pashazadeh, M. Study of Chemical Composition and Antimicrobial Properties of Rosemary (*Rosmarinus Officinalis*) Essential Oil on *Staphylococcus aureus* and *Escherichia coli* In Vitro. *Int. J. Life Sci. Biotechnol.* **2020**. [CrossRef]
55. Bachir, R.G.; Benali, M. Antibacterial Activity of the Essential Oils from the Leaves of Eucalyptus Globulus against *Escherichia coli* and *Staphylococcus aureus*. *Asian Pac. J. Trop. Biomed.* **2012**, *2*, 739–742. [CrossRef]
56. Predoi, D.; Iconaru, S.; Buton, N.; Badea, M.; Marutescu, L. Antimicrobial Activity of New Materials Based on Lavender and Basil Essential Oils and Hydroxyapatite. *Nanomaterials* **2018**, *8*, 291. [CrossRef] [PubMed]
57. Saraiva, M. In Vitro Evaluation of Antioxidant, Antimicrobial and Toxicity Properties of Extracts of Schinopsis Brasiliensis Engl. (Anacardiaceae). *Afr. J. Pharm. Pharmacol.* **2011**, *5*, 1724–1731. [CrossRef]
58. Silva, A.C.O.; Santana, E.F.; Saraiva, A.M.; Coutinho, F.N.; Castro, R.H.A.; Pisciottano, M.N.C.; Amorim, E.L.C.; Albuquerque, U.P. Which Approach Is More Effective in the Selection of Plants with Antimicrobial Activity? *Evid.-Based Complementary Altern. Med.* **2013**, *2013*, 1–9. [CrossRef]
59. Christoph, F.; Kaulfers, P.-M.; Stahl-Biskup, E. A Comparative Study of the in Vitro Antimicrobial Activity of Tea Tree Oils s.l. with Special Reference to the Activity of β-Triketones. *Planta Med.* **2000**, *66*, 556–560. [CrossRef]
60. Cox, S.D.; Mann, C.M.; Markham, J.L.; Bell, H.C.; Gustafson, J.E.; Warmington, J.R.; Wyllie, S.G. The Mode of Antimicrobial Action of the Essential Oil of *Melaleuca alternifolia* (Tea Tree Oil): S.D. COX ET AL. *J. Appl. Microbiol.* **2001**, *88*, 170–175. [CrossRef] [PubMed]
61. Mohsen, E.H.K.; Hossein, J.; Behrooz, A.B.; Mohammad, N. Antimicrobial Activity of Rosemary Essential Oil and Its Interaction with Common Therapeutic Antibiotics on Some Gram Positive and Gram Negative Bacteria. *Iran. J. Infect. Dis. Trop. Med.* **2020**, *24*, 25–34.
62. Elaissi, A.; Rouis, Z.; Mabrouk, S.; Salah, K.B.H.; Aouni, M.; Khouja, M.L.; Farhat, F.; Chemli, R.; Harzallah-Skhiri, F. Correlation Between Chemical Composition and Antibacterial Activity of Essential Oils from Fifteen Eucalyptus Species Growing in the Korbous and Jbel Abderrahman Arboreta (North East Tunisia). *Molecules* **2012**, *17*, 3044–3057. [CrossRef] [PubMed]
63. Vaghasiya, Y.; Nair, R.; Chanda, S. Antibacterial and Preliminary Phytochemical and Physico-Chemical Analysis of *Eucalyptus citriodora* Hk Leaf. *Nat. Prod. Res.* **2008**, *22*, 754–762. [CrossRef]
64. Adaszyńska-Skwirzyńska, M.; Szczerbińska, D. Use of Essential Oils in Broiler Chicken Production—A Review. *Ann. Anim. Sci.* **2017**, *17*, 317–335. [CrossRef]
65. Kunicka-Styczyńska, A.; Sikora, M.; Kalemba, D. Antimicrobial Activity of Lavender, Tea Tree and Lemon Oils in Cosmetic Preservative Systems: Antimicrobial Action of Oils in Cosmetics. *J. Appl. Microbiol.* **2009**, *107*, 1903–1911. [CrossRef]
66. Bosnić, T.; Softić, D.; Grujić-Vasić, J. Antimicrobial Activity of Some Essential Oils and Major Constituents of Essential Oils. *Acta Med. Acad.* **2006**, *35*, 9–14.
67. Hanamanthagouda, M.S.; Kakkalameli, S.B.; Naik, P.M.; Nagella, P.; Seetharamareddy, H.R.; Murthy, H.N. Essential Oils of Lavandula Bipinnata and Their Antimicrobial Activities. *Food Chem.* **2010**, *118*, 836–839. [CrossRef]

antibiotics
MDPI

Article

Determination of Pharmacokinetic and Pharmacokinetic-Pharmacodynamic Parameters of Doxycycline against *Edwardsiella ictaluri* in Yellow Catfish (*Pelteobagrus fulvidraco*)

Ning Xu [1,2,3], Miao Li [2], Xiaohui Ai [1,3,4,*] and Zhoumeng Lin [2,*]

1 Yangtze River Fisheries Research Institute, Chinese Academy of Fishery Sciences, Wuhan 430223, China; xuning@yfi.ac.cn
2 Institute of Computational Comparative Medicine (ICCM), Department of Anatomy and Physiology, College of Veterinary Medicine, Kansas State University, Manhattan, KS 66506, USA; miaoli@ksu.edu
3 Hu Bei Province Engineering and Technology Research Center of Aquatic Product Quality and Safety, Wuhan 430223, China
4 Key Laboratory of Control of Quality and Safety for Aquatic Products, Ministry of Agriculture and Rural Affairs, Beijing 100141, China
* Correspondence: aixh@yfi.ac.cn (X.A.); zhoumeng@ksu.edu (Z.L.)

Abstract: This study aimed to examine the pharmacokinetics of doxycycline (DC) in yellow catfish (*Pelteobagrus fulvidraco*) and to calculate related pharmacokinetic–pharmacodynamic (PK/PD) parameters of DC against *Edwardsiella ictaluri*. The minimum inhibitory concentration of DC against *E. ictaluri* was determined to be 500 μg/L. As the increase of oral dose from 10 to 40 mg/kg, the area under the concentration vs. time curve from 0 to 96 h (AUC_{0-96}) values were considerably increased in gill, kidney, muscle and skin, and plasma, except in liver. C_{max} values exhibited a similar dose-dependent increase trend in plasma and tissues except in liver, but other PK parameters had no apparent dose-dependence. The PK/PD parameter of the ratio of AUC_{0-96} to minimum inhibitory concentration (AUC_{0-96h}/MIC) was markedly increased in plasma and tissues dose-dependently except in liver, but %T > MIC values were increased only moderately at some dose groups. After receiving the same dose with disparate time intervals from 96 to 12 h, the AUC_{0-96h}/MIC was distinctly increased in plasma and tissues, but the %T > MIC had a decreasing trend. When administering 20 mg/kg with a time interval of 96 h, the AUC_{0-96h}/MIC values were consistently >173.03 h and the %T > MIC values were above 99.47% in plasma and all tissues. These results suggest that administration of DC at 20 mg/kg every 96 h is a preferable regimen in yellow catfish.

Keywords: doxycycline; pharmacokinetics; pharmacokinetic–pharmacodynamic (PK/PD) parameters; *Edwardsiella ictaluri*; yellow catfish

Citation: Xu, N.; Li, M.; Ai, X.; Lin, Z. Determination of Pharmacokinetic and Pharmacokinetic-Pharmacodynamic Parameters of Doxycycline against *Edwardsiella ictaluri* in Yellow Catfish (*Pelteobagrus fulvidraco*). *Antibiotics* **2021**, *10*, 329. https://doi.org/10.3390/antibiotics10030329

Academic Editor: Nikola Puvača

Received: 20 February 2021
Accepted: 18 March 2021
Published: 21 March 2021

1. Introduction

Yellow catfish (*Pelteobagrus fulvidraco*) is a predominant cultured fish species in China with a total production of more than 0.48 million tons per year [1]. To pursue a high yield, the culture density of yellow catfish per 1 m^3 is increased continuously, which makes it easy to cause an outbreak of bacterial diseases, especially *Edwardsiella ictaluri* infection. Clinical manifestations of *Edwardsiellosis* are mainly classified as an acute type and a chronic type [2,3]. The acute type has a higher mortality that is infected from the digestive tract to blood and various organs to cause organ hyperemia, hemorrhage, inflammation, denaturation, necrosis, and ulceration. The typical symptom is a sick fish hanging in the water with head up, tail down, sometimes in spasmodically spiral swimming, and leading to death. The chronic type has a longer course than the acute type. The pathogen invades the olfactory bulb through the nasal cavity, then travels to the brain, and finally reaches the skull through the meninges and the skin of head. The typical symptoms are skin necrosis and ulceration and the formation of an open ulcer on the head, known as "head hole disease" [3]. Due to the widespread infection in the fish body of *E. ictaluri*, an aquatic drug with a high permeability is needed to cure the disease. In clinical therapy, the first selected drug is sulfadiazine, which can penetrate the blood–brain barrier to reach the brain, but its therapeutic efficacy is rapidly decreasing because of serious drug resistance [4]. Fortunately, it has been found that doxycycline (DC) is an ideal choice among the approved drugs due to its good penetration properties in the tissues [5–7].

Doxycycline (DC), a member of second-generation tetracyclines, has been extensively used in global aquaculture due to better chemical properties of plasma half-lives, lipid solubility, and antibiotic activity than its analogs [8,9]. DC is also approved in aquaculture against *Aeromonas hydrophila*, *E. ictaluri*, *Fibrobacter columnaris*, *Pseudomonas fluorescens*, and *Vibrio vulnificus* in China [2,10–13]. Currently, multiple pharmacokinetic (PK) and residue depletion studies of DC are available in tilapia [14] and grass carp [15,16]. These studies reported that DC had a plasma elimination half-life of >20 h in grass carp following a single oral dose at 20 mg/kg, and of 39 h in tilapia following a single intravenous dose at 20 mg/kg; these relatively long plasma half-lives were in part caused by enterohepatic recycling [14–16]. For the purpose of fish health, it is important to establish an efficient therapeutic regimen for specific fish species based on pharmacokinetic–pharmacodynamic (PK/PD) studies. Some PK/PD studies have been performed in veterinary animals for optimizing DC's therapeutic regimen. For example, a PK/PD study of DC was carried out in *Mycoplasma gallisepticum*, which causes chronic respiratory disease in chickens using an in vitro dynamic model [17]. The estimated %T > MIC values for 0log10 (CFU/mL), 2log10 (CFU/mL) reduction, and 3log10 (CFU/mL) reduction were 32.48%, 45.68%, and 54.36%, respectively. This study showed good effectiveness and time-dependent characteristics of DC against *M. gallisepticum* in vitro [17]. Zhang and colleagues reported DC's optimum dosage regime against *Haemophilus parasuis* in pigs based on PK/PD integration modeling [18]. According to values of $AUC_{0-24\,h}$/MIC, the doses predicted to obtain bacteriostatic, bactericidal, and elimination effects for *H. parasuis* over 24 h were 5.25, 8.55, and 10.37 mg/kg for the 50% target attainment rate (TAR), and 7.26, 13.82, and 18.17 mg/kg for 90% TAR, respectively [18]. However, there are no PK/PD studies reported in any specific fish species. Furthermore, limited PK/PD information on DC concerning *E. ictaluri* is available in yellow catfish.

The objective of this study was to investigate the pharmacokinetics of DC in yellow catfish at different oral doses and to calculate related PK/PD parameters of DC against *E. ictaluri*. The results will provide useful information to optimize the dosing regimen of DC against *E. ictaluri* in yellow catfish.

2. Results

2.1. *In Vitro Susceptibility Assay*

The average MIC of DC against *E. ictaluri* was 500 μg/L in yellow catfish plasma.

2.2. *Analytical Method Validation*

The limit of detection and the limit of quantification of DC were determined to be 25.0 and 50.0 μg/L (or μg/kg), respectively, in plasma and tissues. The matrix-match calibration curves were established across spiked concentrations from 50 to 2000 μg/L or μg/kg in plasma and tissues, and a good linearity was achieved with the coefficient of correlation R^2 = 0.999. If DC's concentrations in some samples were found to be more than the upper limit of quantification, the remaining samples were repeatedly determined after diluting with the corresponding blank samples. The results of mean recovery rates for DC ranged from 67.2% to 83.7% in plasma and tissues (Table 1). The percentages of relative standard deviations for inter-day and intra-day precision were ≤10% (Table 1).

Table 1. Accuracy and precision of the method for doxycycline in fortified muscle and skin, liver, kidney, gill, and plasma samples of yellow catfish (*Pelteobagrus fulvidraco*).

Tissues or Plasma	Spiked Level (μg/kg or μg/L)	Recovery (%)	Within-Day RSD (%)	Between-Day RSD (%)
Muscle and Skin	50	77.3	4.4	5.1
	500	83.7	3.8	4.6
	5000	80.2	4.7	5.8
Liver	50	71.4	3.1	4.9
	500	72.7	4.0	6.2
	5000	67.2	4.3	5.8
Kidney	50	68.2	5.2	7.3
	500	71.7	2.7	4.5
	5000	79.7	2.2	3.7
Gill	50	80.3	3.5	5.5
	500	81.7	2.8	4.1
	5000	72.6	3.7	5.6
Plasma	50	82.7	4.5	5.7
	500	82.5	3.9	6.3
	5000	77.2	4.7	6.1

RSD: Relative standard deviation.

2.3. PK Profile of DC in Yellow Catfish

The DC concentration vs. time profiles in plasma and tissues of yellow catfish after a single oral administration at different doses of 10, 20, and 40 mg/kg are shown in Figure 1. All raw concentration data of DC are provided in supplementary Tables S1–S3. Generally, DC concentrations in plasma and tissues were increased along with the rise of the given dose level from 10 to 40 mg/kg, especially in gill. An interesting finding was a multiple-peak phenomenon in the concentration-time curves of plasma and tissues. From 0.5 to 48 h post-dosing of 10 mg/kg, the concentrations of DC in plasma and tissues fluctuated, and then gradually decayed (Figure 1 and Table S1). At 20 mg/kg, the levels in plasma and tissues also fluctuated from 0.5 to 48 h and then displayed a decreased trend (Figure 1 and Table S2). After a given dose of 40 mg/kg, the time period of the concentration undulation was further enlarged from 0.08 to 72 h (Figure 1 and Table S3). Overall, the time range of concentration fluctuation at lower doses in various tissues was shorter than that at the highest dose.

Table 2 shows all calculated PK parameters. With the increase of the given dose from 10 to 40 mg/kg, the C_{max} values were increased from 0.66 to 151.94 mg/kg in gill, from 1.03 to 15.40 mg/kg in kidney, from 0.18 to 2.84 mg/kg in muscle and skin, and from 0.44 to 6.99 mg/L in plasma, except in liver, which was firstly increased from 1.08 to 34.81 mg/kg, then decreased to 24.95 mg/kg. The $AUC_{0\text{-}96}$ values exhibited similar increasing trends in gill, kidney, muscle and skin, and plasma, but not in liver. The values of λ_z, $T_{1/2\ \lambda z}$, T_{max}, V_z_F, and CL_F did not present apparent dose-dependence. The AUC_%extrap values were higher than 20% in plasma and muscle and skin in all dose groups and in all tissues in the 10 mg/kg dose group.

Table 2. The pharmacokinetic parameters of doxycycline in gill, kidney, liver, muscle and skin, and plasma of yellow catfish (*Pelteobagrus fulvidraco*) after a single oral dose of 10, 20, and 40 mg/kg, respectively.

Parameters	Unit	Gill			Kidney			Liver			Muscle and Skin			Plasma		
		10	20	40	10	20	40	10	20	40	10	20	40	10	20	40
λz	1/h	0.012	0.043	0.029	0.015	0.023	0.005	0.005	0.042	0.021	0.008	0.008	0.005	0.007	0.009	0.014
T1/2 λz	h	56.55	16.27	23.53	45.15	29.60	143.26	142.52	16.49	32.6	90.28	82.31	147.18	106.38	80.81	51.34
T_{max}	h	0.50	0.50	0.50	1.00	0.50	2.00	1.00	24.00	1.00	6.00	4.00	12.00	6.00	4.00	12.00
C_{max}	mg/kg (L)	0.66	120.74	151.94	1.03	11.64	15.40	1.08	34.81	24.95	0.18	2.30	2.84	0.44	4.67	6.99
$AUC_{0\text{-}96}$	h*mg/L	44.69	708.96	1207.18	57.23	260.95	471.78	54.65	1615.75	790.04	15.22	86.52	126.48	27.86	192.10	223.56
AUC_%extrap	%	35.30	5.40	7.29	31.48	15.00	57.32	63.85	4.42	13.57	50.54	47.75	60.82	51.71	38.42	28.01
Vz_F	L/kg	NA	NA	NA	NA	NA	NA	NA	NA	NA	NA	NA	NA	26.60	7.47	9.54
Cl_F	L/h/kg	NA	NA	NA	NA	NA	NA	NA	NA	NA	NA	NA	NA	0.17	0.06	0.13

Notes: λz, the terminal rate constant; T1/2 λz, the terminal half-life; T_{max}, the time to reach the peak concentration; C_{max}, the peak concentration; $AUC_{0\text{-}96}$, the area under concentration time curve from 0 to 96 h; AUC_%extrap, percentage of AUC from time 0 to infinity due to extrapolation from the last observed time point to infinity; Cl_F, the total body clearance per fraction of dose absorbed; Vz_F, the volume of distribution based on the terminal phase per fraction of dose absorbed; NA, not available or not applicable; *, a multiplication sign.

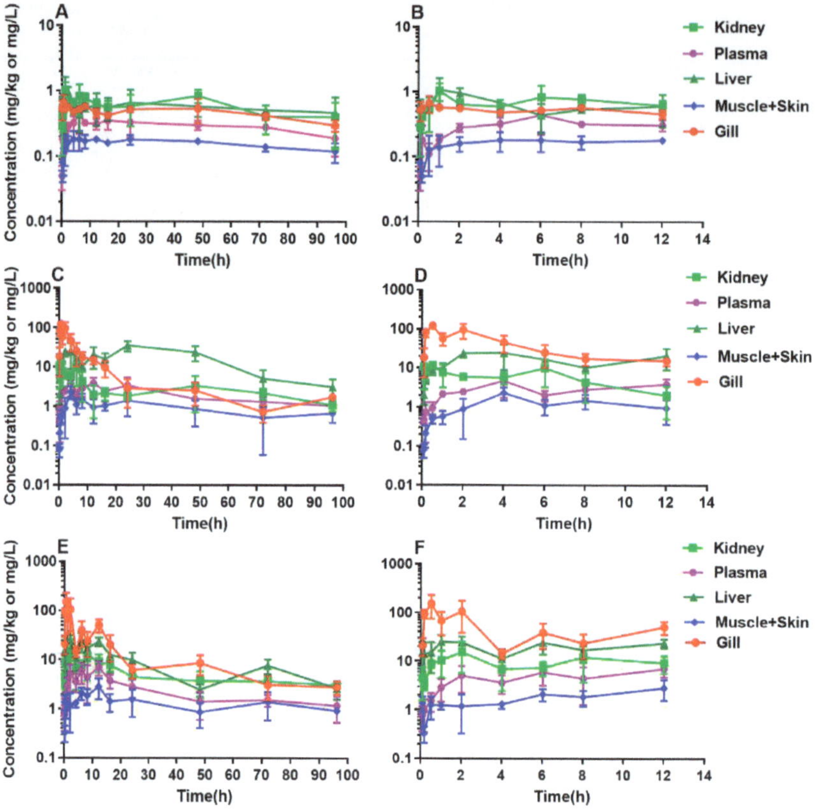

Figure 1. Semi-logarithmic plots of plasma and tissue concentration-time profiles of doxycycline in yellow catfish (*Pelteobagrus fulvidraco*) following an oral dose at 10 (**A**,**B**), 20 (**C**,**D**), or 40 mg/kg (**E**,**F**) at 24 °C. **A**, **C**, and **E**: For all sampling time points; **B**, **D**, and **F**: For a part of the sampling points from 0.083 to 12 h. Sample size: $n = 6$.

2.4. PK/PD Integration for DC in Plasma and Tissues

Table 3 presents the PK/PD parameters of $AUC_{0\text{–}96h}$/MIC and %T > MIC by the integration of PK data and the MIC value using a non-parametric superposition approach. As the increase of the oral dose level from 10 to 40 mg/kg, the values of $AUC_{0\text{–}96h}$/MIC were notably increased in plasma and tissues except for liver. The values of %T > MIC were markedly increased along with the dose increase from 10 to 20 mg/kg. Once the dose was over the threshold of 20 mg/kg, they remained constant in plasma and each tissue. At the scenario of an identical oral dose with changing the administration interval from 96 to 12 h, the values of $AUC_{0\text{–}96h}$/MIC were considerably increased. For example, at a dose of 10 mg/kg, its values raised from 55.72 to 265.29 h in plasma, 89.37 to 425.79 h in gill, from 114.47 to 555.15 h in kidney, from 109.30 to 516.17 h in liver, and 30.43 to 143.61 h in muscle and skin. However, the values of %T > MIC had a declining trend. Furthermore, the values of %T > MIC were below 78.0% at an oral dose of 10 mg/kg. When the administration dose was increased to 20 mg/kg, %T > MIC ranged from 99.5% to 100.0% in plasma and tissues at an administration interval of 96 h, but showed no improvement along with the decrease of dose intervals.

Table 3. The pharmacokinetic–pharmacodynamic parameters of doxycycline in gill, kidney, liver, muscle and skin, and plasma of yellow catfish (*Pelteobagrus fulvidraco*) given an oral dose of 10, 20, and 40 mg/kg at administration intervals of 96, 24, and 12 h, respectively.

Tissues and Plasma	Time Intervals (h)	Oral Doses (mg/kg)					
		10		20		40	
		$AUC_{0\text{–}96}$/MIC (h)	%T > MIC (%)	$AUC_{0\text{–}96}$/MIC (h)	%T > MIC (%)	$AUC_{0\text{–}96}$/MIC (h)	%T > MIC (%)
Gill	96	89.37	43.99	1471.91	100.00	2414.36	100.00
	24	234.19	35.78	5037.98	96.00	7744.17	100.00
	12	425.79	21.94	9768.54	100.00	14677.36	100.00
Kidney	96	114.47	69.44	521.90	100.00	943.55	99.99
	24	304.91	65.56	1433.19	96.00	2707.67	99.99
	12	555.15	34.85	2660.07	94.84	4990.22	63.72
Liver	96	109.30	78.02	3231.50	99.98	1580.08	100.00
	24	284.60	71.70	9277.55	96.00	4548.55	100.00
	12	516.17	34.03	17116.13	23.59	8467.98	60.95
Muscle and Skin	96	30.43	NA	173.03	99.47	252.95	99.89
	24	79.25	NA	479.16	96.00	666.29	95.56
	12	143.61	NA	878.61	43.24	1213.31	40.54
Plasma	96	55.72	NA	384.21	99.90	447.12	99.94
	24	146.31	25.95	1087.35	96.00	1331.33	99.94
	12	265.29	12.99	1999.88	35.16	2461.86	53.31

Notes: $AUC_{0\text{–}96}$/MIC, the ratio of $AUC_{0\text{–}96}$ to minimum inhibitory concentration; %T > MIC, the percentage of time profile of DC concentration more than minimum inhibitory concentration to total time; NA, not available or not applicable.

3. Discussion

E. ictaluri is an important pathogen in global aquaculture, particularly in the culture of yellow catfish and channel catfish, and it causes a great economical loss every year. However, the therapeutic information of the concerned drug based on PK/PD indices is scarce. In this study, we evaluated the PK/PD parameters of a candidate drug of DC against *E. ictaluri* in yellow catfish based on the MIC value and PK parameters following different single oral doses at 10, 20, and 40 mg/kg, respectively. This study provides useful information for the effective use of DC in yellow catfish against *E. ictaluri.*

To obtain sufficient pharmacological information on DC, PK studies of DC were performed in yellow catfish at different single oral doses. According to observed results, an obvious multiple-peak phenomenon was found in DC concentration vs. time curves in plasma and tissues, which was consistent with the results in grass carp (*Ctenopharyngodon idella*) and tilapia (*Oreochromis aureus* × *Oreochromis niloticus*) following a single oral dose at 20 mg/kg at 24 °C [14,16]. In addition, DC displayed multiple peaks in PK profiles in ducks [19], pigs [20], and humans [21]. This multiple-peak feature could be partly due to the impact of enterohepatic recycling because DC might form stable complexes with bile and enter the intestine via the biliary excretion to be reabsorbed into liver after digestion [8].

The PK parameter of $T_{1/2\lambda z}$ ranged from 16.27 to 56.55 h in gill, from 29.60 to 143.26 h in kidney, from 16.49 to 142.52 h in liver, from 82.31 to 147.18 h, and from 80.81 to 106.38 h in plasma after a single oral dose at different levels (10, 20, or 40 mg/kg). These data did not present an apparent dose-dependence of $T_{1/2\lambda z}$ with the increased dose of DC but showed a large difference in the same tissue among different given dose levels. These discrepancies may be possibly due to the calculation method used in the software Phoenix. The $T_{1/2\lambda z}$ was calculated using the equation of $T_{1/2\lambda z} = 0.693/\lambda_z$. The value of λ_z is a linear slope of the kinetic profile at the terminal elimination phase. In Phoenix, there are two calculation approaches for λ_z, one is the best slope identified automatically by the Phoenix software, and another is to manually choose three or more time points to perform the calculation [16]. In the present study, the authors chose the former method to calculate λ_z without manual adjustments. In addition, due to the multiple-peak phenomenon, the selected time points for calculation in each tissue were different, which, in part, caused the differences in values of λ_z. Consequently, $T_{1/2\lambda z}$ in the same tissue under disparate doses presented different values.

In addition to the increase of oral dose, the C_{max} also presented an increasing trend in all tissues except in liver. The exact reason for the lack of a dose-dependent increase in the Cmax of liver is unknown. Only the value of C_{max} in gill was higher than grass carp, but the values in other tissues and plasma were all smaller than grass carp by oral administration at the same dose at 24 °C [16]. The calculated T_{max} values ranged from 0.5 to 24 h following different single DC doses of 10, 20, and 40 mg/kg, which did not exhibit apparent regularities in each tissue as the rise of the dose. At the dose of 20 mg/kg, T_{max} values ranged from 0.5 to 24 h in plasma and tissues except for gill. These values were longer than the corresponding values in grass carp receiving the same dose at 24 °C [16]. Moreover, there was also no obvious dose-dependence in V_z_F values and CL_F values accompanying the increase of administration dose. The V_z_F value (7.47 L/kg) at the dose of 20 mg/kg in yellow catfish was notably higher than that in tilapia (2.32 L/kg) [14] and grass carp (0.87 L/kg) [16] following the same oral dose at identical water temperature, suggesting that the distribution of DC in yellow catfish was more widely than tilapia and grass carp. The CL_F value in yellow catfish (0.06 L/h/kg) was larger than the corresponding values in tilapia (0.04 L/h/kg) [14] and grass carp (0.03 L/h/kg) [16]. Finally, the values of $AUC_{0\text{-}96}$ exhibited an increasing trend with the rise of given dose in gill, kidney, muscle and skin, and plasma, but its value was firstly increased (at a dose from 10 to 20 mg/kg) and then decreased (at a dose from 20 to 40 mg/kg) in liver. The exact reasons for this phenomenon are not known. The AUC_%extrap values were consistently higher than 20% in the plasma and muscle and skin for all dose groups and in all tissues in the 10 mg/kg dose group. This is a limitation of this study and these results suggest that the sensitivity of the analytical method was not good enough and/or the sampling duration was not long enough; thus, the calculation of the half-life values could be inaccurate. Future studies using more sensitive detection methods with longer sampling duration are needed to more accurately calculate the half-life of DC in yellow catfish.

For the purpose of reducing the number of experimental animals, this study used a non-parametric superposition approach with the Phoenix software to simulate the PK profiles after multiple oral doses with different time intervals based on the PK parameters from a single oral dose [22]. Phoenix's non-parametric superposition object is based on non-compartmental results describing single-dose data to predict drug concentrations after multiple doses at a steady state. The predictions are on the basis of an accumulation ratio calculated from the terminal slope, which can be used for simple (the same dose was given in a constant interval) or complicated dosing schedules (based on Phoenix WinNonlin User's Guide). The simulated results can help design optimal dosage regimes or predict outcomes of clinical trials when used in conjunction with the semi-compartmental modeling function. In actual PK studies, the non-parametric superposition approach has been extensively used [23–25]. Its assumptions are typically as follows: (a) Application of linear PK to accommodate a change in dose during the multiple dosing regimen; (b) each dose of a drug acts independently of every other dose; (c) the rate of absorption and the average systemic clearance are consistent for each dosing interval [25].

Regarding the pharmacodynamic component of this study, the parameter of MIC for DC against *E. ictaluri* was measured in yellow catfish plasma. It has been reported that the MIC value measured in the broth was conspicuously different from that measured in plasma [26,27]. A study found that the MIC value of enrofloxacin in plasma countering *A. hydrophila* was remarkably higher than that in broth [28]. The authors proposed that, if different MICs were found in broth and plasma, the corresponding adjustment should be performed by a scaling factor when the PK/PD breakpoint indices were used to optimize dosages. Furthermore, the in vitro susceptibility of macrolides and ketolides also manifested a marked enhancement of antibiotic activity against *Pseudomonas aeruginosa* in RPMI 1640 medium [29]. Therefore, the matrix between broth and plasma may influence antimicrobial activity, and it is better to use plasma for dilution and incubation of bacteria to determine the MIC because the composition of plasma is the closest to the in vivo environment.

DC possesses a high lipophilicity and permeability that can result in high concentrations in various tissues after oral administration [8]. This feature is beneficial for treating infectious diseases. Generally, DC is considered a time-dependent drug. A previous study showed that DC presented time-dependent killing for *M. gallisepticum* in an in vitro model [17]. Cunha and co-workers also reported that DC exhibited a time-dependent killing at low concentrations of 2–4 times the MIC, but a concentration-dependent killing at high concentrations of 8–16 times the MIC against *Staphylococcus aureus*, *Streptococcus pneumoniae*, *Escherichia coli*, and *Pasteurella multocida* [30]. However, a PK/PD study of DC against *H. parasuis* directly showed a dose-dependent property [18]. These discrepancies may be caused by different target pathogens. This viewpoint has been proven in the PK/PD study of gentamicin, which displayed a time-dependent kinetic profile for countering *S. aureus*, but a concentration-dependent kinetic profile against *Pseudomonas aeruginosa* [31]. In this study, one limitation was that the in vitro killing curve was not determined. As a result, we were unable to establish the PK/PD correlation based on the sigmoid inhibitory *Emax* model. Nevertheless, the present study provides valuable information on AUC/MIC and %T > MIC using the non-parametric superstition approach based on PK characteristics at different single oral doses.

AUC/MIC and %T > MIC are important PK/PD indices for establishing or optimizing the dosage regimen. In this study, with the increase of the given dose from 10 to 40 mg/kg, AUC/MIC values were considerably increased in plasma and each tissue except for liver. When the given dose was increased from 10 to 20 mg/kg, %T > MIC values were notably increased in plasma and tissues (e.g., gill, increased from 43.99% to 100.0%). However, when the dose was increased from 20 to 40 mg/kg, no obvious changes for %T > MIC occurred in plasma and tissues (e.g., gill, from 100.0% to 100.0%). From these results, the AUC/MIC have a concentration-dependent effect along with the increase of DC dose in plasma and tissues except in liver, but the %T > MIC was only increased moderately at certain dose levels. If the dosage was over a threshold (e.g., 20 mg/kg), it would remain at a constant. Previous studies have demonstrated that the AUC/MIC ratio of 100–125 is recommended to achieve a higher therapeutic efficacy [32–34]. In this study, the ratios of $AUC_{0–96}$/MIC were more than 173.03 in plasma and tissues after oral administration at a dose of 20 mg/kg with the time interval of 96 h. In addition, with the increase of frequency of the given dose from every 96 h to every 12 h, $AUC_{0–96}$/MIC values were increased by 409.7%–563.7% in plasma and tissues. At the given dose of 20 mg/kg with a time interval of 96 h, %T > MIC values were greater than 99.0%. However, along with the increase of administration frequency, %T > MIC values exhibited a declined tendency. These results indicate that the antimicrobial activity of DC is not necessarily proportional to the frequency of administration. Therefore, we speculate that DC presents time-dependence and %T > MIC is a more suitable PK/PD index for DC against *E. ictaluri* in yellow catfish.

4. Materials and Methods

4.1. Chemicals and Reagents

The doxycycline (DC) standard (purity $\geq$ 98%) for instrument analysis was purchased from Dr. Ehrenstorfer GmbH. (Augsburg, Germany). The DC powder (purity $\geq$ 98%) used for oral gavage was purchased from Zhongbo Aquaculture Biotechnology Co. Ltd. (Wuhan, China). The liquid reagents of water, acetonitrile, and formic acid were obtained from Thermo Fisher (Waltham, USA) and J–T Baker (Philipsburg, USA). Ethylenediaminetetraacetic acid disodium (EDTA-Na_2), sodium dihydrogen phosphate, and citric acid monohydrate were ordered from Shanghai Guoyao Company (Shanghai, China). Cleanert C_{18} sorbent (40–60 µm, analytical grade) was purchased from Shanghai CNW Technologies (Shanghai, China). The centrifugal tubes, 1.5-mL vials, and 0.22-µm politetrafluoroetileno membranes were also obtained from Shanghai CNW Technologies (Shanghai, China).

4.2. Microorganism and Culture Medium

The *Edwardsiella ictaluri* strain was provided by Prof. Aihua Li from the Institute of Hydrobiology, Chinese Academy of Sciences (Wuhan, China). Brain–heart infusion broth used for culturing *E. ictaluri* was purchased from Qingdao Haibo Biotechnology Co. Ltd. (Qingdao, China).

4.3. In Vitro Susceptibility Testing

The minimum inhibitory concentration (MIC) was assayed in plasma using a microbroth dilution method based on the Clinical and Laboratory Standards Institute (CLSI) recommended protocol. Briefly, serial 2-fold dilutions of DC from an initial concentration of 128 μg/mL were loaded into a 96-well microplate using plasma. Then the strain with a density of about 5×10^5 CFU/mL in plasma was incubated with the drug for 24 h at 28 °C. The MIC was defined as the lowest concentration inhibiting bacterial growth.

4.4. Fish and Diet

Three hundred yellow catfish (120.2 ± 15.3 g, 48 months of age, male) were purchased from the culture facility of the Yangtze River Fisheries Research Institute (Wuhan, China). Every 18 fish were held in one tank (volume of each tank: 480 L) and acclimatized for 14 d at a water temperature of 24.0 ± 0.8 °C. The fish were fed with antibiotic-free feed that was made by the Nutritional Research Group in Yangtze River Fisheries Research Institute, Chinese Academy of Fishery Sciences, Wuhan, China. The feed contained 45.6% crude proteins, 6.3% crude fat, 8.4% moisture, 4.8% ash, and 0.4% total phosphorus [35]. The parameters of water quality were determined and maintained at the following status: Total ammonia nitrogen levels ≤ 0.74 mg/L, dissolved oxygen levels at 6.0–7.2 mg/L, pH at 7.1 ± 0.2, and nitrite nitrogen levels < 0.06 mg/L. The blank samples including blood, liver, kidney, muscle and skin, and gill were collected from 15 fish to establish the analytical method of ultra-performance liquid chromatography (UPLC) for DC before the formal experiment. All animal experimental protocols were approved by the Fish Ethics Committee of Yangtze River Fisheries Research Institute, Chinese Academy of Fishery Sciences, Wuhan, China.

4.5. Drug Administration and Sampling

The detailed procedures are referred to our recent studies [36,37]. In brief, the fish were divided into three groups that were treated with three different single doses of DC at 10, 20, and 40 mg/kg, respectively, by oral gavage. Before giving the drug, DC powder was used to prepare the solution at a final concentration of 10 mg/mL. The DC solution was administered to each fish using a hard plastic tube attached to a 1-mL micro-injector. After oral gavage, if the fish regurgitated the given DC solution, the fish was removed from the tank and replaced by another. Blood samples were collected from the caudal vessels of each fish at the time points of 0.083, 0.17, 0.5, 1, 2, 4, 6, 8, 12, 16, 24, 48, 72, and 96 h after oral administration. After blood collection, each fish was dissected to collect liver, kidney, muscle and skin, and gill. Plasma samples were obtained by centrifugation of the corresponding blood samples at 1500 g for 5 min, and stored at −20 °C until analysis. The number of the plasma and tissue samples was n = 6 fish at each sampling time point.

4.6. Sample Preparation and Instrument Analysis

The method of sample preparation and the conditions of instrument analysis were also based on our previously reported procedures with some modifications [38]. In brief, 1 g of tissue samples (e.g., liver, kidney, gill, and muscle and skin) or 1 mL of plasma was thawed at room temperature and transferred into a 15-mL plastic tube. Then 5 mL McIlvaine buffer (0.04 mol/L sodium dihydrogen phosphate, 0.06 mol/L citric acid monohydrate, and 0.1 mol/L EDTA-Na_2, pH = 4) was added to each tube and vigorously shaken for 30 s. After standing for 10 min, 4.5 mL of acetonitrile containing 3% formic acid was pipetted to each tube, and then 1 g of NaCl was weighted into them following shaking for 30 s. To ensure the maximum amount of the target compound was extracted from samples, the mixture of sample and extractant was sufficiently mixed by ultrasound for 5 min, and then centrifugated at 3500 g for 5 min. The resulting supernatant was decanted into a 10-mL tube. The above procedures were repeated. The obtained upper layer was combined into the same tube added 200 mg of C_{18} and 1 g of $MgSO_4$ following shaking 30 s, and centrifuged at 3500 g for 5 min to remove impurities. The cleaned extractant was pipetted into a new 10-mL plastic tube and condensed to dryness by a gentle nitrogen stream at 45 °C. The dry extract was reconstituted by 1 mL 10% acetonitrile-water containing 0.1% formic acid. Finally, the mixture was filtrated by a 0.22 nylon member filter and prepared to analyze by UPLC.

All samples were analyzed by a Waters UPLC (Milford, MA, USA) equipped with a binary solvent manager with a binary solvent pump, a sampler manager with an autosampler, and an ultraviolet detector. The detailed analytical conditions were set in line with our previous studies [15,16].

4.7. Calibration Curves and Recovery Rates

The collected blank samples of plasma, muscle and skin, liver, kidney, and gill were fortified with a standard solution of DC to get final concentrations of 50, 100, 500, 2000, 5000, and 20,000 μg/L or μg/kg. Samples were processed as described above, and each concentration was set with three parallels. Five replicates of spiked plasma and tissue samples at 50, 500, and 5000 μg DC /L or /kg were analyzed to calculate the precision and accuracy.

4.8. Pharmacokinetic Analysis

The data of DC concentrations with time profiles in plasma and tissues were analyzed with a non-compartmental approach using Phoenix WinNonlin 8.0 (Certara, Inc., Princeton, NJ, USA). The prediction of PK profiles after multiple oral doses at different time intervals of dosage was performed using the non-parametric superposition approach [25]. The following PK parameters were calculated: λ_z (terminal rate constant), $T_{1/2\lambda z}$ (terminal half-life), T_{max} (time to observed maximal concentration after drug administration), C_{max} (observed maximal concentration), $AUC_{0–96}$ (area under the concentration vs. time curve from 0 to 96 h), AUC_%extrap (percentage of AUC from time 0 to infinity due to extrapolation from the last observed time point to infinity), V_z_F (volume of distribution based on the terminal phase per fraction of dose absorbed), CL_F (total body clearance per fraction of dose absorbed), $AUC_{0–96}$/MIC (the ratio of $AUC_{0–96}$ to minimum inhibitory concentration), and %T > MIC (the percentage of the time profile of DC concentration more than minimum inhibitory concentration to total time).

5. Conclusions

This study determined the PK and PK/PD parameters of DC against *E. ictaluri* in yellow catfish based on MIC and PK studies after a single oral dose of 10, 20, and 40 mg/kg, respectively, along with a predictive methodology of a non-parametric superposition approach. The value of MIC was 500 μg/L in plasma. The increase of the oral dose enlarged the values of $AUC_{0–96}$ in plasma and tissues except for liver, but other PK parameters had no apparent dose-dependence. The PK/PD parameter of $AUC_{0–96h}$/MIC was prominently increased in plasma and each tissue (except liver) along with the rise of the DC dose, but the %T > MIC was only increased moderately at certain doses. Under the same oral dose with differing administration intervals of 96 to 12 h, the $AUC_{0–96h}$/MIC was considerably increased in plasma and tissues, but the %T > MIC had a declined tendency. Finally, at 20 mg/kg with a time interval of 96 h, the %T > MIC reached from 99.5% to 100.0% in plasma and tissues, which could be the preferable dosage regime. Overall, this study provides some fundamental information on PK and PK/PD parameters to support the design of optimal therapeutic regimens of DC against *E. ictaluri* in yellow catfish.

Supplementary Materials: The following are available online at https://www.mdpi.com/2079-6382/10/3/329/s1, Table S1: The concentrations of doxycycline in plasma and tissues of yellow catfish (*Pelteobagrus fulvidraco*) after a single oral dose at 10 mg/kg at 24 °C; Table S2: The concentrations of doxycycline in plasma and tissues of yellow catfish (*Pelteobagrus fulvidraco*) after a single oral dose at 20 mg/kg at 24 °C; Table S3: The doxycycline concentrations in plasma and tissues of yellow catfish (*Pelteobagrus fulvidraco*) after a single oral dose at 40 mg/kg at 24 °C.

Author Contributions: Conceptualization, N.X.; methodology, N.X.; software, N.X. and M.L.; validation, N.X. and Z.L.; formal analysis, N.X.; investigation, N.X.; resources, Z.L. and X.A.; data curation, N.X. and M.L.; writing—original draft preparation, N.X.; writing—review and editing, Z.L.; visualization, N.X.; supervision, Z.L. and X.A.; project administration, X.A.; funding acquisition, X.A. and N.X. All authors have read and agreed to the published version of the manuscript.

Funding: This research was funded by the National Key R&D Program of China given to Dr. Xiaohui Ai and Dr. Ning Xu., grant number 2019YFD0901701.

Institutional Review Board Statement: The study was conducted in accordance with the guidelines of the Declaration of Helsinki, and approved by the Fish Ethics Committee of Yangtze River Fisheries Research Institute, Chinese Academy of Fishery Sciences, Wuhan, China (YFI2020xuning01, 05/04/2020).

Informed Consent Statement: Not applicable.

Data Availability Statement: All raw experimentally measured time versus concentration data of doxycycline in plasma, liver, kidney, gill, and muscle and skin of yellow catfish (*Pelteobagrus fulvidraco*) at different sampling times following a single oral dose of 10, 20, and 40 mg/kg are provided in Tables S1–S3, respectively, in the Supplementary Materials. All other calculated data are presented in the main text of this manuscript.

Acknowledgments: The authors would like to thank Aihua Li from the Institute of Hydrobiology, Chinese Academy of Sciences (Wuhan, China) for providing the experimental strain of *Edwardsiella ictaluri*. The pharmacokinetic analysis was performed at the Institute of Computational Comparative Medicine (ICCM), Department of Anatomy and Physiology, College of Veterinary Medicine at Kansas State University, and the authors would like to thank Certara USA, Inc. (Princeton, NJ) for providing the Phoenix software as a part of the company's Academic Centers of Excellence program.

Conflicts of Interest: The authors declare no conflict of interest.

References

1. CFFA (Ed.) *China Fishery Statistics Yearbook 2018*; China Agriculture Press: Beijing, China, 2018.
2. Geng, Y.; Wang, K.; Chen, D.; Huang, J. Edwardsiella ictalurid and Edwardsiellosis. *Fish. Sci. Technol. Inf.* **2009**, *36*, 236–239.
3. Liao, Y. Study on Pathomorphology and Pathogen Distribution of Edwardsiella ictalurid in Yellow Catfish. Master Thesis, Sichuan Agricultural University, Yaan, China, 2012.
4. Done, H.Y.; Venkatesan, A.K.; Halden, R.U. Does the recent growth of aquaculture create antibiotic resistance threats different from those associated with land animal production in agriculture? *AAPS J.* **2015**, *17*, 513–524. [CrossRef]
5. Cunha, B.A.; Sibley, C.M.; Ristuccia, A.M. Doxycycline. *Ther. Drug Monit.* **1982**, *4*, 115–135. [CrossRef]
6. Salminen, L. Penetration of ocular compartments by tetracyclines. II. An experimental study with doxycycline. *Albrecht Von Graefes Arch. Klin. Exp. Ophthalmol.* **1977**, *204*, 201–207. [CrossRef]
7. Thompson, S.; Townsend, R. Pharmacological agents for soft tissue and bone infected with MRSA: Which agent and for how long? *Injury* **2011**, *42* (Suppl. 5), S7–S10. [CrossRef]
8. Riviere, J.E.; Papich, M.G. Tetracycline Antibiotics. In *Veterinary Pharmacology and Therapeutics*, 10th ed.; Riviere, J.E., Pahich, M.G., Eds.; John Wiley & Sons Inc: Hoboken, NJ, USA, 2018.
9. Arthur, J.R.; Lavilla-Pitogo, C.R.; Subasinghe, R.P. Use of chemicals in aquaculture in Asia. In Proceedings of the Meeting on the Use of Chemicals In Aquaculture in Asia, Iloilo, Philippines, 20–22 May 1996.
10. Liu, R.; Lian, Z.; Hu, X.; Lü, A.; Sun, J.; Chen, C.; Liu, X.; Song, Y.; Yiksung, Y. First report of Vibrio vulnificus infection in grass carp Ctenopharyngodon idellus in China. *Aquaculture* **2019**, *499*, 283–289. [CrossRef]
11. Deng, B.; Fu, L.; Zhang, X.; Zheng, J.; Peng, L.; Sun, J.; Zhu, H.; Wang, Y.; Li, W.; Wu, X.; et al. The Denitrification Characteristics of Pseudomonas stutzeri SC221-M and Its Application to Water Quality Control in Grass Carp Aquaculture. *PLoS ONE* **2014**, *9*, e114886. [CrossRef] [PubMed]
12. Shireman, J.V.; Colle, D.E.; Rottman, R.W. Incidence and treatment of columnaris disease in grass carp brood stock. *Prog. Fish-Cult.* **1976**, *38*, 116–117. [CrossRef]
13. Song, X.; Zhao, J.; Bo, Y.; Liu, Z.; Wu, K.; Gong, C. Aeromonas hydrophila induces intestinal inflammation in grass carp (Ctenopharyngodon idella): An experimental model. *Aquaculture* **2014**, *434*, 171–178. [CrossRef]
14. Yang, F.; Li, Z.L.; Shan, Q.; Zeng, Z.L. Pharmacokinetics of doxycycline in tilapia (Oreochromis aureus × Oreochromis niloticus) after intravenous and oral administration. *J. Vet. Pharmacol. Ther.* **2014**, *37*, 388–393. [CrossRef] [PubMed]
15. Xu, N.; Li, M.; Fu, Y.; Zhang, X.; Ai, X.; Lin, Z. Tissue residue depletion kinetics and withdrawal time estimation of doxycycline in grass carp, *Ctenopharyngodon idella*, following multiple oral administrations. *Food Chem. Toxicol.* **2019**, *131*, 110592. [CrossRef] [PubMed]

16. Xu, N.; Li, M.; Fu, Y.; Zhang, X.; Dong, J.; Liu, Y.; Zhou, S.; Ai, X.; Lin, Z. Effect of temperature on plasma and tissue kinetics of doxycycline in grass carp (*Ctenopharyngodon idella*) after oral administration. *Aquaculture* **2019**, *511*, 734204. [CrossRef]
17. Zhang, N.; Gu, X.; Ye, X.; Wu, X.; Zhang, B.; Zhang, L.; Shen, X.; Jiang, H.; Ding, H. The PK/PD Interactions of Doxycycline against Mycoplasma gallisepticum. *Front. Microbiol.* **2016**, *7*, 653. [CrossRef] [PubMed]
18. Zhang, L.; Li, Y.; Wang, Y.; Sajid, A.; Ahmed, S.; Li, X. Integration of pharmacokinetic-pharmacodynamic for dose optimization of doxycycline against Haemophilus parasuis in pigs. *J. Vet. Pharmacol. Ther.* **2018**, *41*, 706–718. [CrossRef]
19. Yang, F.; Sun, N.; Zhao, Z.S.; Wang, G.Y.; Wang, M.F. Pharmacokinetics of doxycycline after a single intravenous, oral or intramuscular dose in Muscovy ducks (*Cairina moschata*). *Br. Poult. Sci.* **2015**, *56*, 137–142. [CrossRef] [PubMed]
20. Riond, J.L.; Riviere, J.E. Pharmacokinetics and metabolic inertness of doxycycline in young pigs. *Am. J. Vet. Res.* **1990**, *51*, 1271–1275. [PubMed]
21. Fabre, J.; Pitton, J.S.; Kunz, J.P.; Rozbroj, S.; Hungerbühler, R.M. Distribution and excretion of doxycycline in man. *Chemotherapy* **1966**, *11*, 73–85. [CrossRef] [PubMed]
22. Certara. Phoenix WinNonlin—Nonparametric Superposition. 2019. Available online: https://onlinehelp.certara.com/phoenix/8.2/topics/nonparasuper.htm (accessed on 20 March 2021).
23. Antovska, P.; Ugarkovic, S.; Petruševski, G.; Stefanova, B.; Manchevska, B.; Petkovska, R.; Makreski, P. Development and experimental design of a novel controlled-release matrix tablet formulation for indapamide hemihydrate. *Pharm. Dev. Technol.* **2017**, *22*, 851–859. [CrossRef] [PubMed]
24. Kitano, M.; Matsuzaki, T.; Oka, R.; Baba, K.; Noda, T.; Yoshida, Y.; Sato, K.; Kiyota, K.; Mizutare, T.; Yoshida, R. The antiviral effects of baloxavir marboxil against influenza A virus infection in ferrets. *Influenza Other Respi. Viruses* **2020**, *14*, 710–719. [CrossRef]
25. Zeng, D.; Sun, M.; Lin, Z.; Li, M.; Gehring, R.; Zeng, Z. Pharmacokinetics and pharmacodynamics of tildipirosin against pasteurella multocida in a murine lung infection model. *Front. Microbiol.* **2018**, *9*, 1038. [CrossRef] [PubMed]
26. Delis, G.A.; Koutsoviti-Papadopoulou, M.; Siarkou, V.I.; Kounenis, G.; Batzias, G.C. Pharmacodynamics of amoxicillin against Mannheimia haemolytica and Pasteurella multocida and pharmacokinetic/pharmacodynamic (PK/PD) correlation in sheep. *Res. Vet. Sci.* **2010**, *89*, 418–425. [CrossRef] [PubMed]
27. Aliabadi, F.S.; Ali, B.H.; Landoni, M.F.; Lees, P. Pharmacokinetics and PK-PD modelling of danofloxacin in camel serum and tissue cage fluids. *Vet. J.* **2003**, *165*, 104–118. [CrossRef]
28. Shan, Q.; Wang, J.X.; Wang, J.; Ma, L.S.; Yang, F.H.; Yin, Y.; Huang, R.; Liu, S.G.; Li, L.C.; Zheng, G.M. Pharmacokinetic/pharmacodynamic relationship of enrofloxacin against Aeromonas hydrophila in crucian carp (Carassius auratus gibelio). *J. Vet. Pharmacol. Ther.* **2018**, *41*, 887–893. [CrossRef] [PubMed]
29. Buyck, J.; Plesiat, P.; Traore, H.; Vanderbist, F.; Tulkens, P.; Van Bambeke, F. Increased susceptibility of Pseudomonas aeruginosa to macrolides and ketolides in eukaryotic cell culture media and biological fluids due to decreased expression of oprm and increased outer-membrane permeability. *Clin. Infect. Dis.* **2012**, *55*, 534–542. [CrossRef] [PubMed]
30. Cunha, B.A.; Domenico, P.; Cunha, C.B. Pharmacodynamics of doxycycline. *Clin. Microbiol. Infect.* **2000**, *6*, 270–273. [CrossRef] [PubMed]
31. Tam, V.H.; Kabbara, S.; Vo, G.; Schilling, A.N.; Coyle, E.A. Comparative pharmacodynamics of gentamicin against Staphylococcus aureus and Pseudomonas aeruginosa. *Antimicrob. Agents Chemother.* **2006**, *50*, 2626–2631. [CrossRef] [PubMed]
32. Wright, D.H.; Brown, G.H.; Peterson, M.L.; Rotschafer, J.C. Application of fluoroquinolone pharmacodynamics. *J. Antimicrob. Chemother.* **2000**, *46*, 669–683. [CrossRef]
33. Mckellar, Q.A.; Sanchez Bruni, S.F.; Jones, D.G. Pharmacokinetic/pharmacodynamic relationships of antimicrobial drugs used in veterinary medicine. *J. Vet. Pharmacol. Ther.* **2004**, *27*, 503–514. [CrossRef]
34. Ahmad, I.; Huang, L.; Hao, H.; Sanders, P.; Yuan, Z. Application of PK/PD modeling in veterinary field: Dose optimization and drug resistance prediction. *Biomed. Res. Int.* **2016**, *2016*, 5465678. [CrossRef] [PubMed]
35. Tang, Q.; Wang, C.; Xie, C.; Jin, J.; Huang, Y. Dietary available phosphorus affected growth performance, body composition, and hepatic antioxidant property of juvenile yellow catfish Pelteobagrus fulvidraco. *Sci. World J.* **2012**, *2012*, 987570. [CrossRef]
36. Xu, N.; Fu, Y.; Chen, F.; Liu, Y.; Dong, J.; Yang, Y.; Zhou, S.; Yang, Q.; Ai, X. Sulfadiazine pharmacokinetics in grass carp (*Ctenopharyngodon idellus*) receiving oral and intravenous administrations. *J. Vet. Pharmacol. Ther.* **2020**. [CrossRef] [PubMed]
37. Xu, N.; Fu, Y.; Cheng, B.; Liu, Y.; Yang, Q.; Dong, J.; Yang, Y.; Zhou, S.; Song, Y.; Ai, X. The pharmacokinetics of doxycycline in channel catfish (*Ictalurus punctatus*) following intravenous and oral administrations. *Front. Vet. Sci.* **2020**, *7*, 577234. [CrossRef] [PubMed]
38. Xu, N.; Dong, J.; Zhou, W.; Liu, Y.; Ai, X. Determination of doxycycline, 4-epidoxycycline, and 6-epidoxycycline in aquatic animal muscle tissue by an optimized extraction protocol and ultra-performance performance liquid chromatography with ultraviolet detection. *Anal. Lett.* **2019**, *52*, 452–464. [CrossRef]

antibiotics

Article

In-Water Antibiotic Dosing Practices on Pig Farms

Stephen Little [1,*], Andrew Woodward [2], Glenn Browning [1] and Helen Billman-Jacobe [1]

[1] Asia Pacific Centre for Animal Health, Melbourne Veterinary School, Faculty of Veterinary and Agricultural Sciences, National Centre for Antimicrobial Stewardship, University of Melbourne, Parkville, VIC 3010, Australia; glenfb@unimelb.edu.au (G.B.); hbj@unimelb.edu.au (H.B.-J.)
[2] Melbourne Veterinary School, Faculty of Veterinary and Agricultural Sciences, University of Melbourne, Parkville, VIC 3010, Australia; andrew.woodward@unimelb.edu.au
* Correspondence: littles2@student.unimelb.edu.au

Abstract: Pigs reared on many farms are mass-medicated for short periods with antibiotics through their drinking water to control bacterial pathogen loads and, if a disease outbreak occurs, to treat pigs until clinical signs are eliminated. Farm managers are responsible for conducting in-water antibiotic dosing events, but little is known about their dosing practices. We surveyed managers of 25 medium to large single-site and multi-site pig farming enterprises across eastern and southern Australia, using a mixed methods approach (online questionnaire followed by a one-on-one semi-structured interview). We found wide variation in the antibiotics administered, the choice and use of dosing equipment, the methods for performing dosing calculations and preparing antibiotic stock solutions, the commencement time and duration of each daily dosing event, and the frequency of administration of metaphylaxis. Farm managers lacked data on pigs' daily water usage patterns and wastage and the understanding of pharmacology and population pharmacometrics necessary to optimize in-water dosing calculations and regimens and control major sources of between-animal variability in systemic exposure of pigs to antibiotics. There is considerable scope to increase the effectiveness of in-water dosing and reduce antibiotic use (and cost) on pig farms by providing farm managers with measurement systems, technical guidelines, and training programs.

Keywords: swine; drinking water; antibiotic; systemic exposure; metaphylaxis; treatment; dosing pump; dosing regimen; antibiotic resistance

Citation: Little, S.; Woodward, A.; Browning, G.; Billman-Jacobe, H. In-Water Antibiotic Dosing Practices on Pig Farms. *Antibiotics* **2021**, *10*, 169. https://doi.org/10.3390/antibiotics10020169

Academic Editor: Nikola Puvača
Received: 24 December 2020
Accepted: 3 February 2021
Published: 8 February 2021

1. Introduction

On many commercial pig farms, growing pigs are mass-medicated for short periods through their drinking water to manage herd health, productivity, and welfare [1–3]. Drinking water additives may include antibiotics, vaccines, parasiticides, organic acids, electrolytes, minerals, vitamins, amino acids, sweeteners, direct-fed microbials, essential oils, and potential new therapeutic products such as bacteriophages [2]. In-water dosing is well suited for two antibiotic use patterns in pigs; metaphylaxis and treatment. Metaphylaxis is 'the mass treatment of animal populations currently experiencing any level of disease before the onset of blatant disease'. Treatment is the 'administration of an antibiotic to an animal, or group of animals, which exhibits frank clinical disease' [4]. Metaphylactic, in-water antibiotic dosing of pigs is conducted strategically when the target bacterial pathogen load is low. A short dosing period, administered once or at regular intervals, is intended to achieve a microbiological and clinical cure [5]. In-water antibiotic dosing of pigs to treat a disease outbreak is conducted for a short period until clinical signs disappear. A dosing event should result in the majority of pigs in a group attaining the level of systemic exposure to the antibiotic required to successfully eliminate or substantially reduce the quantity of the target pathogen and achieve high clinical efficacy, while minimizing selection for and propagation of resistant pathogens [6].

Antibiotic stewardship programs across food animal production sectors, including the pig industry, have been implemented in recent years in response to the increasing levels of antibiotic resistance found in human and veterinary medicine [7]. Strategies for antibiotic stewardship in pig production have been assisted by an increasing understanding of the antibiotic use patterns and prescribing behaviours of veterinarians and development of prescribing guidelines [8–11]. In Australia, antibiotics are not approved for use as growth promoters in pigs. On Australian pig farms, veterinarians must prescribe antibiotics to be administered and specify doses based on pig bodyweight. However, farm managers are usually responsible for conducting in-water antibiotic dosing events, and this involves making many decisions that may influence the actual dose administered and the subsequent systemic exposure of pigs in the group to the antibiotic. Despite the pivotal role of farm managers in the mass-medication of pigs with antibiotics through their drinking water, little is known about their choice and use of dosing equipment, the methods they use for making dosing calculations and preparing antibiotic stock solutions, the dosing regimens they use, the frequency of administration of metaphylaxis, and their views on successful in-water dosing.

We surveyed the managers of medium to large single-site and multi-site pig farming enterprises across eastern and southern Australia. A response rate of over 90% was achieved by directly contacting participants with the support of the owners and managers of the enterprises. We used a mixed methods approach, collecting and analysing both quantitative and qualitative data within the same study, as used by other researchers investigating antibiotic use [10,12]. A comprehensive online questionnaire was followed by a one-on-one, semi-structured interview with each farm manager. Our focus was on farm managers' in-water antibiotic dosing practices. The pigs' health status and performance, and the efficacy of the medication programmes were not assessed.

We discovered that in-water dosing practices were highly variable across the farms studied and that measurements were not being taken and used to assess the effectiveness of dosing events, optimize in-water dosing calculations and regimens, and control major sources of between-animal variability in systemic exposure of pigs to antibiotics.

2. Results

Twenty-five pig farm managers agreed to participate in the study. The participants' farms were located in South Australia, Victoria, New South Wales, and Queensland. At the time of the study, these farms accommodated 459,167 weaner and grower/finisher pigs. This represents approximately 21% of all growing pigs accommodated in Australia at any one time [13]. The demographics of the sample population (participants and their farms) are presented in Appendix A, Tables A1 and A2.

2.1. Dosing Equipment Used

The majority of farm managers surveyed used proprietary proportional dosing pumps to water medicate growing pigs, as shown in Table 1. The water-powered or electric-powered pumps inject a concentrated stock solution of antibiotic into the pig building's water distribution system at a specified volumetric ratio e.g., one part stock solution to 100 parts water (commonly abbreviated to '1:100'). Managers reported that their choice of dosing equipment was guided by on-farm factors including the layout of drinking water distribution pipelines to buildings, the water pressure, building access to a mains power supply, the antibiotic products being used, the number of pigs to be dosed in each building, and past experiences with different brands and models of dosing pumps.

Table 1. In-water antibiotic dosing equipment used by farm managers on 25 single-site and multi-site pig farming enterprises.

Dosing Equipment Item	Weaner Buildings (No. Farms = 23)	Grower/Finisher Buildings (No. Farms = 24)
Header tank for batch mixing	3 (12%)	1 (4%)
Water-powered proportional dosing pump	8 (32%)	10 (40%)
Electric-powered proportional dosing pump	10 (40%)	9 (36%)
Water-powered and electric-powered proportional dosing pumps	1 (4%) [a]	1 (4%) [a]
Header tank for batch mixing plus electric-powered proportional dosing pump	1 (4%) [b]	2 (8%) [b,c]
Dispenser into liquid-feed system	0 (0%)	1 (4%)

[a] Uses different pumps for different antibiotics; [b] Currently changing buildings from header tanks to electric-powered dosing pumps; [c] Uses header tanks and electric-powered dosing pumps together for treating outbreaks.

Many farm managers using dosing pumps previously used header tanks but had ceased using them because of concerns about (1) a lack of control and accuracy of dosing, (2) risks to workers' health and safety associated with climbing ladders up to tanks, (3) the excessive time required to manage tanks, especially in large sheds, and (4) risks of staff members accidently depriving pigs of water after dosing by forgetting to re-open each tank's inlet valve when the medicated solution was depleted.

Of the four farm managers using header tanks, three left each tank's inlet valve open during dosing to allow water to flow into the top of tank as the medicated solution was drawn out the bottom of the tank. One manager was in the process of changing over to electric-powered dosing pumps. The other three managers had reduced the need for staff to climb ladders up to tanks by installing a canister system at ground level to transport antibiotic up a pipe into each header tank, but intended to change to dosing pumps in the near future.

We clean (header tanks) in between batches. There's always sediment in the bottom of the tank and material left over from the medication process. We know that it's not an ideal system.

Farm managers used proportional dosing pumps in different ways. Some installed them permanently in water lines to service one or more pig buildings. Others chose to re-locate them from building to building as required. On six managers' farms, including two farms where dosing pumps were used to service multiple buildings, the antibiotic had to travel over 100 m from the dosing pump to some buildings. Two managers had opted to water medicate all weaner and grower/finisher buildings on the farm using a dedicated pipe system for medicated water from one or two dosing pumps located at a central point. On these two farms, the antibiotic had to travel a distance of between 70 and 135 m from the dosing pump to the most distant buildings. Farm managers were aware that locating a dosing pump a substantial distance from the pig building it served increased the antibiotic's transit time from the pump to drinkers. However, they had not considered the potential implications of this, including the increased likelihood of degradation of the antibiotic.

That's the trade off when you've got one doser servicing six sheds rather than having the doser at each of the sheds.

Across the farms, three brands of water-powered dosing pump were used: Dosatron (Dosatron International, Tresses, France); Gator-XL (Diemold International, Inc., Fort Myers, FL, USA); and Chemilizer (Hydro Systems, Cincinnati, OH, USA). All farms using electric-powered dosing pumps used the same brand, Select (Dosing Solutions Ltd., Clavering, Saffron Walden, UK). Farm managers' opinions were divided about whether electric-powered or water-powered dosing pumps were better, and which brand of water-powered dosing pump was best. Factors influencing their views were: ease of use, reliability, cost, access to reliable mains power, ease of repair, and the size of the building the pump was required to service. One manager had multiple water-powered dosing pumps, each dedicated to a particular antibiotic. Another manager used a water-powered dosing pump for high volume dosing events and an electric-powered dosing pump for low volume dosing events. Some managers using Select dosing pumps were unclear about the maximum pumped output of different models and the maximum water pressure for which each was suitable. Only one manager using a Select dosing pump valued its inbuilt water flow meter. On most managers' farms, preventative maintenance of dosing pumps was not performed; instead, pumps were repaired when they failed. Only one farm manager regularly calibrated the pumps.

> *I'll take water powered dosing pumps any day. As long as you've got water going through that pump, that pump's going. Your power can go out. Whatever happens, it doesn't make any difference.*

> *On our farm the capacity of water we're trying to put through the machines means that that machine never stops.*

> *(Dosing pump maintenance) is more reactive than proactive because, really, you don't want to change stuff until it's worn out.*

2.2. Antibiotics and Other Additives Administered to Pigs In-Water

Farm managers administered several different registered antibiotics in-water, as shown in Table 2. Antibiotic use in pigs and other animals in Australia is regulated by a statutory agency, the Australian Pesticides and Veterinary Medicines Authority (APVMA) [14]. Pig industry antibiotic usage patterns are not reported to regulatory authorities. We found that most antibiotics used were of low importance in human medicine, consistent with a previous survey of antibiotic use in the Australian pig industry [15].

Table 2. Antibiotics currently and recently administered in-water to pigs on 25 single-site and multi-site pig farming enterprises.

Antibiotic	Product Form	Class	Importance in Human Medicine [a]
Amoxicillin	Powder	β-lactam	Low
Apramycin	Powder	Aminoglycoside	Medium
Chlortetracycline	Powder	Tetracycline	Low
Lincomycin	Powder	Lincosamide	Medium
Lincomycin + Spectinomycin	Powder	Lincosamide + Aminocyclitol	Medium
Neomycin	Powder	Aminoglycoside	Medium
Oxytetracycline	Powder	Tetracycline	Low
Tiamulin	Liquid	Pleuromutilin	Low NHU [b]
Tilmicosin	Liquid	Macrolide	Low
Trimethoprim-sulphadiazine	Powder	Dihydrofolate reductase inhibitor + sulfonamide	Medium
Tylosin	Powder	Macrolide	Low

[a] Based on list of the Australian Strategic and Technical Advisory Group (ASTAG), 2018 [16]; [b] No human use (NHU) of the antibiotic class in Australia.

Amoxicillin was the antibiotic most commonly used for treatment of disease outbreaks in weaners and in grower/finishers (Figure 1). It was also the antibiotic most commonly used for metaphylaxis in weaner pigs, followed by tiamulin. In grower/finisher pigs, lincomycin and tilmicosin were most commonly used for metaphylaxis. Simultaneous in-water dosing with more than one antibiotic was practiced on two farms (amoxicillin + apramycin on one farm and tiamulin + tilmicosin on the other).

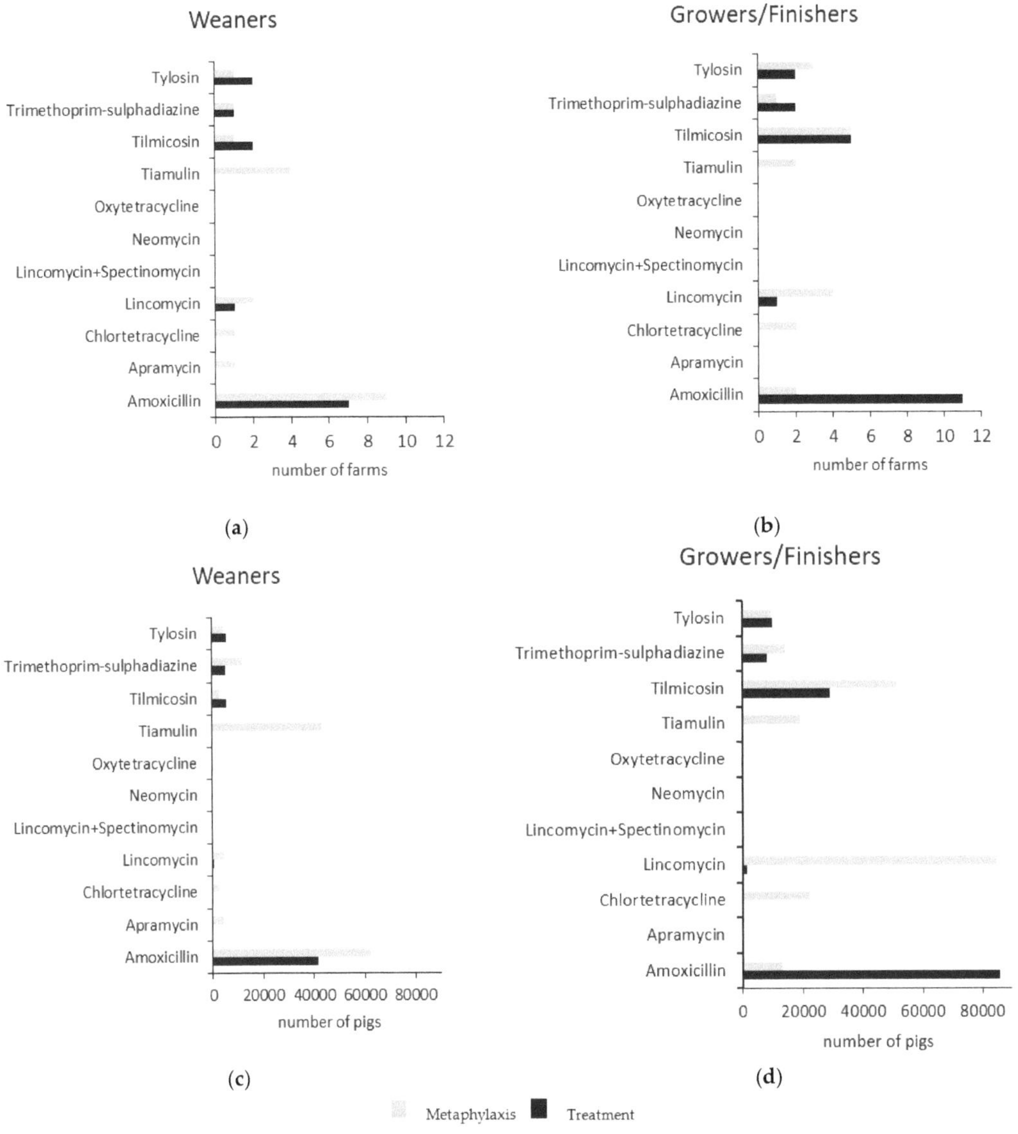

Figure 1. (**a**,**b**) Antibiotics administered in-water to weaner pigs and grower/finisher pigs, respectively, for metaphylaxis and treatment by number of farms. (**c**,**d**) Antibiotics administered in-water to weaner pigs and grower/finisher pigs respectively for metaphylaxis and treatment by number of pigs currently housed on study farms. (25 single-site and multi-site pig farming enterprises, 459,167 growing pigs).

Drinking water was also used to administer non-antibiotic products to pigs. Organic acid products (most commonly Selko®-pH) were administered continuously to weaners as an aid to intestinal health by six managers. However, a further three managers used organic acids periodically to clean pipelines and tanks. One manager used drinking water to administer a proliferative ileitis vaccine (Enterisol), another manager used drinking water to supply electrolytes to newly weaned pigs, and another manager used drinking water to administer sieved weaner manure to maiden gilts as a means of controlling congenital tremors in piglets likely to be caused by a pestivirus.

2.3. In-Water Antibiotic Dosing Calculations

All farm managers reported that they strictly followed the prescription provided by their veterinarians to plan each dosing event. They considered in-water antibiotic dosing to be an important task, and so, where practical, only one or two staff members were authorized and trained to perform dosing calculations and conduct dosing events. The prescription for each antibiotic typically detailed the product name and strength to be used, the number of pigs to be medicated and their average bodyweight (kg), the quantity of product to be administered (kg or litres) based on dose rate (mg/kg bodyweight) of the active constituent, the number of dosing events to be conducted on consecutive days, and the applicable meat withholding period. Additional information that was included on the prescription or was left to the farm manager's discretion included duration and commencement time of each day's dosing event, the injection ratio of the antibiotic stock solution into the water line, and the corresponding volume of stock solution to be prepared based on an estimated volume of water (litres) that the pigs would use over the dosing period. Many managers were provided with a Microsoft Excel spreadsheet by the veterinarian to assist with these calculations.

> *I might have 1000 pigs on arrival, which at say 25 kg, and that gives me 25,000 kg. Then I'll roughly work those 2500 L they'll drink. What I'm doing there is then I'm giving them 2.5 kg of Tilmovet into 25 L of water.*

Pig bodyweights used in most dosing calculations were averages estimated from target weight-for-age growth charts. However, on one farm, sentinel pens in each building were weighed regularly and these values were then used in dosing calculations.

> *If they're going to do a 15-week medication, we know they roughly put on 5 kg per week, so by the time they're 15 weeks they should be around 55 kg. You're going to have some pigs there that are 40 kg, you might have some that are 60. We do an average over the shed.*

The values for water wastage, as a percentage of total water used by pigs, that were factored into dosing calculations varied widely on managers' farms, ranging from 0% to 65%, i.e., some farms made no allowance for wastage, assuming that all the antibiotic mixed in the stock solution or header tank would be consumed by pigs. While managers were able to list many factors which could contribute to water wastage, their assumed water wastage rates in buildings fitted with water troughs/bowls varied widely, as did their assumptions for wastage rates in buildings fitted with nipple/bite drinkers. Fixed water wastage values tended to be applied by prescribing veterinarians across buildings on all farms under their supervision, irrespective of the type of drinker being used by the pigs to be dosed and the prevailing seasonal conditions. Only one farm used different water wastage values for summer and winter months.

Most farm managers did not appear to appreciate how the water wastage rate affected the quantity (and therefore cost) of the antibiotic product that must be administered during a dosing event to ensure that the prescribed dose was ingested by pigs on average. They were also not aware of how factoring an inaccurate water wastage value into a dosing calculation could lead to substantial under-dosing or over-dosing.

2.4. In-Water Antibiotic Dosing Regimens Used

When medicating pigs, farm managers conducted daily in-water dosing events over two or more consecutive days. The duration of metaphylaxis or treatment of outbreaks ranged from 2 to 5 days. Five managers conducted up to five consecutive daily dosing events if required to resolve a disease outbreak (see Appendix B, Figure A1 for summary and descriptive statistics). Selection of the number of daily in-water dosing events was largely at the manager's discretion.

> *Generally the vet's script says 3 to 5 days and then we'll just go off how mortalities are going. If the response is slower we'll go for 5 days, if it responds quicker we'll just do the 3 (days).*

The time of day at which each daily in-water dosing event was commenced was between 6:00 and 12:00. (Median = 7:00). The duration of each daily dosing event varied widely, from 4 to 24 h. (See Appendix B, Figure A2 for summary and descriptive statistics). Ten farm managers always dosed for a period of ≤8 h, commencing between 6:00 and 9:00. These managers tended to be satisfied that most pigs would ingest sufficient quantities of antibiotic before the end of normal staff working hours (typically 15:00) and wanted to supervise the entire event. Seven farm managers always conducted each dosing event over 24 h, effectively dosing continuously for the chosen number of days.

> *Most pigs will have a drink within 8 to 10 h. Every pig has virtually got a hit of amoxicillin.*

> *(By dosing for 24 h) we're picking up the outliers, ones that are a bit scared to go and have a drink, the smaller pigs, ones that possibly are sick and need treatment.*

> *If I'm going to only have it for 8 (hours), I guarantee you then that only means they're going to get it for 5 (hours), and 5 isn't long enough, not to get the dosage of water. During the day, they're normally lying there in the afternoon underneath the sprinkler staying cool. They will normally get up and start eating, it might be 7, 8, 9 o'clock when it starts.*

Fourteen farm managers were able to suggest a value for their pigs' water usage, expressing it in litres per pig per day, percentage of pig bodyweight per day, or litres per day for a given building or the whole farm. When asked when periods of peak water usage occurred each day, managers provided a wide range of responses. Only one manager's response was based on water usage data collected using a water flow metering system (Farm 16). Analysis of water usage data from one of this manager's weaner buildings over a 14-day period is provided as an example (Figure 2). These data demonstrated a bimodal pattern of usage with peaks at approximately 8:00 and 16:30.

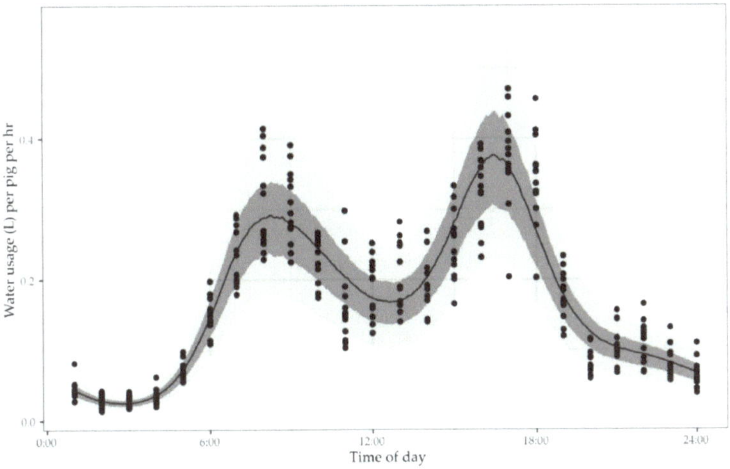

Figure 2. Water usage per pig as a function of time of day over 13 consecutive days (27 August 2020 to 8 September 2020) in a room housing 2150 weaner pigs aged 56 to 69 days of age on Farm 16. The Bayesian hierarchical model for water usage as a smooth function of time of day was generated using the brms package in R. The points are the observations, the solid line the population prediction, and the bands are the 50% and 90% population prediction intervals.

Most farm managers understood that pigs' water usage patterns may alter with climatic conditions. However, only one farm (Farm 11) deliberately altered its dosing event commencement time in summer to align it with the high water usage period observed in the afternoon [17]. Seven managers observed changes in water pressure or flow rates during peak demand periods. Some participants managing concrete/slatted floor buildings noted that during extremely hot weather, pigs tended to become restless and squealed, and lay on wet concrete around the drinkers, obstructing other pigs from gaining access.

2.5. *Preparation of Antibiotic Stock Solutions*

The amoxicillin (as amoxicillin trihydrate) products used were generally found by farm managers to be difficult to dissolve at the high concentrations required for dosing pump stock solutions. Sodium carbonate ('soda ash') was therefore routinely mixed in water with amoxicillin (usually at a ratio of one part soda ash to three parts amoxicillin by weight) to increase the pH of the stock solution, thereby improving its solubility [18]. Thirteen managers using dosing pumps to administer amoxicillin trihydrate products to pigs, used a range of volumetric injection ratios: 1:33 (three farms), 1:50 (two farms), 1:100 (seven farms) and 1:200 (one farm). Six of these managers dosed pigs over ≤8 h, at injection ratios of 1:33 (two farms), 1:50 (one farms), 1:100 (two farms) or 1:200 (one farm), necessitating the preparation of even more concentrated stock solutions. All managers using amoxicillin trihydrate products at an injection ratio of 1:50 to 1:200 used a magnetic stirrer or small submersible pump to continuously agitate the solution. When discussing the mixability of amoxicillin and other antibiotics, most did not distinguish between the product being in solution or in suspension, unless they observed sediment on the bottom of the container. Recommended protocols for preparing and using stock solutions of specific antibiotic products in proportional dosing pumps were not provided by the manufacturers of antibiotic products or dosing pumps, requiring farm managers (and veterinarians) to develop their own methods.

Lincomycin, the second most commonly used antibiotic, was considered to be very easy to mix and well accepted by pigs. Tiamulin and tilmicosin were also considered easy to use, as they were available in liquid form. Other antibiotics were problematic. Managers reported that tylosin tended to clump when mixed in water and could block filters. It also had an unpleasant taste if the fine powder entered the nose or mouth. Five managers who had used oxytetracycline and chlortetracycline found them particularly difficult to use in dosing pumps. Other antimicrobials that managers had experience using were apramycin (1 farm), trimethoprim/sulphadiazine (5 farms), and neomycin (1 farm).

I think amoxil is probably the worst (for solubility).

Lincomycin mixes well. You mix it up and it stays clear.

Lincomycin has a sweet taste, so they just come back for more.

Tylosin leaves a horrible taste in your mouth, the dust.

2.6. *Frequency of Metaphylactic In-Water Dosing by Phase of Production*

There was wide variation in the proportions of total days in the weaner and grower/finisher phases on which pigs on each farm were administered antibiotics in-water for metaphylaxis (Figure 3). Twelve of the 25 farm managers surveyed medicated weaner pigs in-water for metaphylaxis; the other 13 managers only did so for treatment of disease outbreaks. Sixteen managers medicated grower/finisher pigs in-water for metaphylaxis; the other nine managers only used in-water medication for treatment of outbreaks. The highest user of in-water antibiotics per pig (Farm 5) dosed weaner pigs four days per week (two days with amoxicillin followed by two days with chlortetracycline) and dosed grower/finisher pigs for two days per week (alternating amoxicillin and chlortetracycline). There were no significant relationships between the frequency of in-water antibiotic dosing for metaphylaxis in the weaner and grower/finisher phases and (1) the number of weaner and grower/finisher pigs accommodated on farm; (2) type of building (shelters with straw-floor pens vs. conventional buildings with solid/slatted/mesh-floored pens); or (3) production flow (all-in-all-out vs. continuous).

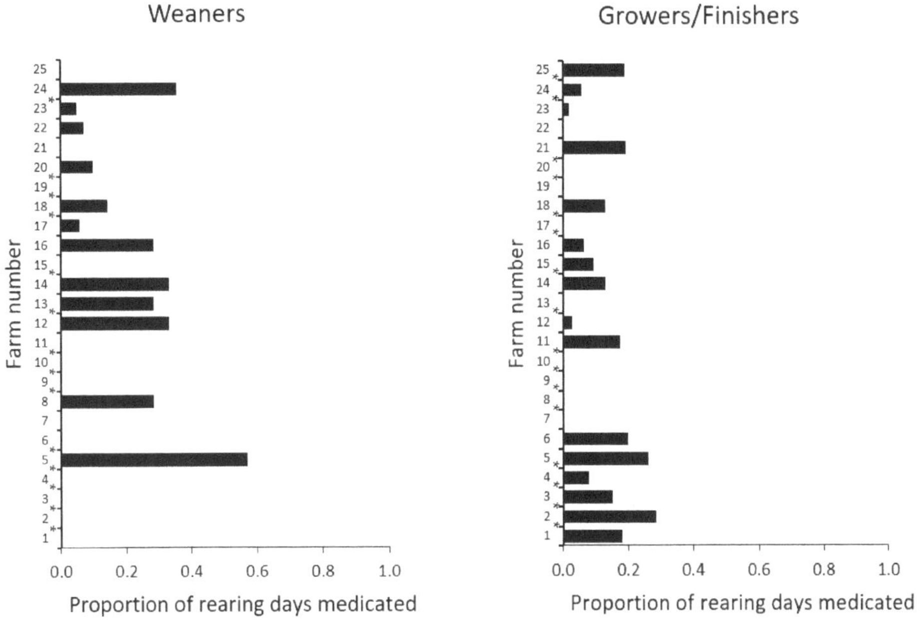

(**a**) (**b**)

Figure 3. (**a**) Proportion of total rearing days on which one or more antibiotics were administered in-water to weaner pigs for metaphylaxis. (**b**) Proportion of total rearing days on which one or more antibiotics were administered in-water to grower/finisher pigs for metaphylaxis. (25 single-site and multi-site pig farming enterprises, 459,167 growing pigs). Descriptive statistics for weaners: median, 0.00; range, 0.00–0.57; Quartile (Q) 1, 0.00; Q3, 0.29; interquartile range (IQR), 0.29. Descriptive statistics for grower/finishers: median, 0.06; range, 0.00–0.29; Q1, 0.00; Q3, 0.18; IQR: 0.18. Note: * symbol indicates that one or more antibiotics were also administered in-feed to pigs on any rearing days.

Although continuous in-feed administration of antibiotics is legally permitted in Australia, on 11 managers' farms, antibiotics were not administered to weaners in feed, and on 10 farms they were not administered to grower/finishers in feed. Some other farms had actively scaled back in-feed administration of antibiotics to pigs or intended to do so. Two managers were setting up dosing equipment in buildings not yet equipped for water medication to make this possible. One manager was proud that, having ceased in-feed medication some years ago, their farm now needed to use very little in-water medication to manage herd health.

About five years ago the company decided to do no feed medication whatsoever. Now I'm hardly doing any water medication.

2.7. Farm Managers' Views on Successful In-Water Antibiotic Dosing

Farm managers' views on successful in-water antibiotic dosing were formed largely by their experiences during disease outbreaks treating sick pigs. Disease outbreaks were a source of considerable concern for managers and their staff, as they were difficult to predict and tended to occur suddenly. Managers judged the success of in-water dosing primarily on the speed with which morbidity and mortalities within a group of sick pigs were reduced after dosing commenced. The frequency of disease outbreaks, pig growth rates, and the uniformity of pig size and body weight were also considered.

During the interviews, farm managers were asked to rate, on a 10-point ordinal scale, how satisfied they were (with 1 being not satisfied at all, and 10 being completely satisfied) that the majority of growing pigs in each building that were water medicated had ingested the dose of antibiotic prescribed by the veterinarian. Twenty managers provided a score. The median score was 7.5 (range, 4–9.5). One manager gave a lower score for dosing to treat pigs in outbreaks (5/10) than for metaphylaxis (7/10) as he felt he had less control in outbreak situations.

Many farm managers did not readily relate the antibiotic dose prescribed by the veterinarian (expressed in mg antibiotic/kg pig bodyweight) to a quantity of antibiotic that needed to be ingested by each pig over a daily in-water dosing event. Managers were not aware that the inhibitory actions of antibiotics differ, with some being time-dependent, some being concentration-dependent, and some being both time and concentration-dependent. Several managers held the view that pigs only needed to ingest some antibiotic during the dosing event for it to be effective in controlling or curing disease.

> *The pig only has to drink a litre of water during that six-hour period to get its full medication. It doesn't matter if it gets that in one mouthful or goes back several times during the day and has a two or three goes at it.*

However, one manager demonstrated an understanding of the sources of variation in systemic exposure of pigs within a group to the antibiotic and why, in a disease outbreak in a building, some pigs would die despite in-water dosing with an appropriate antibiotic:

> *There's 1000 pigs in the shed. Let's say 900 of them got a drink. Out of that 900 let's say 600 got the right volume. Out of that 600, let's say 200 of them didn't absorb it and it didn't have the right effect.*

Farm managers suggested a number of factors that could influence the consistency of the dose of antibiotic ingested by pigs in a group during an in-water dosing event. These included:

- Changes in the concentration of the antibiotic in the water over time
- The duration of the dosing period
- Lags in delivery of antibiotic to drinkers in pens further from the dosing pump or header tank
- Variation in the volume of medicated water consumed by pigs due to:
    - Some weanling pigs being slow to start eating and drinking after placement
    - Large pigs consuming more water than smaller pigs
    - Healthy pigs consuming more water than sick pigs
    - Dominant pigs consuming more water than subordinate pigs
    - Pigs' ease of access to drinkers in the pen (the number of drinkers per pen and/or the position of the drinkers in the pen)
    - Differences in the palatability of different antibiotic products
- Differences in environmental conditions in different sections of building—e.g., cooler south side vs. warmer northern side, due to the tracking of the sun
- The design of the building—the building shape and dimensions, the distances pigs in each pen must walk to feeders and drinkers

In interview discussions with farm managers on many aspects of in-water antibiotic dosing and the in-water and in-feed medication programmes in use on managers' farms, concerns about antibiotic resistance and the need to preserve the potency of antibiotics through good antibiotic stewardship were not raised by any participants. Nevertheless, all managers reported that a reduction in antibiotic use was a worthy objective for their farm and the pig industry as a whole.

3. Discussion

There were two main findings from our study: (1) in-water antibiotic dosing practices varied widely across farms in the antibiotics administered, in the choice and use of dosing equipment, in the methods used for dosing calculations, in the dosing regimens used, in the methods for preparation of antibiotic stock solutions, and in the frequency of metaphylactic dosing of pigs in weaner and grower/finisher phases; and (2) with insufficient measured data and understanding of pharmacology and population pharmacometrics, farm managers were unable to assess the effectiveness of dosing events, optimize in-water dosing calculations and regimens, and control major sources of between-animal variability in systemic exposure of pigs to antibiotics.

3.1. Sub-Optimal In-Water Antibiotic Dosing Practices That May Have Contributed to Many Pigs Not Having Sufficient Exposure to Antibiotic

For in-water dosing to successfully reduce pathogen load and achieve high clinical efficacy while minimizing selection and propagation of resistant pathogens in each pig, the antibiotic concentration at the site of infection needs to rise rapidly above the minimum inhibitory concentration (MIC) and attain a target value for the pharmacokinetic/pharmacodynamic (PK/PD) index appropriate for the antibiotic based on its inhibitory action [19]. For example, for amoxicillin (a time-dependent antibiotic), the PK/PD target should be >40% of time 24 h > MIC [20]. On many farms surveyed, the probability that most pigs (e.g., 90%) in a group medicated by in-water dosing would have this level of systemic exposure is likely to be reduced, given the frequency of sub-optimal dosing practices.

Many farm managers who participated in the study used amoxicillin trihydrate and some used trimethoprim-sulphadiazine or chlortetracycline hydrochloride for metaphylactic and/or treatment dosing. Several managers described challenges in dissolving these products in dosing pump stock solution containers or header tanks. This was unsurprising, as these three antimicrobials have much lower solubilities in water than other commonly used antimicrobials [21]. Antimicrobials must be fully dissolved and remain in solution at close to the target concentration for the entire dosing period if the prescribed dose is to be ingested, absorbed, and distributed within each pig [22]. Shorter dosing periods and/or low injection ratios require the amoxicillin stock solution to be very highly concentrated, far in excess of amoxicillin's solubility threshold, so it is likely that those managers who chose to use a lower injection ratio (e.g., 1:100 or 1:200) and/or a shorter dosing period (≤ 8 h) injected substantial quantities of suspended amoxicillin particles (rather than amoxicillin in solution) into the water pipeline early in the dosing event and thus under-dosed many pigs, even though they used sodium carbonate to improve its solubility and continuous agitated the stock solution. [2,21].

On those farms where dosing pumps were located substantial distances from the buildings they served, the transit time for an antibiotic from the dosing pump to the drinkers may be considerable. This time may provide an opportunity for substantial degradation of the antibiotic if it is exposed to factors that adversely affect its stability over time, such as low water pH, high water hardness, metal piping, the presence of chlorine, metal ions, pH modifiers, and another antibiotic with which it reacts [23–25]. On those farms where managers did not perform preventative maintenance on dosing pumps, one would expect failures to have occurred more often during dosing events, resulting in many (or all) pigs not having the required exposure to the antibiotic.

While the solubility thresholds of commonly used antibiotics are not exceeded when solutions are prepared for dosing using header tanks, some variation in the concentration of an antibiotic held in a header tank may occur over time if the solution is not continuously agitated [26]. The three farm managers using header tanks who dosed with each tank's inlet valve left open would be very unlikely to achieve PK/PD targets, as this practice results in a progressive dilution over the dosing period and thus a decline in the concentration of the antibiotic in the water supplied to the pigs.

The water wastage values used by farm managers (and veterinarians) in their dosing calculations are likely to be inaccurate, as managers lacked access to systems to measure these values in farm buildings prior to dosing events. If the water wastage rate was under-estimated, most (or all) pigs would be under-dosed and therefore not have the required exposure to the antibiotic. Water wastage by pigs has been found in experimental studies to vary widely, from 9% to 60% of total water usage, depending on a range of factors, including water flow rates, drinker design and position, room temperature, levels of competition between pigs, diet, and water quality [27–30].

In our study, the dosing regimens used by farm managers varied widely in commencement time and duration. The number of consecutive days over which each series of in-water dosing events was conducted also varied. Most managers understood that the dose of antibiotic ingested by pigs was a function of the concentration of antibiotic in the water and the volume of water consumed by each pig hour-by-hour. However, they appeared to not understand that matching commencement of a daily dosing event with the beginning of a period of moderate to high water consumption would result in high hourly rates of antibiotic ingestion by pigs over the first few hours, leading to a more rapid rise in the plasma concentration of the antibiotic and earlier attainment of the PK-PD target for the antibiotic. This approach is consistent with the 'front-loaded' dosing regimens used in human critical care medicine, in which a 'loading dose' is administered to a patient prior to continuous intravenous infusion in order to reach the desired PK/PD target more rapidly [31–33]. An added advantage of this approach is that it helps to minimize the length of time that the plasma concentration of antibiotic lies in the 'mutant selection window' just above the MIC, thereby reducing selection for and propagation of resistant pathogens [19,34,35]. We are not aware of any commercially available proportional dosing pumps that can automatically administer an initial loading dose. However, this may be advantageous.

The wide range of responses about the periods of peak water usage each day was consistent with recent studies showing that pig water consumption patterns vary widely between animals and within animals over time [17,29,36,37]. Access to a water flow metering system, allowing the average water usage patterns of a group of pigs to be determined for several days prior to each dosing event, would enable farm managers (and veterinarians) to select the optimal time of the day to commence dosing. This could particularly help those managers conducting in-water dosing events over short periods, i.e., $\leq$8 h, and those administering low metaphylactic doses over 24 h, to increase the probability that most pigs attain the PK/PD target for the antibiotic (a brief summary of how specific in-water dosing practices would be expected to impact on systemic exposure to an antibiotic is available online in Supplementary Materials).

There is little evidence to guide decisions about the optimal duration of antibiotic therapy in humans or other animals, or specifically in pigs. Past recommendations were largely arbitrary. While human studies comparing morbidity and mortality after shorter or longer courses of antibiotic therapy have yielded inconsistent results, a recent systematic review concluded that reductions in the duration of antibiotic therapy could play an important role in antibiotic stewardship and was feasible for the treatment of many human infectious diseases [38]. Further studies are required in pigs to develop guidelines for the duration of dosing.

Several studies have investigated patterns of antibiotic use in pig production across pig producing countries [15,39–46]. However, this is the first large-scale study that has specifically explored use of in-water antibiotics on commercial pig farms. Without knowledge of the antibiotic dose rate (mg/kg bodyweight) used in each dosing event, we were unable to quantify in-water antibiotic use as 'treatment incidence' (TI) based on the number of used daily doses (UDD_{pig}) [44]. However, the large variation in the frequency of metaphylactic in-water dosing between farms in our study is consistent with recent studies of oral antibiotic use on pig farms in Australia and other countries [3,15,44,46,47]. On the farms participating in our study, antibiotics were used with higher frequency in the grower/finisher phase than in the weaner phase. This contrasts with other studies [41,47–49]. Farm managers' apparent lack of awareness and concern about antibiotic resistance is consistent with studies in Canada, the UK, and Europe in which pig farmers were found to be more concerned about financial matters and managing herd health than antibiotic resistance [50]. It may also reflect a view among farm managers that managing antibiotic resistance is the responsibility of veterinarians.

3.2. Consequences of Sub-Optimal In-Water Antibiotic Dosing Practices on Pig Farms

If sub-optimal in-water antibiotic dosing practices, as found on many farms surveyed, led to most pigs in a group medicated not having sufficient systemic exposure to the antibiotic to eliminate (or substantially reduce the quantity of) the target pathogen, it is plausible that the pathogen load in the pigs would remain high and a disease outbreak may occur, necessitating urgent in-water antibiotic dosing at a high dose rate [5,35] (Figure 4). If this dosing also failed to eliminate or substantially reduce the pathogen load in most pigs, then there may be a repeating cycle of disease outbreaks requiring urgent in-water treatment dosing. Antibiotic use (and cost) per pig produced on these farms may be further increased if, through a desire by farm managers and veterinarians to manage risk to pig health, welfare, and productivity, metaphylactic in-water dosing is conducted more frequently using moderate to high doses, and/or in-feed medication is introduced, or increased. Increased antibiotic use may have further consequences, including increased selection for and propagation of resistant pathogens and increased dissemination of antibiotics in effluent to the environment. If a farm's in-water dosing practices are such that many pigs in a group do not ingest a sufficient dose of antibiotic during an in-water dosing event, then many pigs may also not ingest a sufficient quantity of a non-antibiotic additive with dose-dependent efficacy if it were administered in water. This warrants future investigation.

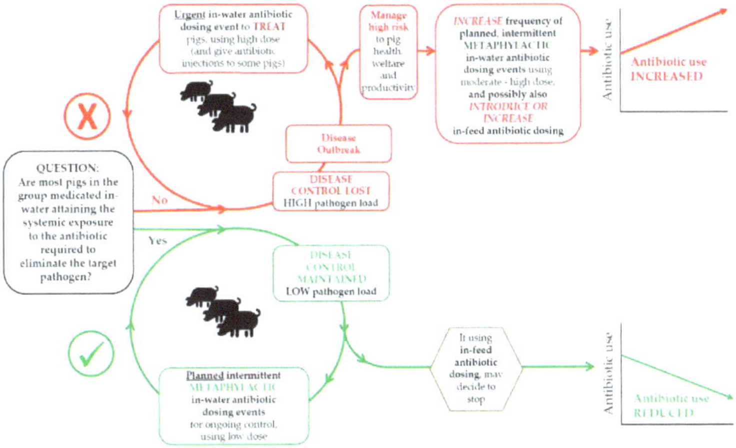

Figure 4. Schematic showing possible pathways resulting in increased antibiotic use (red) or reduced antibiotic use (green) in pigs, based on whether most pigs in the medicated group have sufficient systemic exposure to the antibiotic to eliminate the target pathogen.

3.3. Limitation of the Study

The survey successfully integrated qualitative and quantitative data on the in-water antibiotic dosing practices of a sample of Australian pig farm managers. However, the survey has limitations. Our sample was not randomly selected from the population of Australian pig farm managers. This is explained in Materials and Methods. The survey was focused on pig farm managers' in-water dosing practices and physical characteristics of each farm relevant to in-water dosing. We did not survey veterinarians to collect data on pigs' health status and performance, the prescribing behaviour of veterinarians, or the efficacy of the medication programmes implemented. Our survey should be considered as a first step in gaining a detailed understanding of in-water antibiotic dosing practices used by pig farm managers. Practices may differ in each country. Further research is therefore needed to compare our findings on the in-water antibiotic dosing practices of pig farm managers with those in other countries.

3.4. Conclusions

There is considerable scope to improve in-water antibiotic dosing practices on commercial pig farms, and thereby increase the effectiveness of in-water dosing and reduce antibiotic use (and cost) on farms. To enable farm managers (and veterinarians) to achieve these outcomes, they would require access to (1) on-farm measuring systems that provide easily interpretable data on the water wastage and daily water usage pattern of each group of pigs being dosed; and (2) technical guidelines and training on in-water antibiotic dosing based on key principles of antibiotic pharmacology and population pharmacometrics. Development and extension of the technical guidelines and training programs would need to be led by industry, supported by commercial pig enterprises, and involve a multidisciplinary development and training team of pig veterinarians, pharmacologists, and other professionals with relevant expertise. With these measurement systems, technical guidelines and training in place, veterinarians would be better able to work with farm managers in designing and conducting in-water dosing and perform regular audits of farms' in-water dosing systems and practices.

4. Materials and Methods

Farm managers were recruited for this study using a purposive sampling method that aimed to obtain a sample population of farm managers of medium to large single-site and multi-site pig farming enterprises across Australia. To be eligible to participate in the study, a person was required to be a pig farm manager responsible for management of the water system and in-water antibiotic dosing of growing pigs. Their farm must have operated for at least six months, have more than 500 weaner and grower pigs, participated in the Australian Pork Industry Quality Assurance Program, reared growing pigs indoors (in concrete-floored rooms/sheds or in straw-floored shelters), and water medicated weaner and/or grower/finisher pigs with antibiotics for metaphylaxis and treatment of bacterial diseases. The cohort of farms included in the study was non-random, but representative of the Australian pig industry, comprising approximately 21% of all growing pigs accommodated in Australia at any time. Each farm manager was contacted directly by telephone and invited to participate in the survey. They were then emailed a detailed handout explaining the study's aims and design and a consent form for signature and return prior to commencement.

The study used a mixed-methods approach. An initial quantitative phase comprised an online questionnaire. Once completed, a qualitative phase followed, comprising a one-on-one semi-structured interview. The online questionnaire and the interview were designed to each be completed by participants in less than 45 min. The online questionnaire (available online in pdf format in Supplementary Materials) was designed to provide an understanding of variability across farms regarding the features of the buildings in which growing pigs were reared, drinking water supply systems, and water medication dosing systems and programmes. It used recommended design features to make it more effective and user-friendly [51,52]. The questionnaire was created and managed in REDCap (Research Electronic Data Capture), a secure web-based application for building and managing online surveys (Vanderbilt University, Nashville, Tennessee, USA). Participants were required to respond to all questions and asked to complete the questionnaire within two weeks of receipt using a web-link. The most demanding part of the questionnaire was that seeking characteristics of two weaner buildings and two grower/finisher buildings on the farm, as respondents needed to consult farm records and make some measurements.

This part was therefore positioned near the beginning of the questionnaire. This appeared to assist users. Thorough pre-testing was conducted with colleagues and farm managers and refinements were made to improve the questionnaire's clarity and ease of use before it was deployed.

Each farm manager was interviewed within four weeks of completing the online questionnaire. Each interview was conducted using an interview guide based on a review of the literature and previous discussions by the lead author (S.L.) with farm managers and veterinarians. The interview guide (available online in Supplementary Materials) comprised mostly open questions to facilitate discussion of the design and function of the farm's drinking water distribution system, the pigs' daily water usage patterns, the provision of water to pigs in specific buildings, and the in-water medication dosing process used. Two pilot interviews were conducted, and the interview guide was reviewed and revised prior to use. The changes made were mainly to terminology.

Quantitative data collected from each farm manager in the online questionnaire were used in the interview to tailor questions to each participant and encouraged richer, more detailed responses from participants. Every effort was made not to direct or influence the participant's responses. All interviews were conducted by S.L. Interviews were initially conducted face-to-face on the farm at a time convenient for the participant. However, due to logistical challenges and more stringent biosecurity measures imposed by farms during the study to manage the risk of African swine fever, later interviews were conducted by telephone. Each interview was recorded on a digital recorder (audio only) with the permission of each participant to facilitate later qualitative analysis.

Questionnaire responses captured in REDCap from each participant were exported into Excel, de-identified, and then subjected to statistical analysis in Excel and R. Interviews were transcribed verbatim from audio recordings into text documents and de-identified. Transcripts were then entered into the qualitative data analysis software package NVivo version 12 (QSR International Pty. Ltd., Melbourne, Victoria, Australia) and openly coded and analysed by the interviewer using qualitative data analysis principles and thematic analysis [53]. Coding of transcripts was done manually. This was an iterative process, with nodes being refined as more data were coded. The final coding framework used in NVivo is available online in Supplementary Materials. Sentiment analysis was performed in NVivo using automatic coding. Selected comments made by participants in the interviews that the lead author found illustrative were included in the Results section.

Supplementary Materials: The following are available online at https://www.mdpi.com/2079-6382/10/2/169/s1: S1: Online questionnaire created and managed in REDCap (pdf version); S2: Semi-structured interview guide; S3: Final coding framework [NVivo] used to analyse interview transcripts; and S4: Summary table 'Specific in-water dosing practices, their consequences and the expected impact on pigs' systemic exposure to an antibiotic administered through their drinking water'.

Author Contributions: Conceptualisation, S.L., H.B.-J. and G.B.; investigation, S.L.; methodology, S.L.; software, S.L., A.W.; validation, S.L. and H.B.-J.; formal analysis, S.L. and A.W.; resources, H.B.-J.; data curation, S.L.; writing—original draft preparation, S.L.; writing—review and editing, H.B.-J., A.W., G.B.; visualisation, S.L., H.B.-J., A.W.; supervision, H.B.-J.; project administration, G.B.; funding acquisition, G.B. All authors have read and agreed to the published version of the manuscript.

Funding: This research was supported by a National Health and Medical Research Council Centre for Research Excellence grant for the National Centre for Antibiotic Stewardship. S.B. Little 0000-0002-3715-3225.

Institutional Review Board Statement: The study was conducted with the approval of the University of Melbourne Veterinary and Agricultural Sciences Human Ethics Advisory Group (I.D. No. 1853192.1, approved 22 November 2018 and amended 11 June 2019) and was conducted in compliance with its conditions.

Informed Consent Statement: Informed consent was obtained from all subjects involved in the study.

Data Availability Statement: The data presented in this study are available on request from the corresponding author. The data are not publicly available due to conditions of the ethics agreement.

Acknowledgments: The authors wish to thank the pig farm managers who kindly participated in this research study. We also wish to thank the pig farming enterprises that supported this study.

Conflicts of Interest: The authors declare no conflict of interest. The funders had no role in the design of the study; in the collection, analyses, or interpretation of data; in the writing of the manuscript, or in the decision to publish the results.

Appendix A

Table A1. Demographics of the 25 pig farm managers who participated in the study.

Characteristic	Study Participants N
Gender:	
Male	23
Female	2
Age:	
<25	0
25–34	1
35–44	5
45–54	9
>55	10
Years working in pig industry:	
<2	0
2–5	1
6–10	3
>10	21
Years managing current farm:	
<2	6
2–5	3
6–10	4
>10	12

Table A2. Characteristics of the 25 pig farms studied.

Characteristic	Study Farms %
Location [state of Australia]:	
South Australia	36%
Victoria	32%
New South Wales	24%
Queensland	8%
Animals on farm:	
Sows, boars and growing pigs	48%
Growing pigs only	52%
Single- or multiple-site configuration:	
Single	72%
Multiple	28%
Weaner pig buildings described in questionnaire:	
Type:	
Solid/slatted/mesh-floored pens in conventional buildings	61%
Straw-floor pens in eco-shelters	39%
Age of buildings:	
<2 years	22%
3–10 years	0%
11–20 years	34%
20 years	44%

Table A2. *Cont.*

Characteristic	Study Farms %
Grower/finisher pig buildings described in questionnaire:	
Type:	
Solid/slatted/mesh-floored pens in conventional buildings	30
Straw-floor pens in eco-shelters	17
Age of buildings:	
<2 years	12%
3–10 years	6%
11–20 years	30%
20 years	52%
Pig flow in weaner buildings	
All-in-all-out by room or building	94%
Continuous flow	6%
Pig flow in grower/finisher buildings	
All-in-all-out by room or building	78%
Continuous flow	22%

Appendix B

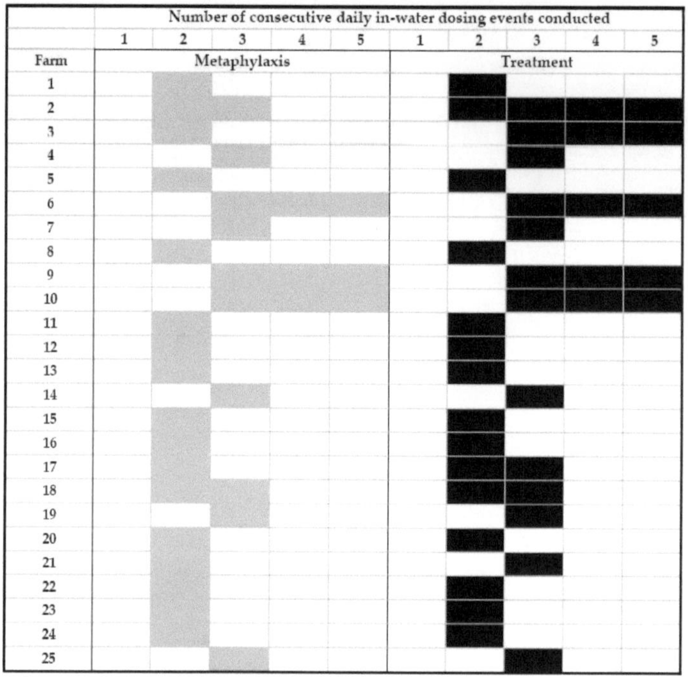

	Metaphylaxis		Treatment	
	Min.	Max.	Min.	Max.
Median	2	2	2	3
Range	1	3	1	3
Minimum	2	2	2	2
Maximum	3	5	3	5
Quartile 1	2	2	2	2
Quartile 3	3	3	3	3
Interquartile range	1	1	1	1

Figure A1. Summary and descriptive statistics for the number of consecutive daily in-water antibiotic dosing events conducted for metaphylaxis and treatment of clinical disease on the 25 pig farms studied.

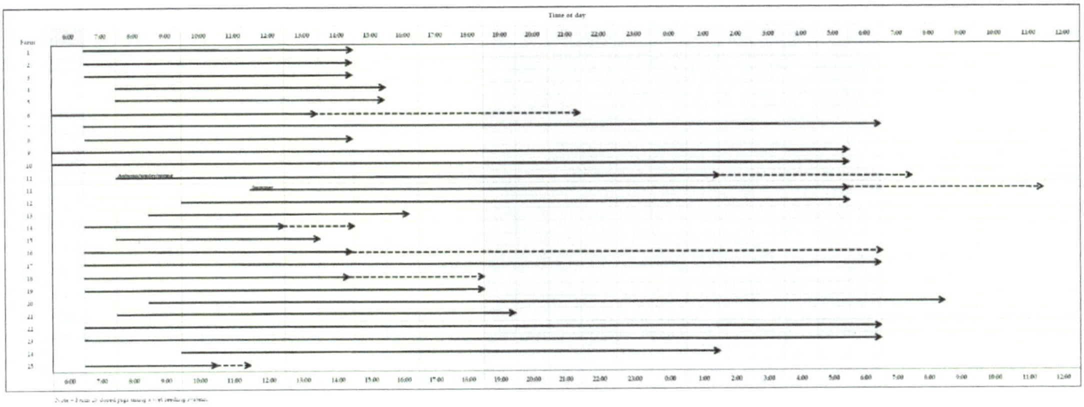

	Start time	Duration (hours)	
		Minimum	Maximum
Median	7:00	10	[illegible]
Minimum	[illegible]	4	4
Maximum	12:00	24	24
Quartile 1	7:00	5	5
Quartile 3	9:00	23	24
Interquartile range	[illegible]	[illegible]	[illegible]

Figure A2. Summary and descriptive statistics for start time and duration of each daily in-water antibiotic dosing event on the 25 pig farms studied.

References

1. Grandin, F.C.; Lacroix, M.Z.; Gayrard, V.; Viguié, C.; Mila, H.; Toutain, P.-L.; Picard-Hagen, N. Session 12: Residues and Contaminants. *J. Vet. Pharmacol. Ther.* **2018**, *41*, 43–45. [CrossRef]
2. Edwards, L. Drinking Water Quality and Its Impact on the Health and Performance of Pigs. Co-Operative Research Centre for High Integrity Australian Pork. Innovation Project 2A-118. 2018. Available online: http://porkcrc.com.au/wp-content/uploads/2018/08/2A-118-Drinking-Water-Quality-Final-Report.pdf (accessed on 12 December 2020).
3. Fertner, M.E.; Boklund, A.; Dupont, N.; Toft, N. Changes in group treatment procedures of Danish finishers and its influence on the amount of administered antimicrobials. *Prev. Vet. Med.* **2016**, *126*, 89–93. [CrossRef]
4. Page, S.; Gautier, P. Use of antimicrobial agents in livestock. *Rev. Sci. Tech. l'OIE* **2012**, *31*, 145–188. [CrossRef]
5. Vasseur, M.V.; Lacroix, M.Z.; Toutain, P.-L.; Bousquet-Melou, A.; Ferran, A.A. Infection-stage adjusted dose of beta-lactams for parsimonious and efficient antibiotic treatments: A Pasteurella multocida experimental pneumonia in mice. *PLoS ONE* **2017**, *12*, e0182863. [CrossRef] [PubMed]
6. Toutain, P.-L.; Lees, P. WS04 The population PK/PD approach for a rational use of anti-infective drugs to minimize resistance. *J. Vet. Pharmacol. Ther.* **2006**, *29*, 26–29. [CrossRef]
7. Patel, S.J.; Wellington, M.; Shah, R.M.; Ferreira, M.J. Antibiotic Stewardship in Food-Producing Animals: Challenges, Progress, and Opportunities. *Clin. Ther.* **2020**, *42*, 1649–1658. [CrossRef] [PubMed]
8. Coyne, L.A.; Latham, S.M.; Williams, N.J.; Dawson, S.; Donald, I.J.; Pearson, R.B.; Smith, R.F.; Pinchbeck, G.L. Understanding the culture of antimicrobial prescribing in agriculture: A qualitative study of UK pig veterinary surgeons. *J. Antimicrob. Chemother.* **2016**, *71*, 3300–3312. [CrossRef]
9. Coyne, L.; Latham, S.; Dawson, S.; Donald, I.; Pearson, R.; Smith, R.; Williams, N.; Pinchbeck, G.; La, C.; Sm, L.; et al. Antimicrobial use practices, attitudes and responsibilities in UK farm animal veterinary surgeons. *Prev. Vet. Med.* **2018**, *161*, 115–126. [CrossRef]
10. Coyne, L.; Latham, S.M.; Dawson, S.; Donald, I.J.; Pearson, R.B.; Smith, R.F.; Williams, N.J.; Pinchbeck, G.L. Exploring Perspectives on Antimicrobial Use in Livestock: A Mixed-Methods Study of UK Pig Farmers. *Front. Vet. Sci.* **2019**, *6*, 257. [CrossRef]
11. Cutler, R.; Gleeson, B.; Page, S.; Norris, J.; Browning, G.; Australian Veterinary Association Ltd and Animal Medicines Australia. Antimicrobial prescribing guidelines for pigs. *Aust. Vet. J.* **2020**, *98*, 105–134. [CrossRef]
12. Hardefeldt, L.Y.; Gilkerson, J.R.; Billman-Jacobe, H.; Stevenson, M.A.; Thursky, K.; Bailey, K.E.; Browning, G.F. Barriers to and enablers of implementing antimicrobial stewardship programs in veterinary practices. *J. Vet. Intern. Med.* **2018**, *32*, 1092–1099. [CrossRef] [PubMed]
13. Australian Pork Limited. Import, Export, and Domestic Production Report. June 2020. Available online: http://australianpork.com.au/wp-content/uploads/2020/08/ImportExport-Dom-Prod-Jun-report-1.pdf (accessed on 12 December 2020).
14. Australian Pesticides and Veterinary Medicines Authority. PubCRIS. Available online: https://portal.apvma.gov.au/pubcris (accessed on 12 December 2020).

15. Jordan, D.; Chin, J.-C.; Fahy, V.; Barton, M.; Smith, M.; Trott, D. Antimicrobial use in the Australian pig industry: Results of a national survey. *Aust. Vet. J.* **2009**, *87*, 222–229. [CrossRef]
16. Australian Strategic and Technical Advisory Group on AMR. Importance Ratings and Summary of Antibacterial Uses in Human and Animal Health in Australia. Commonwealth of Australia Canberra, Australia. Available online: https://www.amr.gov.au/resources/importance-ratings-and-summary-antibacterial-uses-human-and-animal-health-australia (accessed on 12 December 2020).
17. Brumm, M.C. *Patterns of Drinking Water Use in Pork Production Facilities*; Nebraska Swine Report; University of Nebraska: Lincoln, NE, USA, 2006; pp. 10–14.
18. Félix, I.; Moreira, L.; Chiavone-Filho, O.; Mattedi, S. Solubility measurements of amoxicillin in mixtures of water and ethanol from 283.15 to 298.15 K. *Fluid Phase Equilibria* **2016**, *422*, 78–86. [CrossRef]
19. Lees, P.; Pelligand, L.; Ferran, A.; Bousquet-Melou, A.; Toutain, P.-L. Application of pharmacological principles to dosage design of antimicrobial drugs. *Pharmacol. Matters* **2015**, 22–24.
20. Rey, J.F.; Laffont, C.M.; Croubels, S.; De Backer, P.; Zemirline, C.; Bousquet, E.; Guyonnet, J.; Ferran, A.A.; Bousquet-Melou, A.; Toutain, P.-L. Use of Monte Carlo simulation to determine pharmacodynamic cutoffs of amoxicillin to establish a breakpoint for antimicrobial susceptibility testing in pigs. *Am. J. Vet. Res.* **2014**, *75*, 124–131. [CrossRef]
21. Little, S.B.; Crabb, H.K.; Woodward, A.P.; Browning, G.F.; Billman-Jacobe, H. Review: Water medication of growing pigs: Sources of between-animal variability in systemic exposure to antimicrobials. *Animals* **2019**, *13*, 3031–3040. [CrossRef]
22. Crea, F.; Cucinotta, D.; De Stefano, C.; Milea, D.; Sammartano, S.; Vianelli, G. Modeling solubility, acid–base properties and activity coefficients of amoxicillin, ampicillin and (+)6-aminopenicillanic acid, in NaCl(aq) at different ionic strengths and temperatures. *Eur. J. Pharm. Sci.* **2012**, *47*, 661–677. [CrossRef] [PubMed]
23. Dorr, P.; Madson, D.; Wayne, S.; Scheidt, A.B.; Almond, G.W. Impact of pH modifiers and drug exposure on the solubility of pharmaceutical products commonly administered through water delivery systems. *JSHAP* **2009**, *17*, 217–222.
24. Jerzsele, A.; Nagy, G.; Lehel, J.; Semjen, G. Oral bioavailability and pharmacokinetic profile of the amoxicillin-clavulanic acid combination after intravenous and oral gavage administration in broiler chickens. *J. Vet. Pharmacol. Ther.* **2009**, *32*, 506–509. [CrossRef] [PubMed]
25. Acero, J.L.; Benitez, F.J.; Real, F.J.; Roldan, G. Kinetics of aqueous chlorination of some pharmaceuticals and their elimination from water matrices. *Water Res.* **2010**, *44*, 4158–4170. [CrossRef] [PubMed]
26. Canning, P.; Bates, J.; Skoland, K.; Coetzee, J.; Wulf, L.; Rajewski, S.; Wang, C.; Gauger, P.; Ramirez, A.; Karriker, L.A. Variation in water disappearance, daily dose, and synovial fluid concentrations of tylvalosin and 3-*O*-acetyltylosin in commerical pigs during five day water medication with tylvalosin under field conditions. *J. Vet. Pharmacol. Ther.* **2018**, *41*, 632–636. [CrossRef] [PubMed]
27. Li, Y.Z.; Chénard, L.; Lemay, S.P.; Gonyou, H.W. Water intake and wastage at nipple drinkers by growing-finishing pigs1. *J. Anim. Sci.* **2005**, *83*, 1413–1422. [CrossRef] [PubMed]
28. Meiszberg, A.M.; Johnson, A.K.; Sadler, L.J.; A Carroll, J.; Dailey, J.W.; Krebs, N. Drinking behavior in nursery pigs: Determining the accuracy between an automatic water meter versus human observers12. *J. Anim. Sci.* **2009**, *87*, 4173–4180. [CrossRef]
29. Andersen, H.-L.; Dybkjær, L.; Herskin, M. Growing pigs' drinking behaviour: Number of visits, duration, water intake and diurnal variation. *Animals* **2014**, *8*, 1881–1888. [CrossRef]
30. Wang, M.; Yi, L.; Liu, J.; Zhao, W.; Wu, Z. Water consumption and wastage of nursery pig with different drinkers at different water pressures in summer. *Trans. Chin. Soc. Agric. Eng.* **2017**, *33*, 161–166.
31. De Waele, J.J.; Lipman, J.; Carlier, M.; Roberts, J.A. Subtleties in practical application of prolonged infusion of β-lactam antibiotics. *Int. J. Antimicrob. Agents* **2015**, *45*, 461–463. [CrossRef]
32. Osthoff, M.; Siegemund, M.; Balestra, G.; Abdul-Aziz, M.H.; Roberts, M.S. Prolonged administration of β-lactam antibiotics—A comprehensive review and critical appraisal. *Swiss Med. Wkly.* **2016**, *146*, w14368. [CrossRef]
33. Roberts, J.A.; Paul, S.K.; Akova, M.; Bassetti, M.; De Waele, J.J.; Dimopoulos, G.; Kaukonen, K.-M.; Koulenti, D.; Martin, C.; Montravers, P.; et al. DALI: Defining Antibiotic Levels in Intensive Care Unit Patients: Are Current -Lactam Antibiotic Doses Sufficient for Critically Ill Patients? *Clin. Infect. Dis.* **2014**, *58*, 1072–1083. [CrossRef]
34. Gianvecchio, C.; Lozano, N.A.; Henderson, C.; Kalhori, P.; Bullivant, A.; Valencia, A.; Su, L.; Bello, G.; Wong, M.; Cook, E.; et al. Variation in Mutant Prevention Concentrations. *Front. Microbiol.* **2019**, *10*, 42. [CrossRef]
35. Paterson, I.K.; Hoyle, A.; Ochoa, G.; Baker-Austin, C.; Taylor, N.H. Optimising Antibiotic Usage to Treat Bacterial Infections. *Sci. Rep.* **2016**, *6*, 37853. [CrossRef] [PubMed]
36. Soraci, A.L.; Amanto, F.; Tapia, M.O.; De La Torre, E.; Toutain, P.-L. Exposure variability of fosfomycin administered to pigs in food or water: Impact of social rank. *Res. Vet. Sci.* **2014**, *96*, 153–159. [CrossRef]
37. Rousseliere, Y.; Hemonic, A.; Marcon, M. Individual monitoring of the drinking behavior of weaned piglets. *JRP* **2016**, *48*, 355–356.
38. Pezzani, M.D.; Be, G.; Cattaneo, P.; Zaffagnini, A.; Gobbi, F.; Rodari, P.; Bisoffi, Z.; Tacconelli, E. Evidence Based Review on Optimal Duration of Antibiotic Therapy for Bacterial Infections to Support Antimicrobial Stewardship Recommendations. WHO Secretariat Report. 2019, pp. 1–28. Available online: https://www.who.int/selection_medicines/committees/expert/22/applications/ABWG_optimal_duration_AB.pdf (accessed on 12 December 2020).
39. Rosengren, L.B.; Waldner, C.L.; Reid-Smith, R.J.; Harding, J.C.; Gow, S.P.; Wilkins, W.L. Antimicrobial use through feed, water, and injection in 20 swine farms in Alberta and Saskatchewan. *Can. J. Vet. Res.* **2008**, *72*, 143–150. [PubMed]

40. Moreno, M.A. Survey of quantitative antimicrobial consumption in two different pig finishing systems. *Vet. Rec.* **2012**, *171*, 325. [CrossRef]
41. Van Rennings, L.; Von Münchhausen, C.; Ottilie, H.; Hartmann, M.; Merle, R.; Honscha, W.; Käsbohrer, A.; Kreienbrock, L. Cross-Sectional Study on Antibiotic Usage in Pigs in Germany. *PLoS ONE* **2015**, *10*, e0119114. [CrossRef]
42. Lekagul, A.; Tangcharoensathien, V.; Yeung, S. Patterns of antibiotic use in global pig production: A systematic review. *Vet. Anim. Sci.* **2019**, *7*, 100058. [CrossRef]
43. Jensen, V.; Jacobsen, E.; Bager, F. Veterinary antimicrobial-usage statistics based on standardized measures of dosage. *Prev. Vet. Med.* **2004**, *64*, 201–215. [CrossRef]
44. Timmerman, T.; Dewulf, J.; Catry, B.; Feyen, B.; Opsomer, G.; De Kruif, A.; Maes, D. Quantification and evaluation of antimicrobial drug use in group treatments for fattening pigs in Belgium. *Prev. Vet. Med.* **2006**, *74*, 251–263. [CrossRef]
45. Stevens, K.B.; Gilbert, J.; Strachan, W.D.; Robertson, J.; Johnston, A.M.; Pfeiffer, D.U. Characteristics of commercial pig farms in Great Britain and their use of antimicrobials. *Vet. Rec.* **2007**, *161*, 45–52. [CrossRef] [PubMed]
46. Van Der Fels-Klerx, H.J.; Puister-Jansen, L.F.; Van Asselt, E.D.; Burgers, S.L.G.E. Farm factors associated with the use of antibiotics in pig production1. *J. Anim. Sci.* **2011**, *89*, 1922–1929. [CrossRef] [PubMed]
47. Callens, B.; Persoons, D.; Maes, D.; Laanen, M.; Postma, M.; Boyen, F.; Haesebrouck, F.; Butaye, P.; Catry, B.; Dewulf, J. Prophylactic and metaphylactic antimicrobial use in Belgian fattening pig herds. *Prev. Vet. Med.* **2012**, *106*, 53–62. [CrossRef]
48. Jensen, V.F.; De Knegt, L.; Andersen, V.D.; Wingstrand, A. Temporal relationship between decrease in antimicrobial prescription for Danish pigs and the "Yellow Card" legal intervention directed at reduction of antimicrobial use. *Prev. Vet. Med.* **2014**, *117*, 554–564. [CrossRef] [PubMed]
49. Sjolund, M.; Postma, M.; Collineau, L.; Lösken, S.; Backhans, A.; Belloc, C.; Emanuelson, U.; Beilage, E.; Stärk, K.; Dewulf, J. Quantitative and qualitative antimicrobial usage patterns in farrow-to-finish pig herds in Belgium, France, Germany and Sweden. *Prev. Vet. Med.* **2016**, *130*, 41–50. [CrossRef]
50. Visschers, V.H.M.; Backhans, A.; Collineau, L.; Iten, D.; Loesken, S.; Postma, M.; Belloc, C.; Dewulf, J.; Emanuelson, U.; Beilage, E.G.; et al. Perceptions of antimicrobial usage, antimicrobial resistance and policy measures to reduce antimicrobial usage in convenient samples of Belgian, French, German, Swedish and Swiss pig farmers. *Prev. Vet. Med.* **2015**, *119*, 10–20. [CrossRef] [PubMed]
51. Taylor-Powell, E.; Marshall, M.G. *Questionnaire Design: Asking Questions with a Purpose*; UW-Extension Cooperative Extension Service: Madison, WI, USA, 1996; pp. 1–18.
52. Andrews, D.; Nonnecke, B.; Preece, J. Electronic Survey Methodology: A Case Study in Reaching Hard-to-Involve Internet Users. *Int. J. Hum.-Comput. Interact.* **2003**, *16*, 185–210. [CrossRef]
53. Braun, V.; Clarke, V. Using thematic analysis in psychology. *Qual. Res. Psychol.* **2006**, *3*, 77–101. [CrossRef]

antibiotics MDPI

Article

Third Generation Cephalosporin Resistant *Enterobacterales* Infections in Hospitalized Horses and Donkeys: A Case–Case–Control Analysis

Anat Shnaiderman-Torban [1], Dror Marchaim [2,3,†], Shiri Navon-Venezia [4,5,†], Ori Lubrani [1], Yossi Paitan [6,7], Haya Arielly [6] and Amir Steinman [1,*,†]

1 Koret School of Veterinary Medicine (KSVM), The Robert H. Smith Faculty of Agriculture, Food and Environment, The Hebrew University of Jerusalem, Rehovot 7610001, Israel; ashnaiderman@gmail.com (A.S.-T.); ori.lubrani@mail.huji.ac.il (O.L.)
2 Unit of Infection Control, Shamir (Assaf Harofeh) Medical Center, Zerifin, Beer Yaakov 70300, Israel; drormarchaim@shamir.gov.il
3 Sackler School of Medicine, Tel-Aviv University, Tel-Aviv 69978, Israel
4 Department of Molecular Biology, Faculty of Natural Science, Ariel University, Ariel 40700, Israel; shirinv@ariel.ac.il
5 The Miriam and Sheldon Adelson School of Medicine, Ariel University, Ariel 40700, Israel
6 Department of Clinical Microbiology and Immunology, Sackler Faculty of Medicine, Tel Aviv University, Tel Aviv 6997801, Israel; yossi.paitan@clalit.org.il (Y.P.); Ariellyhaya@clalit.org.il (H.A.)
7 Clinical Microbiology Lab, Meir Medical Center, Kfar Saba 4428164, Israel
* Correspondence: amirst@savion.huji.ac.il; Tel.: +972-3-9688544
† These authors contributed equally to this paper.

Abstract: In human medicine, infections caused by third-generation cephalosporin-resistant *Enterobacterales* (3GCRE) are associated with detrimental outcomes. In veterinary medicine, controlled epidemiological analyses are lacking. A matched case–case–control investigation (1:1:1 ratio) was conducted in a large veterinary hospital (2017–2019). In total, 29 infected horses and donkeys were matched to 29 animals with third-generation cephalosporin-susceptible *Enterobacterales* (3GCSE) infections, and 29 uninfected controls (overall $n = 87$). Despite multiple significant associations per bivariable analyses, the only independent predictor for 3GCRE infection was recent exposure to antibiotics (adjusted odds ratio (aOR) = 104, $p < 0.001$), but this was also an independent predictor for 3GCSE infection (aOR = 22, $p < 0.001$), though the correlation with 3GCRE was significantly stronger (aOR = 9.3, $p = 0.04$). In separated multivariable outcome models, 3GCRE infections were independently associated with reduced clinical cure rates (aOR = 6.84, $p = 0.003$) and with 90 days mortality (aOR = 3.6, $p = 0.003$). *Klebsiella* spp. were the most common 3GCRE (36%), and $bla_{CTX\text{-}M\text{-}1}$ was the major β-lactamase (79%). Polyclonality and multiple sequence types were evident among all *Enterobacterales* (e.g., *Klebsiella pneumoniae*, *Escherichia coli*, *Enterobacter cloacae*). The study substantiates the significance of 3GCRE infections in equine medicine, and their independent detrimental impact on cure rates and mortality. Multiple *Enterobacterales* genera, subtypes, clones and mechanisms of resistance are prevalent among horses and donkeys with 3GCRE infections.

Keywords: cephalosporins; extended-spectrum β-lactamase; equine; resistance; case–case–control

Citation: Shnaiderman-Torban, A.; Marchaim, D.; Navon-Venezia, S.; Lubrani, O.; Paitan, Y.; Arielly, H.; Steinman, A. Third Generation Cephalosporin Resistant *Enterobacterales* Infections in Hospitalized Horses and Donkeys: A Case–Case–Control Analysis. *Antibiotics* **2021**, *10*, 155. https://doi.org/10.3390/antibiotics10020155

Academic Editor: Nikola Puvača

Received: 18 January 2021
Accepted: 1 February 2021
Published: 4 February 2021

1. Introduction

Third-generation cephalosporin-resistant *Enterobacterales* (3GCRE) are spreading worldwide [1]. Resistance is mainly due to the production of plasmid-mediated extended-spectrum β-lactamases (ESBLs) and AmpC β-lactamases, as well as the hyper-production of chromosomal Amp-C β-lactamases [2]. In human medicine, infections caused by 3GCRE are often associated with a delay in the initiation of appropriate antibiotic therapy, and therefore with worse clinical outcomes [3], since delays in the initiation of appropriate therapy are the strongest modifiable independent predictor for mortality in adult inpatients with severe sepsis [4]. In well-designed analyses in humans, these infections were independently associated with higher mortality rates, increased hospital charges, and longer lengths of hospital stay (LOS) [3]. This was further demonstrated in high-risk human patients, where infection with ESBL-producing *Enterobacterales* (ESBL-PE) has been shown to affect the clinical outcome by leading to an increased rate of inadequate initial therapy and a higher mortality [5]. A major concern regarding 3GCRE infections, and specifically ESBL-PE infections, is co-resistances to additional classes of therapeutical options, i.e., fluoroquinolones, aminoglycosides, trimethoprim-sulfamethoxazole. This further contributes to the epidemiological significance of these infections, both in human and in veterinary medicine [6,7].

Third-generation cephalosporins are critically important veterinary antimicrobials, as defined by the World Organization for Animal Health [8]. However, in recent years, there have been increasing reports pertaining to colonization and infections caused by 3GCRE among animals [9]. In equine medicine, reports of 3GCRE and in particular ESBL-PE infections are emerging, both in the community and in healthcare settings [10]. Shedding rates of 3GCRE by healthy horses in farms were reported worldwide, varying from 5.2% to 44% [11–15]. In three different studies, conducted in two different equine hospitals, shedding rates were shown to increase by 2.5–5.1-fold during hospitalization, implying that the nosocomial acquisition and spread of these resistant bacteria is common in certain veterinary facilities [11,16,17]. Moreover, there are numerous reports on various severe and invasive 3GCRE infectious syndromes among horses, e.g., skin and soft tissue infections, surgical site infections, upper respiratory tract infections, and bacteremia [18–21]. Furthermore, in horses, synovial infection with multidrug-resistant (MDR) bacteria was significantly associated with euthanasia [22]. However, the controlled scientific evidence, pertaining to risk factors and outcomes, which are independently associated with 3GCRE infections in equine medicine, is scarce.

In human medicine, the case–case–control methodology is considered today the "gold standard" in terms of analyzing risk factors/predictors in the field of antimicrobial resistance [23]. In this nested matched case-control design, every patient with a resistant pathogen is matched to a patient with a susceptible pathogen and to a patient with no pathogen (i.e., uninfected control). This methodology enables us to point out the specific predictors independently associated with the resistance determinant, while "diluting" the impact of the infection itself (i.e., by either a resistant or a susceptible strain). In veterinary medicine, as far as we know, there are no reported case–case–control studies in the field of antimicrobial resistance among animals. Our study aims were to conduct a matched case–case–control investigation, to study the predictors and outcomes, which are independently associated with 3GCRE infections among horses and donkeys.

2. Results

2.1. Population Characteristics

During the study period, there were 1564 admissions of horses and 56 admissions of donkeys recorded at the Koret School of Veterinary Medicine, Veterinary Teaching Hospital (KSVM-VTH) (Table S1). Overall, 232 clinical specimens were submitted to the bacteriological lab, of which 32 specimens (14%), which were obtained from 29 animals, grew 3GCRE. The 29 patients with 3GCRE infection ("resistant cases") were then matched to 29 patients with third-generation cephalosporin-susceptible *Enterobacterales* (3GCSE) infection ("susceptible cases"), and to 29 patients with no infection ("uninfected controls"). In total, 87 animals were enrolled (82 horses and 5 donkeys). The median age of the entire cohort was 2.75 years (range 0–24), the main breed was Arabian (48.3%, $n = 42/87$), 2.3% were geriatric ($n = 2/87$), 41.4% were neonates ($n = 36/87$), 10.3% were shelter residents ($n = 9/87$), 59.8% were females ($n = 52/87$), and out of 17 adult males, 64.7% were castrated ($n = 11/17$, i.e., 18 males were neonatal colts and were therefore not castrated and not included in the denominator for this calculation). Specifically for the donkeys, all five were adults, three were females and two were not castrated males. Eight percent (7/87) of all patients were hospitalized in the preceding three months, and the median length of stay was eight days (range: 2–181 days).

2.2. Predictors of 3GCRE Infections

Table 1 summarizes selected bivariable analyses conducted between the three groups of patients.

Table 1 depicts a summarization of the bivariable analyses conducted between the three study groups. Most predictors associated with a 3GCRE infection in bivariable analysis were also associated with 3GCSE infection, including recent surgeries, recent invasive procedures and recent exposure to multiple classes of antibiotics. In the multivariable matched model of patients with 3GCRE infection vs. uninfected controls, the only independent predictor remaining in the model was recent exposure to antibiotics (adjusted odds ratio (aOR) = 104, 95% CI 9.778–1106.182, $p < 0.001$). However, recent exposure to antibiotics remained also the only predictor associated with 3GCSE infection (aOR = 22, 95% CI 5.086–92.303, $p < 0.001$). In a matched multivariable model of patients with 3GCRE infection vs. patients with 3GCSE infection, recent exposure to antibiotics was significantly and independently associated with 3GCRE infection (aOR = 9.3, 95% CI 1.06–80.934, $p = 0.04$).

Table 1. Selected bivariable analyses comparing risk factors of patients infected with 3GCRE, patients infected with susceptible *Enterobacterales* and uninfected control patients ($n = 29$ in each group).

Parameter		3GCRE [1] No. (Valid % [3])	3GCSE [2] No. (Valid % [3])	Uninfected No. (Valid % [1])	3GCRE vs. Uninfected		3GCSE vs. Uninfected		3GCRE vs. 3GCSE	
					OR (95% CI)	*p*-Value	OR (95% CI)	*p*-Value	OR (95% CI)	*p*-Value
Demographics										
Age (Years), Median (Range)		2.25 (0–24)	3 (0–20)	3 (0–17)		0.93		0.756		0.786
Age Group	Neonates (<30 days)	12 (41.4)	12 (41.4)	12 (41.4)	1 (0.35–2.844)	>0.99	1.0 (0.352–2.844)	>0.99	1 (0.352–2.844)	>0.99
	Elderly (>20 years)	1 (3.4)	1 (3.4)	0	1.036 (0.97–1.11)	>0.99	1.036 (0.97–1.11)	>0.99	1 (0.06–16.791)	>0.99
Weight (Kg), Median (Range)/ mean ±SD		125 (22–520)	118 (40–118)	200 (30–614)		0.859		0.94		0.92
Female Gender		19 (65.5)	21 (72.4)	12 (41.4)	0.372 (0.128–1.077)	0.065	0.269 (0.09–0.808)	**0.017**	1.382 (0.452–4.225)	0.57
Castrated Adult Male [4]		2 (66.7)	3 (60)	6 (66.7)	1 (0.063–15.988)	>0.99	0.75 (0.078–7.21)	>0.99	1.333 (0.067–26.618)	>0.99
Pregnant Mare		4 (28.6)	5 (41.7)	2 (25)	1.2 (0.166–8.659)	>0.99	2.143 (0.299–15.355)	0.642	0.56 (0.11–2.8620	0.683
Shelter Resident		4 (13.8)	2 (6.9)	3 (10.3)	1.387 (0.282–6.83)	>0.99	0.642 (0.099–4.159)	>0.99	2.16 (0.363–12.84)	0.670
Recent exposure to healthcare environments and/or settings										
Recent Hospitalization (<3 months)		6 (20.7)	1 (3.4)	0 (0)	1.3 (1.053–1.605)	**0.023**	1.036 (0.967–1.109)	>0.99	7.304 (0.819–65.114)	0.102
Surgery Prior (<3 months) to the Date of Event [5]		16 (55.2)	12 (42.9)	0 (0)	2.231 (1.49–3.34)	**<0.001**	1.75 (1.27–2.412)	**<0.001**	1.641 (0.576–4.675)	0.352
Urologic Procedure During Hospitalization, Prior to the Date of Event [5]		14 (48.3)	11 (39.3)	2 (6.9)	12.6 (2.517–63.063)	**0.001**	8.735 (1.721–44.328)	**0.004**	1.442 (0.5.4–4.128)	0.494
Upper Airways Procedure During Hospitalization, Prior to the Date of Event [5]		9 (31)	3 (10.7)	1 (3.4)	12.6 (1.476–107.543)	**0.005**	3.36 (0.328–34.415)	0.352	3.75 (0.895–15.715)	0.06
Plasma Therapy During Hospitalization, Prior to the Date of Event [5]		10 (34.5)	4 (14.3)	0 (0)	1.526 (1.172–1.988)	**0.001**	1.167 (1.003–1.357)	0.052	3.281 (0.868–12.4)	0.116
Feeding/Nasogastric Tube During Hospitalization, Prior to the Date of Event [5]		16 (57.1)	14 (46.4)	9 (32.1)	2.815 (0.946–8.376)	0.06	1.83 (0617–5.423)	0.247	1.538 (0.536–4.416)	0.422
Prior MDRO [6] Isolation (<1 year)		2 (6.9)	0 (0)	0 (0)	1.074 (0.973–1.186)	0.491	a	a	1.074 (0.973–1.186)	0.492
Prior ESBL Isolation (<1 year)		0 (0)	0 (0)	0 (0)	a	a	a	a	a	a

Table 1. *Cont.*

Parameter	3GCRE [1] No. (Valid % [3])	3GCSE [2] No. (Valid % [3])	Uninfected No. (Valid % [1])	3GCRE vs. Uninfected		3GCSE vs. Uninfected		3GCRE vs. 3GCSE	
				OR (95% CI)	*p*-Value	OR (95% CI)	*p*-Value	OR (95% CI)	*p*-Value
Background conditions and co-morbidities prior to the date of event [3]									
Chronic Lung Disease	2 (6.9)	3 (10.3)	0 (0)	1.074 (0.973–1.186)	0.491	1.115 (0.986–1.262)	0.237	0.642 (0.099–4.159)	>0.99
Neurologic Disease [7]	6 (20.7)	1 (3.4)	4 (13.8)	1.63 (0.408–6.521)	0.487	0.223 (0.023–2.132)	0.352	7.304 (0.819–65.114)	0.102
Immunosuppression [8]	7 (24.1)	1 (3.6)	1 (3.4)	8.909 (1.019–77.905)	0.052	1.037 (0.062–17.429)	>0.99	8.591 (0.981–75.221)	0.052
Hyperlactatemia [9]	4 (66.7)	4 (40)	4 (36.4)	3.5 (0.431–28.447)	0.335	1.167 (0.2–6.805)	>0.99	3 (0.361–24.919)	0.608
Azotemia [10]	7 (25.9)	4 (40)	10 (35.7)	0.63 (0.198–2.003)	0.432	0.3 (0.0815–1.113)	0.064	2.1 (0.537–8.217)	0.281
Antimicrobial therapy prior (< 3 months) to the date of event [5]									
Any Antibiotic Treatment	28 (96.6)	20 (71.4)	3 (10.3)	242.667 (23.722–2482.349)	**<0.001**	21.667 (5.086–92.303)	**<0.001**	11.2 (1.296–96.787)	**0.012**
Penicillins	20 (71.4)	15 (53.6)	1 (3.4)	70 (8.1–604.917)	**<0.001**	32.308 (3.845–271.441)	**<0.001**	2.167 (0.717–6.55)	0.168
Fluoroquinolone	6 (21.4)	3 (11.1)	0 (0)	1.273 (1.049–1.544)	**0.01**	1.125 (0.985–1.285)	0.106	2.182 (0.486–9.796)	0.469
Aminoglycoside	23 (82.1)	9 (32.1)	1 (3.4)	128 (14.034–1182.052)	**<0.001**	13.263 (1.55–113.47)	**0.005**	9.711 (2.78–33.92)	**<0.001**
Polymyxin	6 (37.5)	9 (56.3)	0 (0)	1.6 (1.095–2.339)	**0.006**	2.286 (1.311–3.984)	**<0.001**	0.467 (0.113–1.92)	0.288
Metronidazole	4 (14.3)	5 (17.9)	0 (0)	1.167 (1.003–1.357)	0.052	1.217 (1.024–1.447)	**0.023**	0.767 (0.183–3.216)	>0.99
Cephalosporins	4 (14.3)	2 (7.1)	0 (0)	1.167 (1.003–1.357)	0.052	1.077 (0.972–1.193)	0.237	2.167 (0.363–12.922)	0.669
Acute illness indices at the date of event [5]									
Sepsis [11]	10 (34.5)	6 (20.7)	0 (0)	1.526 (1.172–1.988)	**0.001**	1.261 (1.047–1.518)	**0.023**	2.018 (0.62–6.569)	0.24

[1] 3GCRE: Third-generation cephalosporin-resistant *Enterobacterales*. [2] 3GCSE: Third-generation cephalosporin-susceptible *Enterobacterales*. [3] Data are presented as valid percent, i.e., after removing the missing values from the denominator. [4] Only adult males included. Neonates were not included. [5] The date of event was defined as the date on which the first sign or symptom of the infection was documented, or the date of culture among patients with no sign or symptom documentation. [6] Isolates were defined as multidrug-resistant based on established criteria [24]. [7] Neurologic disease included any of the following: perinatal asphyxia syndrome, meningitis and radial nerve paralysis. [8] Immunosuppression was defined if one of the following criteria was positive: neutropenia on admission (neutrophil count < 2.9 cells/µL [25]), corticosteroids treatment (<1 month) or chemotherapy (<3 months). [9] Hyperlactatemia was defined as blood lactate levels >2.06 mmol/dL [26]. [10] Azotemia was defined as a baseline creatinine >1.9 mg/dL [27]. [11] Sepsis was defined based on established criteria [25,28]. [a] Analysis cannot be computed since at least one of the values is missing.

2.3. Clinical Outcomes of 3GCRE Infections

In bivariable outcome analyses, 3GCRE infections were significantly associated with in-hospital mortality, 14-days mortality, 90-days mortality, 1-year mortality, upper airway procedure following the infection, surgery following the infection, and longer LOS (after excluding the patients who died), and was significantly associated with clinical failure (Table 2). In separate multivariable models for each of these variables, 3GCRE infection remained independently associated with failure of clinical cure (aOR = 6.84, 95% CI 1.919–24.39, $p = 0.003$), 90-days mortality (aOR = 3.623, 95% CI 1.107–11.863, $p = 0.003$) and with surgery following the infection (aOR = 3.364, 95% CI 1.169–9.685, $p = 0.025$). In a sub-analysis that included only patients with 3GCRE or 3GCSE infection, 3GCRE infection was independently and negatively associated with the administration of appropriate antibiotic therapy throughout the course of illness (OR = 0.041, 95% CI 0.009–0.187, $p < 0.001$), and in terms of the number of days for which the appropriate antimicrobials were administered ($p < 0.001$) (Table 2).

Table 2. Selected bivariable analyses comparing outcomes of patients with 3GCRE infection, patients with 3GCSE infections, and uninfected control patients (n = 29 in each group).

Parameter	3GCRE [1] No. (Valid % [1])	3GCSE [2] No. (Valid % [3])	Uninfected No. (Valid % [1])	3GCRE vs. Uninfected		3GCSE vs. Uninfected		3GCRE vs. 3GCSE	
				OR (95% CI)	p-Value	OR (95% CI)	p-Value	OR (95% CI)	p-Value
Total length of stay (LOS) after excluding the patients who died in hospital, days, median (range)	17.5 (2–181)	9 (2–59)	4 (2–17)		**<0.001**		**<0.001**		**0.027**
LOS from date of event [4] to discharge after excluding the patients who died in-hospital, days, median (range)	11.5 (1–181)	8 (0–59)	4 (2–17)		**0.002**		0.068		0.11
Additional hospitalization in the following 3 months	2 (10.5)	4 (17.4)	2 (8)	1.353 (0.173–10.592)	>0.99	2.421 (0.399–14.688)	0.407	0.559 (0.091–3.446)	0.673
Clinical failure [5]	14 (51.9)	6 (21.4)	1 (3.4)	**30.3 (3.57–250)**	**<0.001**	7.634 (0.855–66.667)	0.052	**3.77 (1.157–12.195)**	**0.024**
Bacteriological cure [10]	3 (60)	1 (50)		a	a	a	a	1.5 (0.055–40.633)	>0.99
Surgery following the date of event [4]	18 (64.3)	15 (57.7)	7 (26.9)	**4.725 (1.537–14.552)**	**0.005**	**3.231 (1.081–9.656)**	**0.033**	1.463 (0.504–4.24)	0.483
Urologic procedure following the date of event [4]	18 (62.1)	15 (57.7)	7 (26.9)	**4.295 (1.42–12.997)**	**0.008**	**3.231 (1.081–9.656)**	**0.033**	1.33 (0.466–3.792)	0.594
Upper airways procedures following the date of event [4]	5 (17.2)	12 (41.4)	13 (44.8)	0.256 (0.076–0.86)	**0.045**	0.869 (0.307–2.458)	0.791	**0.295 (0.088–0.994)**	**0.043**
Feeding tube/nasogastric tube following the date of event [4]	16 (59.3)	15 (55.6)	25 (86.2)	0.233 (0.063–0.858)	**0.023**	**0.2 (0.055–0.734)**	**0.011**	1.164 (0.395–3.425)	0.783
In hospital mortality	9 (31)	0 (10.3)	0 (0)	**1.45 (1.136–1.851)**	**0.002**	1.083 (0.97–1.21)	0.49	3.9 (0.933–16.31)	0.052
14-days mortality [6]	8 (30.8)	4 (16)	0 (0)	**1.444 (1.118–1.866)**	**0.004**	1.19 (1.003–1.413)	0.11	2.333 (0.602–9.049)	0.214
90-days mortality [6]	12 (48)	5 (20.8)	2 (8)	**8.462 (1.61–44.53)**	**0.002**	3.026 (0.527–17.394)	0.247	3.257 (0.932–11.38)	0.059
1-year mortality [6,7]	11 (47.8)	5 (20.8)	5 (18.5)	**4.062 (1.166–14.154)**	**0.024**	1.158 (0.29–4.617)	>0.99	**3.508 (0.996–12.359)**	**0.046**
Appropriate therapy [8] (given 2 days before to 5 days after culture date)	3 (11.5)	19 (76)		a	a	a	a	**0.041 (0.009–0.187)**	**<0.001**
Days of appropriate therapy [8], median (range)/mean ± SD	0 (0–16)	7.1±5.9		a	a	a	a		**<0.001**
Days to appropriate therapy [8], median (range)	0 (0–1)	0 (0–5)		a	a	a	a		0.929

[1] 3GCRE: Third-generation cephalosporin-resistant *Enterobacterales*. [2] 3GCSE: Third-generation cephalosporin-susceptible *Enterobacterales*. [3] Data are presented as valid percent, i.e., after removing the missing values from the denominator. [4] The date of event was captured as the beginning of the first clinical sign or symptom which defines infection, which was associated with the culture of interest. [5] Clinical failure was defined as non-recovery (for infections, non-recovery from infectious syndrome; for uninfected, non-recovery from the disease leading to hospitalization). [6] Mortality from culture date. [7] One-year mortality data were captured following a telephone interview with the owner. [8] Appropriate therapy was defined according to in vitro susceptibilities (of the microbiology lab report). [a] Analysis cannot be computed since at least one of the values is missing.

2.4. GCRE Samples Description, Species Distribution and Resistance Rates

There were 39 3GCRE isolates, recovered from 32 clinical specimens, obtained from 29 patients. Twenty-one (65.6%) cultures were polymicrobial. Ten samples (31.25%) were collected from hospitalized equids during the first 48 hours of hospitalization, i.e., suggesting acquisition in the community [29]. The two most prevalent infectious syndromes were umbilical cord [30] and surgical-site infections (i.e., SSI; Figure 1). SSIs were following either laparotomy or orthopedic surgery (50% each). Of the 39 3GCRE isolates (Figure 2), the major pathogens were *Klebsiella* spp. (n = 14/39, 35.89%), *Enterobacter* spp. (n = 13/39, 33.33%), and *Escherichia coli* (n = 5/39, 12.82%). The resistance rates of the isolates to the commonly prescribed agents in veterinary medicine, in addition to β-lactams, are depicted in Figure 3. Nearly all isolates (38/39, 97.43%) were categorized as MDR organisms (MDRO) [24].

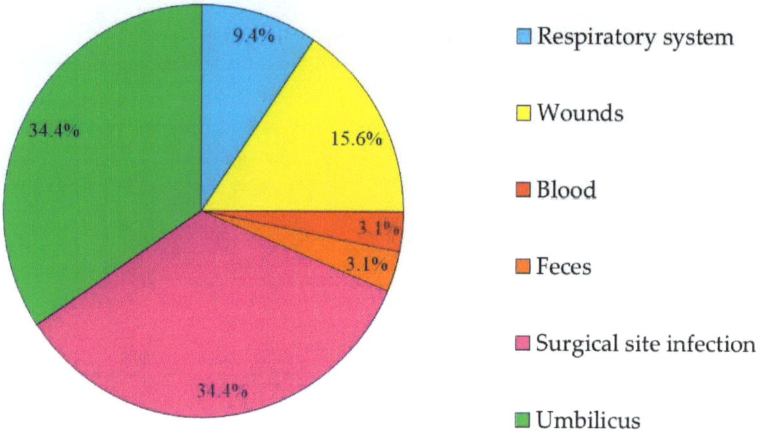

Figure 1. The distribution according to the source (body-site) from which the 3GCRE pathogen was isolated (*n* = 32 cultures).

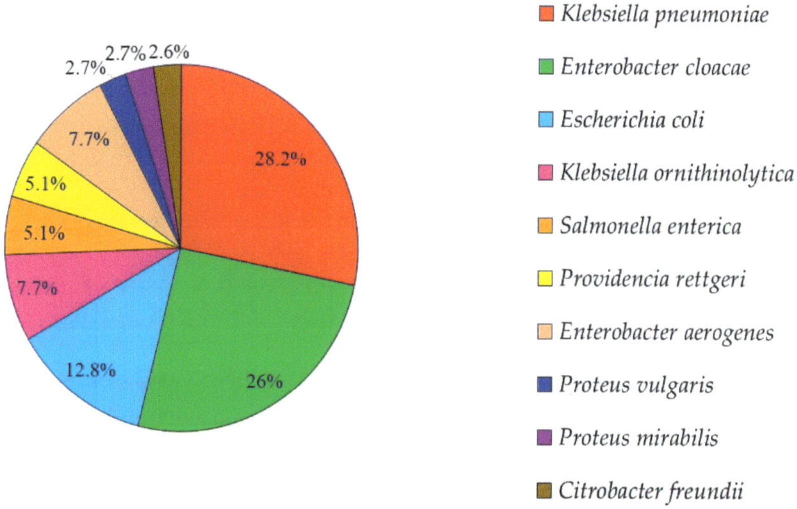

Figure 2. 3GCRE species distribution (*n* = 39 pathogens).

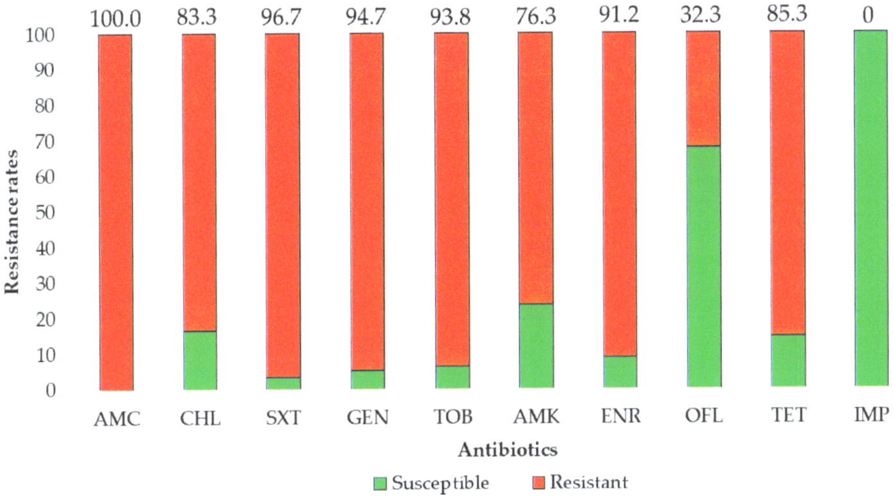

Figure 3. Resistance rates of 3GCRE pathogens (n = 39) towards commonly prescribed agents. AMC, amoxicillin-clavulonate; CHL, chloramphenicol; SXT, trimethoprim-sulfamethoxazole; GEN, gentamicin; TOB, tobramycin; AMK, amikacin; ENR, enrofloxacin; OFL, ofloxacin; TET, tetracycline; IMP, imipenem.

2.5. Molecular Characteristics of 3GCRE Isolates

Of the 39 3GCRE isolates, 26 (66.67%) were identified as ESBL producers via phenotypic tests. Nineteen of those (n = 19/26, 73.1%) were available for further molecular analyses. Of those, 17 isolates (89.5%) were $bla_{\text{CTX-M}}$ producers; i.e., the majority were $bla_{\text{CTX-M-1}}$ (n = 15/17, 88.2%), followed by $bla_{\text{CTX-M-9}}$ (n = 2/17, 11.8%).

The multi locus sequence type (MLST) of the three major species (*K. pneumoniae*, *E. cloacae*, *E. coli*) revealed the presence of polyclonality and diverse groups of sequence types (ST). The six *K. pneumoniae* isolates belonged to ST35 (umbilical infection, SSI—one isolate of each), ST13 (two isolates originated from umbilical infections), ST985 (one isolate from a wound), and ST528 (one isolate from an umbilicus). The three *E. coli* isolates were ST38 (blood), ST361 (umbilicus), and ST2179 (respiratory tract). The four *E. cloacae* were ST182 (wound), ST66 (respiratory tract), and ST254 and ST135 (umbilicus both).

3. Discussion

In 2016, the World Health Organization (WHO) declared infections resulting from MDRO to pose one of the major challenges and threats to humanity [31]. In equine medicine, the incidence of MDRO infections has risen exponentially in recent years [32], along with scrutiny, awareness and assessment for the proper usage of antimicrobials, infection control measures, the development of practice standards, and incorporating the routine use of clinical microbiology practices [33]. *Enterobacterales* are a major group of MDRO recognized by the WHO [31]. This group of pathogens became resistant to ESBL agents (i.e., 3GCRE), which are among the most common, efficacious and bactericidal antimicrobial agents. In order to implement established measures in infection control and antimicrobial stewardship (AMS), i.e., to curb the continued emergence and spread of these 3GCRE pathogens, detailed and controlled epidemiological analyses in veterinary hospitals are warranted. Therefore, a matched case–case–control investigation was executed in a large university-affiliated veterinary hospital, to explore the clinical and molecular epidemiology of 3GCRE infections among equids. The matched case–case–control design is considered today the "gold standard" methodology in investigating risk factors in the field of MDRO emergence and transmission. This design enables us to explore the independent predictors for the emergence of the MDRO, while controlling for multiple biases and confounders associated with "the infection"in general [23]. In order to tailor appropriately and implement a successful prevention strategy, a controlled analysis isolating the true independent predictors associated with the emergence of the resistance determinant per se is warranted.

In this case–case–control investigation, 29 animals (24 horses and 5 donkeys) with 3GCRE infection were matched to 29 animals with 3GCSE infections, and 29 uninfected controls (overall $n = 87$). In bivariable analyses (Table 1), there were multiple significant associations with 3GCRE infections, as compared to uninfected controls, e.g., recent hospitalizations, previous recent invasive procedures, plasma therapy, and recent exposure to antibiotics (specifically to penicillins, fluoroquinolones, aminoglycosides and polymyxins). In multivariable analysis, only exposure to antimicrobials remained an independent predictor of 3GCRE infection. However, in the multivariable model of 3GCSE infections vs. uninfected controls, exposure to antimicrobials was also the only independent predictor of 3GCSE infection, implying this is a predictor for infection in general, not a predictor for the emergence or acquisition of the resistance determinant. It must be noted though that the association with recent exposure to antimicrobials was much stronger among the 3GCRE group, and in a multivariable model of patients with 3GCRE infection vs. patients with 3GCSE infection, exposure to antimicrobials was an independent predictor for 3GCRE infection (aOR = 9.3, 95% CI 1.1–81).

In general, there are two modes by which an animal could acquire an MDRO: (1) patient-to-patient transmission (e.g., from another animal, through staff, from the proximal environment, from shared equipment); or (2) the emergence of resistance, wherein the susceptible isolates that patients harbor acquire resistance mechanisms through mobile genetic elements (e.g., ESBL), or by expressing an MDR phenotype mediated by chromosomal genes due to certain stressors (e.g., AmpC) [34]. Preventing or curbing patient-to-patient transmission in human medicine is achieved through barrier precautions and infection control practices, e.g., hand hygiene, isolation precautions, cohorting with dedicated staff, environmental cleaning, surveillance programs to identify asymptomatic carriage, and sometime decolonization protocols whenever relevant [34]. This is also relevant to equine medicine, and has received attention mainly due to outbreaks with methicillin-resistant *Staphylococcus aureus* (MRSA), which have the potential to result in zoonotic transmission to veterinary personnel and pet owners [35]. In such an outbreak, which occurred a decade ago in our hospital, the strict implementation of many of these measures resulted in the cessation of the outbreak, and indeed six months after the intervention, both personnel and hospitalized horses were all MRSA-negative, and the intervention was considered successful [36]. In contrast, tackling the emergence of resistance requires the enforcing of adherence to AMS policies and programs, which is also relevant in equine medicine where the implementation of AMS is required, and indeed is evolving, although much more is required [32]. The fact that exposure to antibiotics was the only independent predictor associated with infection in general, and specifically with 3GCRE infection, implies that stewardship guidelines and practices are not yet sufficiently implemented. As depicted in the results, over 31% of the animals were admitted with 3GCRE infections from non-acute care settings, i.e., community-onset infections. This is not unexpected, since in a recent study, in the same veterinary hospital, on admission 19.6% of the horses were ESBL-PE shedders, and 20.8% of horses on farms were also ESBL-PE shedders [11]. This implies that AMS intervention, policies, monitoring and guidelines should be implemented in the community (horse farms and private practitioners) as well, in order to prevent the continued emergence and spread of resistances among animals (and humans). This study highlights again the importance of investing in AMS in veterinary medicine, specifically in community settings and farms.

There were multiple negative outcomes associated with 3GCRE infections in bivariate analyses (Table 2), as was previously reported in human studies [37]. Infections caused by 3GCRE were negatively associated with appropriate therapy administration and with the number of appropriate therapy days. In a recent human study, a delay in instituting appropriate therapy was an independent predictor for prolonged LOS, increased hospitalization costs, and mortality [38,39]. In our study, in multivariable separate models, 3GCRE was independently associated with a higher clinical failure rate, with surgery following the infection, and with 90-day mortality. This again emphasizes, as in the human studies [3], the epidemiological significance and relevance of 3GCRE infections in equine medicine.

Our findings reflect the complex molecular epidemiology and characteristics associated with 3GCRE infections among hospitalized equids. We have found a variety of bacterial species, i.e., 69% of samples were polymicrobial. In detailed molecular investigations, even the same bacteria which were analyzed belonged to multiple clones, including clones which were previously reported in equine isolates, e.g., *E. coli* sequence types (STs) 38, 361 [18] and 2179 [40], and *E. cloacae* STs 135 [41] and 254 [42]. Additional clones reported herein were previously reported among humans, but not among horses, i.e., *E. cloacae* STs 66 [43] and 182 [44], and *K. pneumoniae* STs 13, 35 [45], 528 [46] and 985 [47]. Some of these STs were identified as MDR international human clones. For example, *E. coli* ST38 is an emerging clone in Germany [48], *E. cloacae* ST66 was isolated from human hospitals in Japan, France, Spain and Israel [43], and *K. pneumoniae* ST35 was isolated from China and Yemen [49,50]. This ST dissemination has major implications for human medicine and the "one health" approach, due to the close human–horse proximities and interactions [51].

The most prevalent culture sites were the umbilicus and SSI. In human medicine, only a few reports describe 3GCRE umbilical infections [52–54]. In contrast, in neonatal foals, several studies have described or reported 3GCRE isolation from the umbilicus [16,18,55,56]. Umbilical remnant infections in foals can be successfully diagnosed and treated; however, they can also lead to potentially fatal complications by seeding bacteria to other parts of the body [57]. Umbilical remnant infection should always be considered in a foal with a patent urachus, which can be either acquired or congenital, and can act as an opening for bacterial invasion [57]. Care of the umbilical remnant and the environment in which the foal lives, the adequate passive transfer of immunity postpartum and intrauterine infection prepartum, are important factors in the development of umbilical remnant infection [57]. In terms of the pathophysiology, this resembles vertical transmission in humans, and highlights the fact that the neonate acquired the 3GCRE pathogen at birth (when labor occurred in outpatient settings), and not in healthcare. The management of umbilical infections is challenging among foals, due to the presumably low penetration of antibiotics into the infected tissue. This also promotes the emergence of resistance among offending isolates [55]. According to our knowledge, this is the first epidemiological investigation of 3GCRE infections among foals.

The study has several limitations. It is a retrospective chart-based study; therefore, some medical information may have been missing or incorrectly recorded. In addition, the study was conducted in a single center, and therefore the findings could not be generalizable automatically to other centers. The study also suffers from the small sample size of patients with 3GCRE infections; although the case–case–control design enabled us to increase somewhat its strength, many of the multivariable models were unstable, and this impacted the risk factors and outcomes analyses.

4. Materials and Methods

4.1. Study Design

A retrospective matched case–case–control investigation pertaining to horses and donkeys of all age groups was conducted at the Koret School of Veterinary Medicine, Veterinary Teaching Hospital (KSVM-VTH), Israel, from June 2017 to January 2019. KSVM-VTH is the only veterinary teaching hospital in Israel and has a large animal department that could contain up to 40 hospitalized horses. The study was approved by the Internal Research Committee of the KSVM-VTH, Israel (Protocol KSVM-VTH/15_2015). The investigation consisted of three groups of patients: (1) 3GCRE-infected patients, (2) 3GCSE-infected patients, and (3) uninfected control patients. Only the first 3GCRE for each patient was included in the final analysis (i.e., patient-unique cases). Resistant cases were defined as patients suffering from an infection (i.e., no asymptomatic carriers were included) due to an *Enterobacterales* spp., non-susceptible to ≥1 third-generation cephalosporines (e.g., ceftriaxone, ceftiofur, cefpodoxime, ceftazidime). Susceptible cases were defined as patients suffering from an infection caused by *Enterobacterales* spp., susceptible to all third-generation cephalosporins. The uninfected control group consisted of patients without any infectious syndrome, and with no *Enterobacterales* isolated. A 3GCSE case and an uninfected control were matched to each 3GCRE case (1:1:1 ratio). The matching criteria (in order of importance [23]) included the following: animal species (equine vs. assinus), bacterial species, age group (neonate/adult/geriatric), clinical syndrome, and time at risk (i.e., days from admission date to culture date). For uninfected controls, the time at risk was captured as the total length of stay [23]. A neonate was defined as an animal ≤30 days old [58] and a geriatric animal was defined as age ≥20 years [59]. The date of event was captured as the beginning of the first clinical sign or symptom of infection that was associated with the culture of interest. Appropriate therapy was defined as per the in vitro susceptibilities report given from 48 hours prior to the culture date and up to five days following the culture date [60]. Days to appropriate therapy were defined as the number of calendar days from culture to the first dose of "appropriate" therapy (as defined above). Data were extracted from medical records, including demographic data, recent exposures to health care environments and settings, background conditions, medical treatments, invasive procedures (in the past three months), empiric antibiotic regimens (i.e., from two days prior to culture date to three days following culture date), main antibiotic regimens (i.e., 3–14 days following culture date) and outcomes. Immunosuppression was defined as ≥1 of the following: neutropenia, or glucocorticoids/chemotherapy exposures in the previous three months. One-year mortality data were captured following a telephone interview with the owner.

4.2. Bacterial Isolates Collection, Identification and Susceptibility Testing

All study isolates were subjected to Vitek-2 (BioMérieux, Inc., Marcy-l'Etoile, France) for species identification and phenotypic susceptibility testing (AST-N270 Vitek 2 card). Susceptibility to ofloxacin and imipenem was determined by using the disc diffusion assay (Oxoid, Basingstoke, UK). ESBL production testing was determined according to the Clinical and Laboratory Standards Institute (CLSI) benchmarks and guidelines [61]. Isolates were defined as MDR based on established criteria [24].

4.3. Molecular Characterization of ESBL-PE

Isolates were examined for the presence of the $bla_{CTX\text{-}M}$ group by using a multiplex polymerase chain reaction (PCR) from ESBL-PE DNA lysates, as previously described [62]. Strains identified as *E. coli*, *K. pneumoniae* or *Enterobacter cloacae* were genotyped using an enterobacterial repetitive intergenic consensus (ERIC) PCR amplification using the following primer: 5-AAGTAAGTGACTGGGGTGAGCG-3′ [63]. Strains showing a distinct ERIC PCR pattern were further analyzed by MLST as previously described (IDGenomics, Seattle, WA, USA) [64–66].

4.4. Statistical Analyses

Statistical analyses were performed using SPSS software (IBM; Version 24; SPSS Inc., Chicago, IL, USA). Data distribution was determined according to the skewness, kurtosis, and the Shapiro–Wilk's test. Continuous variables were analyzed using t-tests or Mann–Whitney U-tests. Categorical variables were analyzed using the Fisher's exact test or the Pearson chi-square test. In all analyses, $p \leq 0.05$ indicated significance. Univariable and multivariable matched analyses determine the predictors of 3GCRE infection (vs. uninfected controls) and of 3GCSE infection (vs. uninfected controls). According to the case–case–control methodology, the eventual independent predictors of 3GCRE infection would be only those predictors associated with 3GCRE infection, but not with 3GCSE infection [23]. Logistic regression models were conducted by using the backwards stepwise method. Univariable and multivariable outcomes analyses (logistic regression) were conducted while enforcing the case type parameter (i.e., the 3GCRE group vs. the groups of 3GCSE and of the uninfected controls combined) in each outcome model.

5. Conclusions

This case–case–control study reveals and quantifies the clinical and epidemiological importance and significance of 3GCRE infections in equine medicine, and in equine hospitals. Larger studies in additional centers and countries are warranted. Antibiotic stewardship programs, both in hospitals and community settings, are mandatory in order to curb the continued dissemination and spread of 3GCRE pathogens.

Supplementary Materials: The following are available online at https://www.mdpi.com/2079-6382/10/2/155/s1. Table S1: Descriptive statistics for the entire study population (n = 1620 horses and donkeys).

Author Contributions: Conceptualization: A.S., S.N.-V. and A.S.-T.; methodology: D.M., Y.P., H.A., A.S.-T.; software: D.M., A.S.-T.; validation: A.S., S.N.-V. and A.S.-T.; formal analysis: A.S., S.N.-V. and A.S.-T.; investigation: A.S.-T., O.L.; resources: A.S., S.N.-V., and Y.P.; data curation: A.S.-T., O.L.; writing—original draft preparation: A.S.-T., A.S., S.N.-V., D.M; writing—review and editing: all authors; visualization: A.S., S.N.-V., D.M. and A.S.-T.; supervision, project administration and funding acquisition: A.S., S.N.-V. and D.M. All authors have read and agreed to the published version of the manuscript.

Funding: This research received no external funding.

Institutional Review Board Statement: The study was approved by the Internal Research Committee of the KSVM-VTH, Israel (Protocol KSVM-VTH/15_2015).

Informed Consent Statement: Not applicable.

Data Availability Statement: Data is contained within the article or Supplementary Material.

Acknowledgments: The authors would like to thank the clinicians and technicians of the Koret School of Veterinary Medicine—Veterinary Teaching Hospital, large animal department for their assistance in sample collection.

Conflicts of Interest: The authors declare no conflict of interest.

References

1. Singh, R.; Singh, A.P.; Kumar, S.; Giri, B.S.; Kim, K.-H. Antibiotic Resistance in Major Rivers in the World: A Systematic Review on Occurrence, Emergence, and Management Strategies. *J. Clean. Prod.* **2019**, *234*, 1484–1505. [CrossRef]
2. Lee, J.H.; Bae, I.K.; Lee, S.H. New Definitions of Extended-Spectrum β-Lactamase Conferring Worldwide Emerging Antibiotic Resistance. *Med. Res. Rev.* **2012**, *32*, 216–232. [CrossRef] [PubMed]
3. Schwaber, M.J.; Carmeli, Y. Mortality and Delay in Effective Therapy Associated with Extended-Spectrum Beta-Lactamase Production in Enterobacteriaceae Bacteraemia: A Systematic Review and Meta-Analysis. *J. Antimicrob. Chemother.* **2007**, *60*, 913–920. [CrossRef]
4. Paul, M.; Shani, V.; Muchtar, E.; Kariv, G.; Robenshtok, E.; Leibovici, L. Systematic Review and Meta-Analysis of the Efficacy of Appropriate Empiric Antibiotic Therapy for Sepsis. *Antimicrob. Agents Chemother.* **2010**, *54*, 4851–4863. [CrossRef]
5. Biehl, L.M.; Schmidt-Hieber, M.; Liss, B.; Cornely, O.A.; Vehreschild, M.J.G.T. Colonization and Infection with Extended Spectrum Beta-Lactamase Producing Enterobacteriaceae in High-Risk Patients - Review of the Literature from a Clinical Perspective. *Crit. Rev. Microbiol.* **2016**, *42*, 1–16. [CrossRef] [PubMed]
6. Coque, T.M.; Baquero, F.; Cantón, R. Increasing Prevalence of ESBL-Producing Enterobacteriaceae in Europe. *Eurosurveillance* **2008**, *13*, 19044.
7. Dupouy, V.; Abdelli, M.; Moyano, G.; Arpaillange, N.; Bibbal, D.; Cadiergues, M.-C.; Lopez-Pulin, D.; Sayah-Jeanne, S.; de Gunzburg, J.; Saint-Lu, N.; et al. Prevalence of Beta-Lactam and Quinolone/Fluoroquinolone Resistance in Enterobacteriaceae From Dogs in France and Spain—Characterization of ESBL/PAmpC Isolates, Genes, and Conjugative Plasmids. *Front. Vet. Sci.* **2019**, *6*, 279. [CrossRef]
8. World Organization for Animal Health. Available online: https://www.oie.int/scientific-expertise/veterinary-products/antimicrobials/ (accessed on 17 January 2021).

9. Walther, B.; Tedin, K.; Lübke-Becker, A. Multidrug-Resistant Opportunistic Pathogens Challenging Veterinary Infection Control. *Vet. Microbiol.* **2017**, *200*, 71–78. [CrossRef] [PubMed]
10. Steinman, A.; Navon-Venezia, S. Antimicrobial Resistance in Horses. *Animals* **2020**, *10*, 1161. [CrossRef]
11. Shnaiderman-Torban, A.; Navon-Venezia, S.; Dor, Z.; Paitan, Y.; Arielly, H.; Abu Ahmad, W.; Kelmer, G.; Fulde, M.; Steinman, A. Extended-Spectrum β-Lactamase-Producing Enterobacteriaceae Shedding in Farm Horses Versus Hospitalized Horses: Prevalence and Risk Factors. *Animals* **2020**, *10*, 282. [CrossRef] [PubMed]
12. de Lagarde, M.; Fairbrother, J.M.; Arsenault, J. Prevalence, Risk Factors, and Characterization of Multidrug Resistant and ESBL/AmpC Producing Escherichia Coli in Healthy Horses in Quebec, Canada, in 2015–2016. *Animals* **2020**, *10*, 523. [CrossRef] [PubMed]
13. Hordijk, J.; Farmakioti, E.; Smit, L.A.M.; Duim, B.; Graveland, H.; Theelen, M.J.P.; Wagenaar, J.A. Fecal Carriage of Extended-Spectrum-β-Lactamase/AmpC-Producing Escherichia Coli in Horses. *Appl. Environ. Microbiol.* **2020**, *86*. [CrossRef]
14. Sukamawinata, E.; Sato, W.; Mitoma, S.; Kanda, T.; Kusano, K.; Kambayashi, Y.; Sato, T.; Ishikawa, Y.; Goto, Y.; Uemura, R.; et al. Extended-Spectrum β-Lactamase-Producing Escherichia Coli Isolated from Healthy Thoroughbred Racehorses in Japan. *J. Equine Sci.* **2019**, *30*, 47–53. [CrossRef] [PubMed]
15. Anyanwu, M.U.; Ugwu, I.C.; Onah, C.U. Occurrence and Antibiogram of Generic Extended-Spectrum Cephalosporin-Resistant and Extended-Spectrum β-Lactamase-Producing Enterobacteria In Horses. *Maced. Vet. Rev.* **2018**, *41*, 123–132. [CrossRef]
16. Shnaiderman-Torban, A.; Paitan, Y.; Arielly, H.; Kondratyeva, K.; Tirosh-Levy, S.; Abells-Sutton, G.; Navon-Venezia, S.; Steinman, A. Extended-Spectrum β-Lactamase-Producing Enterobacteriaceae in Hospitalized Neonatal Foals: Prevalence, Risk Factors for Shedding and Association with Infection. *Animals* **2019**, *9*, 600. [CrossRef]
17. Schoster, A.; van Spijk, J.; Damborg, P.; Moodley, A.; Kirchgaessner, C.; Hartnack, S.; Schmitt, S. The Effect of Different Antimicrobial Treatment Regimens on the Faecal Shedding of ESBL-Producing Escherichia Coli in Horses. *Vet. Microbiol.* **2020**, *243*, 108617. [CrossRef]
18. Shnaiderman-Torban, A.; Navon-Venezia, S.; Dahan, R.; Dor, Z.; Taulescu, M.; Paitan, Y.; Edery, N.; Steinman, A. CTX-M-15 Producing Escherichia Coli Sequence Type 361 and Sequence Type 38 Causing Bacteremia and Umbilical Infection in a Neonate Foal. *J. Equine Vet. Sci.* **2020**, *85*, 102881. [CrossRef] [PubMed]
19. Loncaric, I.; Cabal Rosel, A.; Szostak, M.P.; Licka, T.; Allerberger, F.; Ruppitsch, W.; Spergser, J. Broad-Spectrum Cephalosporin-Resistant Klebsiella Spp. Isolated from Diseased Horses in Austria. *Animals* **2020**, *10*, 332. [CrossRef] [PubMed]
20. Hann, M.; Timofte, D.; Isgren, C.M.; Archer, D.C. Bacterial Translocation in Horses with Colic and the Potential Association with Surgical Site Infection: A Pilot Study. *Vet. Rec.* **2020**, *187*, 68. [CrossRef] [PubMed]
21. Walther, B.; Klein, K.-S.; Barton, A.-K.; Semmler, T.; Huber, C.; Wolf, S.A.; Tedin, K.; Merle, R.; Mitrach, F.; Guenther, S.; et al. Extended-Spectrum Beta-Lactamase (ESBL)-Producing Escherichia Coli and Acinetobacter Baumannii among Horses Entering a Veterinary Teaching Hospital: The Contemporary "Trojan Horse". *PLOS ONE* **2018**, *13*, e0191873. [CrossRef]
22. Gilbertie, J.M.; Schnabel, L.V.; Stefanovski, D.; Kelly, D.J.; Jacob, M.E.; Schaer, T.P. Gram-Negative Multi-Drug Resistant Bacteria Influence Survival to Discharge for Horses with Septic Synovial Structures: 206 Cases (2010–2015). *Vet. Microbiol.* **2018**, *226*, 64–73. [CrossRef] [PubMed]
23. Kaye, K.S.; Harris, A.D.; Samore, M.; Carmeli, Y. The Case–case–control Study Design: Addressing the Limitations of Risk Factor Studies for Antimicrobial Resistance. *Infect. Control Hosp. Epidemiol.* **2005**, *26*, 346–351. [CrossRef]
24. Magiorakos, A.-P.; Srinivasan, A.; Carey, R.B.; Carmeli, Y.; Falagas, M.E.; Giske, C.G.; Harbarth, S.; Hindler, J.F.; Kahlmeter, G.; Olsson-Liljequist, B.; et al. Multidrug-Resistant, Extensively Drug-Resistant and Pandrug-Resistant Bacteria: An International Expert Proposal for Interim Standard Definitions for Acquired Resistance. *Clin. Microbiol. Infect. Off. Publ. Eur. Soc. Clin. Microbiol. Infect. Dis.* **2012**, *18*, 268–281. [CrossRef]
25. Sheats, M.K. A Comparative Review of Equine SIRS, Sepsis, and Neutrophils. *Front. Vet. Sci.* **2019**, *6*, 69. [CrossRef] [PubMed]
26. Roy, M.-F.; Kwong, G.P.S.; Lambert, J.; Massie, S.; Lockhart, S. Prognostic Value and Development of a Scoring System in Horses With Systemic Inflammatory Response Syndrome. *J. Vet. Intern. Med.* **2017**, *31*, 582–592. [CrossRef] [PubMed]
27. Savage, V.L.; Marr, C.M.; Bailey, M.; Smith, S. Prevalence of Acute Kidney Injury in a Population of Hospitalized Horses. *J. Vet. Intern. Med.* **2019**, *33*, 2294–2301. [CrossRef]
28. Brewer, B.D.; Koterba, A.M.; Carter, R.L.; Rowe, E.D. Comparison of Empirically Developed Sepsis Score with a Computer Generated and Weighted Scoring System for the Identification of Sepsis in the Equine Neonate. *Equine Vet. J.* **1988**, *20*, 23–24. [CrossRef]
29. Edwardson, S.; Cairns, C. Nosocomial Infections in the ICU. *Anaesth. Intensive Care Med.* **2019**, *20*, 14–18. [CrossRef]
30. Oreff, G.L.; Tatz, A.J.; Dahan, R.; Segev, G.; Berlin, D.; Kelmer, G. Surgical Management and Long-Term Outcome of Umbilical Infection in 65 Foals (2010–2015). *Vet. Surg.* **2017**, *46*, 962–970. [CrossRef]
31. Willyard, C. The Drug-Resistant Bacteria That Pose the Greatest Health Threats. *Nature* **2017**, *543*, 15. [CrossRef]
32. Weese, J.S. Antimicrobial Use and Antimicrobial Resistance in Horses. *Equine Vet. J.* **2015**, *47*, 747–749. [CrossRef]
33. Prescott, J.F. Outpacing the Resistance Tsunami: Antimicrobial Stewardship in Equine Medicine, an Overview. *Equine Vet. Educ.* **2020**. [CrossRef]
34. Adler, A.; Friedman, N.D.; Marchaim, D. Multidrug-Resistant Gram-Negative Bacilli: Infection Control Implications. *Infect. Dis. Clin. N. Am.* **2016**, *30*, 967–997. [CrossRef]
35. Singh, A.; Walker, M.; Rousseau, J.; Monteith, G.J.; Weese, J.S. Methicillin-Resistant Staphylococcal Contamination of Clothing Worn by Personnel in a Veterinary Teaching Hospital. *Vet. Surg. VS* **2013**, *42*, 643–648. [CrossRef]

36. Schwaber, M.J.; Navon-Venezia, S.; Masarwa, S.; Tirosh-Levy, S.; Adler, A.; Chmelnitsky, I.; Carmeli, Y.; Klement, E.; Steinman, A. Clonal Transmission of a Rare Methicillin-Resistant Staphylococcus Aureus Genotype between Horses and Staff at a Veterinary Teaching Hospital. *Vet. Microbiol.* **2013**, *162*, 907–911. [CrossRef]
37. Gallagher, J.C.; Kuriakose, S.; Haynes, K.; Axelrod, P. Case–case–control Study of Patients with Carbapenem-Resistant and Third-Generation-Cephalosporin-Resistant Klebsiella Pneumoniae Bloodstream Infections. *Antimicrob. Agents Chemother.* **2014**, *58*, 5732–5735. [CrossRef] [PubMed]
38. Bonine, N.G.; Berger, A.; Altincatal, A.; Wang, R.; Bhagnani, T.; Gillard, P.; Lodise, T. Impact of Delayed Appropriate Antibiotic Therapy on Patient Outcomes by Antibiotic Resistance Status From Serious Gram-Negative Bacterial Infections. *Am. J. Med. Sci.* **2019**, *357*, 103–110. [CrossRef]
39. Tacconelli, E.; Cataldo, M.A.; Mutters, N.T.; Carrara, E.; Bartoloni, A.; Raglio, A.; Cauda, R.; Mantengoli, E.; Luzzaro, F.; Pan, A.; et al. Role of Place of Acquisition and Inappropriate Empirical Antibiotic Therapy on the Outcome of Extended-Spectrum β-Lactamase-Producing Enterobacteriaceae Infections. *Int. J. Antimicrob. Agents* **2019**, *54*, 49–54. [CrossRef] [PubMed]
40. Leigue, L.; Warth, J.F.G.; Melo, L.C.; Silva, K.C.; Moura, R.A.; Barbato, L.; Silva, L.C.; Santos, A.C.M.; Silva, R.M.; Lincopan, N. MDR ST2179-CTX-M-15 Escherichia Coli Co-Producing RmtD and AAC(6′)-Ib-Cr in a Horse with Extraintestinal Infection, Brazil. *J. Antimicrob. Chemother.* **2015**, *70*, 1263–1265. [CrossRef]
41. Haenni, M.; Saras, E.; Ponsin, C.; Dahmen, S.; Petitjean, M.; Hocquet, D.; Madec, J.-Y. High Prevalence of International ESBL CTX-M-15-Producing Enterobacter Cloacae ST114 Clone in Animals. *J. Antimicrob. Chemother.* **2016**, *71*, 1497–1500. [CrossRef]
42. Börjesson, S.; Greko, C.; Myrenås, M.; Landén, A.; Nilsson, O.; Pedersen, K. A Link between the Newly Described Colistin Resistance Gene Mcr-9 and Clinical Enterobacteriaceae Isolates Carrying BlaSHV-12 from Horses in Sweden. *J. Glob. Antimicrob. Resist.* **2020**, *20*, 285–289. [CrossRef] [PubMed]
43. Izdebski, R.; Baraniak, A.; Herda, M.; Fiett, J.; Bonten, M.J.M.; Carmeli, Y.; Goossens, H.; Hryniewicz, W.; Brun-Buisson, C.; Gniadkowski, M. MLST Reveals Potentially High-Risk International Clones of Enterobacter Cloacae. *J. Antimicrob. Chemother.* **2015**, *70*, 48–56. [CrossRef]
44. Torres-González, P.; Valle, M.B.; Tovar-Calderón, E.; Leal-Vega, F.; Hernández-Cruz, A.; Martínez-Gamboa, A.; Niembro-Ortega, M.D.; Sifuentes-Osornio, J.; Ponce-de-León, A. Outbreak Caused by Enterobacteriaceae Harboring NDM-1 Metallo-β-Lactamase Carried in an IncFII Plasmid in a Tertiary Care Hospital in Mexico City. *Antimicrob. Agents Chemother.* **2015**, *59*, 7080–7083. [CrossRef]
45. Marcade, G.; Brisse, S.; Bialek, S.; Marcon, E.; Leflon-Guibout, V.; Passet, V.; Moreau, R.; Nicolas-Chanoine, M.-H. The Emergence of Multidrug-Resistant Klebsiella Pneumoniae of International Clones ST13, ST16, ST35, ST48 and ST101 in a Teaching Hospital in the Paris Region. *Epidemiol. Infect.* **2013**, *141*, 1705–1712. [CrossRef]
46. Nagasaka, Y.; Kimura, K.; Yamada, K.; Wachino, J.-I.; Jin, W.; Notake, S.; Yanagisawa, H.; Arakawa, Y. Genetic Profiles of Fluoroquinolone-Nonsusceptible Klebsiella Pneumoniae Among Cephalosporin-Resistant K. Pneumoniae. *Microb. Drug Resist.* **2014**, *21*, 224–233. [CrossRef]
47. Loucif, L.; Kassah-Laouar, A.; Saidi, M.; Messala, A.; Chelaghma, W.; Rolain, J.-M. Outbreak of OXA-48-Producing Klebsiella Pneumoniae Involving a Sequence Type 101 Clone in Batna University Hospital, Algeria. *Antimicrob. Agents Chemother.* **2016**, *60*, 7494–7497.
48. Kremer, K.; Kramer, R.; Neumann, B.; Haller, S.; Pfennigwerth, N.; Werner, G.; Gatermann, S.; Schroten, H.; Eckmanns, T.; Hans, J.B. Rapid Spread of OXA-244-Producing Escherichia Coli ST38 in Germany: Insights from an Integrated Molecular Surveillance Approach; 2017 to January 2020. *Eurosurveillance* **2020**, *25*, 2000923. [CrossRef]
49. Alsharapy, S.A.; Gharout-Sait, A.; Muggeo, A.; Guillard, T.; Cholley, P.; Brasme, L.; Bertrand, X.; Moghram, G.S.; Touati, A.; De Champs, C. Characterization of Carbapenem-Resistant Enterobacteriaceae Clinical Isolates in Al Thawra University Hospital, Sana'a, Yemen. *Microb. Drug Resist.* **2019**, *26*, 211–217. [CrossRef]
50. Shen, Z.; Gao, Q.; Qin, J.; Liu, Y.; Li, M. Emergence of an NDM-5-Producing Hypervirulent Klebsiella Pneumoniae Sequence Type 35 Strain with Chromosomal Integration of an Integrative and Conjugative Element, ICEKp1. *Antimicrob. Agents Chemother.* **2020**, *64*, e01675-19. [CrossRef]
51. Royden, A.; Ormandy, E.; Pinchbeck, G.; Pascoe, B.; Hitchings, M.D.; Sheppard, S.K.; Williams, N.J. Prevalence of Faecal Carriage of Extended-Spectrum β-Lactamase (ESBL)-Producing Escherichia Coli in Veterinary Hospital Staff and Students. *Vet. Rec. Open* **2019**, *6*, e000307. [CrossRef]
52. Uzunović, S.; Ibrahimagić, A.; Hodžić, D.; Bedenić, B. Molecular Epidemiology and Antimicrobial Susceptibility of AmpC- and/or Extended-Spectrum (ESBL) ß-Lactamaseproducing Proteus Spp. Clinical Isolates in Zenica-Doboj Canton, Bosnia and Herzegovina. *Med. Glas. Off. Publ. Med. Assoc. Zenica-Doboj Cant. Bosnia Herzeg.* **2016**, *13*, 103–112.
53. Uzunović, S.; Bedenić, B.; Budimir, A.; Kamberović, F.; Ibrahimagić, A.; Delić-Bikić, S.; Sivec, S.; Meštrović, T.; Varda Brkić, D.; Rijnders, M.I.A.; et al. Emergency (Clonal Spread) of Methicillin-Resistant Staphylococcus Aureus (MRSA), Extended Spectrum (ESBL)—And AmpC Beta-Lactamase-Producing Gram-Negative Bacteria Infections at Pediatric Department, Bosnia and Herzegovina. *Wien. Klin. Wochenschr.* **2014**, *126*, 747–756. [CrossRef] [PubMed]
54. Kaftandzhieva, A.; Kotevska, V.; Jankoska, G.; Kjurcik-Trajkovska, B.; Cekovska, Z.; Petrovska, M. Extended-Spectrum Beta-Lactamase-Producing E. Coli and Klebsiella Pneumoniae in Children at University Pediatric Clinic in Skopje. *Maced. J. Med. Sci.* **2009**, *2*, 36–41. [CrossRef]
55. Rampacci, E.; Passamonti, F.; Bottinelli, M.; Stefanetti, V.; Cercone, M.; Nannarone, S.; Gialletti, R.; Beccati, F.; Coletti, M.; Pepe, M. Umbilical Infections in Foals: Microbiological Investigation and Management. *Vet. Rec.* **2017**, *180*, 543-543. [CrossRef]

56. Willis, A.T.; Magdesian, K.G.; Byrne, B.A.; Edman, J.M. Enterococcus Infections in Foals. *Vet. J. Lond. Engl. 1997* **2019**, *248*, 42–47. [CrossRef]
57. Elce, Y.A. Infections in the equine abdomen and pelvis: Perirectal abscesses, umbilical infections, and peritonitis. *Vet. Clin. North Am. Equine Pract.* **2006**, *22*, 419–436. [CrossRef]
58. Wohlfender, F.D.; Barrelet, F.E.; Doherr, M.G.; Straub, R.; Meier, H.P. Diseases in Neonatal Foals. Part 1: The 30 Day Incidence of Disease and the Effect of Prophylactic Antimicrobial Drug Treatment during the First Three Days Post Partum. *Equine Vet. J.* **2009**, *41*, 179–185. [CrossRef]
59. McGowan, C. Welfare of Aged Horses. *Animals* **2011**, *1*, 366–376. [CrossRef]
60. Pogue, J.M.; Kaye, K.S.; Cohen, D.A.; Marchaim, D. Appropriate Antimicrobial Therapy in the Era of Multidrug-Resistant Human Pathogens. *Clin. Microbiol. Infect.* **2015**, *21*, 302–312. [CrossRef]
61. CLSI. *Autoverification of Medical Laboratory Results for Specific Disciplines*, 1st ed.; CLSI Guideline AUTO15; Clinical and Laboratory Standards Institute: Wayne, PA, USA, 2019.
62. Woodford, N.; Fagan, E.J.; Ellington, M.J. Multiplex PCR for Rapid Detection of Genes Encoding CTX-M Extended-Spectrum β-Lactamases. *J. Antimicrob. Chemother.* **2006**, *57*, 154–155. [CrossRef]
63. Versalovic, J.; Koeuth, T.; Lupski, J.R. Distribution of Repetitive DNA Sequences in Eubacteria and Application to Fingerprinting of Bacterial Genomes. *Nucleic Acids Res.* **1991**, *19*, 6823–6831. [CrossRef]
64. Miyoshi-Akiyama, T.; Hayakawa, K.; Ohmagari, N.; Shimojima, M.; Kirikae, T. Multilocus Sequence Typing (MLST) for Characterization of Enterobacter Cloacae. *PLoS ONE* **2013**, *8*, e66358. [CrossRef]
65. Diancourt, L.; Passet, V.; Verhoef, J.; Grimont, P.A.D.; Brisse, S. Multilocus Sequence Typing of Klebsiella Pneumoniae Nosocomial Isolates. *J. Clin. Microbiol.* **2005**, *43*, 4178–4182. [CrossRef]
66. Wirth, T.; Falush, D.; Lan, R.; Colles, F.; Mensa, P.; Wieler, L.H.; Karch, H.; Reeves, P.R.; Maiden, M.C.J.; Ochman, H.; et al. Sex and Virulence in Escherichia Coli: An Evolutionary Perspective. *Mol. Microbiol.* **2006**, *60*, 1136–1151. [CrossRef] [PubMed]

antibiotics

MDPI

Article

The Spectrum of Antimicrobial Activity of Cyadox against Pathogens Collected from Pigs, Chicken, and Fish in China

Muhammad Kashif Maan, Zhifei Weng, Menghong Dai, Zhenli Liu, Haihong Hao, Guyue Cheng, Yulian Wang, Xu Wang and Lingli Huang *

National Reference Laboratory of Veterinary Drμg Residues/MOA Key Laboratory of Food Safety Evaluation, Huazhong Agricultural University, Wuhan 430070, China; kashif.maan@uvas.edu.pk (M.K.M.); hzauwengzhifei@163.com (Z.W.); daimenghong@mail.hzau.edu.cn (M.D.); liuzhli009@mail.hzau.edu.cn (Z.L.); haohaihong@mail.hzau.edu.cn (H.H.); chengguyue@mail.hzau.edu.cn (G.C.); wangyulian@mail.hzau.edu.cn (Y.W.); wangxu@mail.hzau.edu.cn (X.W.)
* Correspondence: huanglingli@mail.hzau.edu.cn

Abstract: Cyadox has potential use as an antimicrobial agent in animals. However, its pharmacodynamic properties have not been systematically studied yet. In this study, the in vitro antibacterial activities of cyadox were assayed, and the antibacterial efficacy of cyadox against facultative anaerobes was also determined under anaerobic conditions. It was shown that *Clostridium perfringens* and *Pasteurella multocida* (MIC = 0.25 and 1 μg/mL) from pigs, *Campylobacter jejuni* and *Pasteurella multocida* from poultry, *E. coli*, *Streptococcus* spp., and *Flavobacterium columnare* from fish were highly susceptible to cyadox (MIC= 1 and 8 μg/mL). However, *F. columnare* has no killing effect for drug tolerance. Under in vitro anaerobic conditions, the antibacterial activity of cyadox against most facultative anaerobes was considerably enhanced Under anaerobic conditions for the facultative anaerobes, susceptible bacteria were *P. multocida*, *Aeromonas spp.* (including *A. hydrophila*, *A. veronii*, *A. jandaei*, *A. caviae*, and *A. sobria*, excluding *A. punctata*), *E. coli*, *Salmonella* spp. (including *S. choleraesui*, *S. typhimurium*, and *S. pullorum*), *Proteus mirabilis*, *Vibrio fluvialis*, *Yersinia ruckeri*, *Erysipelothrix*, *Acinetobacter baumannii*, and *Streptococcus agalactiae* (MICs were 0.25~8 μg/mL, MBCs were 1–64 μg/mL). Intermediate bacteria were *Enterococcus* spp. (including *E. faecalis* and *E. faecium*), *Yersinia enterocolitica*, and *Streptococcus* spp. (MICs mainly were 8~32 μg/mL, MBCs were 16~128 μg/mL). This study firstly showed that cyadox had strong antibacterial activity and had the potential to be used as a single drug in the treatment of bacterial infectious diseases.

Keywords: cyadox; antimicrobial activity; pathogenic bacteria; clinical breakpoints

Citation: Maan, M.K.; Weng, Z.; Dai, M.; Liu, Z.; Hao, H.; Cheng, G.; Wang, Y.; Wang, X.; Huang, L. The Spectrum of Antimicrobial Activity of Cyadox against Pathogens Collected from Pigs, Chicken, and Fish in China. *Antibiotics* **2021**, *10*, 153. https://doi.org/10.3390/antibiotics10020153

Academic Editors: Nikola Puvača, Chantal Britt and Jonathan Gómez-Raja

Received: 22 December 2020
Accepted: 28 January 2021
Published: 3 February 2021

1. Introduction

Cyadox is a synthetic compound belonging to quinoxaline-1,4-dioxides, which are widely used as an antibacterial agent with a broad spectrum of antimicrobial activity and growth promoters in veterinary medicine [1]. Compared with the other members of quinoxalines such as carbadox and olaquindox, the cyadox is safer [2–5] according to the long term toxicity test, a subchronic oral toxicity test, and a phototoxicity test of cyadox in previous studies [6] and can promote the growth of different animals with more obvious effects such as better growth-enhancing functions in food-producing animals including fish, goats, pigs and poultry with less toxic effects than olaquindox, when used as feed additive [7] in animal feed. Moreover, further studies have demonstrated that cyadox was better as a growth promotor if compared with carbadox and olaquindox [8]. Since carbadox and olaquindox have been banned or limited to be used in food animals due to their toxicities, making cyadox as a substitution product having a capacious prospect in animal husbandry and aquaculture. Cyadox has excellent pharmacokinetic characteristics. Previous studies have shown the distribution and metabolism of Cyadox in swine, and six major metabolites were identified as follows: Disdesoxy- Cyadox (Cy1), Cyadox 4-monoxide (Cy2), N-decyanoacetyl Cyadox (Cy4), Quinocaline-2-carboxylic acid (Cy6), 11, 12-dihydro-bisdesoxycaydox (Cy9), 2-hydromethyl-quinoxaline (Cy12). To fully reflect the pharmacodynamic of cyadox, it is necessary to detect the antibacterial activity of cyadox and its metabolites.

However, there are few studies on the pharmacodynamics of cyadox at present. As a potent antimicrobial agent, Cyadox had been proved to have a wide spectrum of activity against many pathogenic bacteria of pigs, poultry, and fish [9]. In vivo, cyadox reduces diarrhea frequencies of different animals and prevents *E. coli* infection in piglets and broilers [10]. It has high antimicrobial activity in vitro against *E. coli* under anaerobic conditions. MIC values for cyadox in MHB (Mueller–Hinton broth) against *E. coli* were 1 to 4 μg/mL [11]. Some studies showed that cyadox could promote the growth of swine, chicken, and fish [3,12]. However, there are only limited data on the prophylactic schedule in piglets. At present, there is not a scientifically validated dosage for treating *E. coli* diarrhea.

However, the results of previous studies were not sufficient to explain the antimicrobial characteristics of cyadox. Hence, there is a need for a further and complete study to build up the antimicrobial spectrum using the standard method of Clinical and Laboratory Standards Institute (CLSI) approved by the FDA.

The purpose of this study was to evaluate the minimum inhibitory concentration (MIC) and minimal bactericidal concentration (MBC) of cyadox in vitro against different species of bacteria from pigs, poultry, and fishes, most of which were enteric pathogens, and compare the antimicrobial spectrum of cyadox with other commonly used antimicrobial agents. Under anaerobic conditions, the antimicrobial activity of some quinoxalines were different as compared to cyadox because cyadox exhibits much stronger activity in the absence of oxygen [10]. therefore, cyadox may be active against facultative anaerobes under anaerobic conditions. Based upon systematic toxicological and microbiological safety evaluations, cyadox shows much lower toxicity and higher safety than other well-known quinoxalines such as olaquindox and carbadox, which have been banned or strictly limited in their use in food-producing animals because of their potential toxicities [13]. However, it is hopeful that cyadox would be developed as a replacer of olaquindox and carbadox with greater safety and excellent antimicrobial activity. Based on the related guidelines and standards of the Clinical and Laboratory Standards Institute (CLSI), we determined the in vitro antibacterial activities of cyadox and established the antimicrobial spectrum of cyadox comprehensively and systematically in pathogenic bacteria from swine, chicken, and fish in the present study. The deep knowledge about the pharmacodynamics of cyadox will lay a solid foundation for the application of cyadox as a new veterinary drug.

2. Materials and Methods

2.1. Bacteria

Standard strains of *E. Coli*, *Pasteurella multocida*, *Salmonella*, *Erysipelothrix*, *Streptococcus*, *Enterococcus* spp., and *Clostridium perfringen* were obtained from China Veterinary Culture Collection Center (CVCC) and American Type Cell Culture (ATCC). Pathogenic bacteria (including 7 quality control strains and 4 testing strains *Aeromonas veronii*, *Pseudomonas pyocyanea*, *Salmonella typhimurium*, and *Proteus mirabilis*) were obtained directly from the ATCC and MicroBiologics (St Cloud, MN, USA). Other clinical isolates of pigs and chickens (*Escherichia coli* 9 strains, *Pasteurella multocida* 1 strain, *Salmonella pullorum* 8 strains, *Staphylococcus aureus* 3 strains, *Streptococcus* spp. 2 strains) were obtained from State Key Laboratory of Agricultural Microbiology, Huazhong Agricultural University, Wuhan, China. Fish pathogenic bacteria (*Yersinia ruckeri* SC90-2-4, *Aeromonas hydrophila* XS91-4-1, *Aeromonas jandaei* F30-3, *Aeromonas caviae* DMA1-A, *Aeromonas sobria* CR79-1-1, *Aeromonas punctata* 58-20-9, *Edwardsiella ictaluri* HSN-1, *Vibrio fluvialis* WY91-24-3, *Flavobacterim columnare* G4, *Pseudomonas fluorescent* W81-11 and 56-12-10, *Streptococcus agalactiae* XQ-1, and the 4 strains of *Mycobacterium tuberculosis*) were derived from numerous laboratories of State Key Laboratory of Freshwater Ecology and Biotechnology, Institute of Hydrobiology, Chinese Academy of Sciences. Other fish pathogens (*Escherichia coli* 1 strains, *Aeromonas hydrophila* 4 strains, *Aeromonas sobria* 3 strains, *Acinetobacter baumannii* 1 strains, *P. fluorescent* 8 strains, *Staphylococcus aureus* 2 strains) were obtained from the College of Fisheries, Huazhong Agricultural University, Wuhan, China. All the strains were stored at −70 °C in 20% skimmed milk. All the bacteria were inoculated at least twice on MH (Mueller Hinton) agar growth media prior to testing.

2.2. Study Drug and Susceptibility Testing

Cyadox powder (purity percent is ≥98%) was synthesized by the Institute of Veterinary Pharmaceutics (Huazhong Agricultural University, Wuhan, China). For the preparation of the working solution for MIC determination desired amount of cyadox was dissolved in dimethyl sulfoxide (DMSO) at the concentration of 1280 μg/mL as a stock solution. For MIC (Minimum inhibitory Concentration) determination, each bacterial strain was cultured to a logarithmic phase to obtain the turbidity of the 0.5 McFarland standard and then was diluted 100 times with MH broth to obtain a density of 1×10^6 CFU/mL which was used as the inoculum suspension. MIC was defined as the minimum concentration of compound that resulted in no visible growth. MIC determination was performed by the microbroth dilution method according to the CLSI (Clinical and Laboratory Standards Institute, formerly NCCLS) guidelines. The test was performed in a 96-well microtiter plate in a final volume of 100 μL. Each well was inoculated with serially diluted antimicrobial agents and the inoculum suspension (1:1 *v/v*). Different inoculation conditions for different bacteria isolated from livestock and poultry were used for MIC determination. Nonfastidious bacteria (*Escherichia coli, Salmonella* spp., *Yersinia* spp. *Proteus mirabilis, Pseudomonas* spp., *Staphylococcus aureus, Enterococcus* spp.) were cultured in CAMHB (cation-adjusted Mueller-Hinton broth) at 37 °C for 16–20 h according to the CLSI guidelines. Fastidious organisms (*Pasteurella* spp., *Streptococcus* spp., and *Erysipelothrix* spp.) were cultured in the media of CAMHB+LHB (cation-adjusted Mueller–Hinton broth supplemented with 2.5% lysed horse blood) for 18–20 h at 37 °C. Microaerophilic bacteria *Campylobacter jejuni* were cultured in CAMHB+LHB at 42 °C for 24 h under 10% CO_2. Anaerobic bacteria, such as *Clostridium perfringens* were cultured in Brucella broth under 80% N_2-10% CO_2-10% H_2 at 37 °C for 24 h. The inoculation conditions for the bacteria isolated from fish were set according to the CLSI guidelines at a temperature of 28 °C. *Vibrio fluvialis* was cultured in CAMHB with 1% NaCl for 24 h; *E. ictaluri* was cultured in CAMHB for 48 h; *Flavobacterim columnare* was cultured in CAMHB diluted for 24 h; *Streptococcus agalactiae* was cultured in CAMHB supplemented with 2.5% lysed horse blood for 24 h. *E. coli, F. columnare, Aeromonas* spp. (including *A. hydrophila, A. veronii, A. jandaei, A. caviae, A. sobria,* and *A. punctata*), *V. fluvialis, A. baumannii,* and *Y. ruckeri* isolated from fish were cultured in CAMHB for 24 h. *Mycobacterium tuberculosis* was cultured on Lowenstein–Jensen medium (LJ) solidified by coagulation at 83 °C for 40 min and incubated at 37 °C [14]. Quality control was monitored using *Escherichia coli* ATCC 25922, *Enterococcus faecalis* ATCC 29212, *Staphylococcus aureus* ATCC 29213, *Streptococcus pneumoniae* ATCC 49619, *Campylobacter jejuni* ATCC 33560, *Bacteroides fragilis* ATCC 25285, and *Bacteroides thetaiotaomicron* ATCC 29741.

MBC (Minimal Bactericidal Concentration) was determined according to the document M26-AE of CLSI. The lowest concentration of antimicrobial agent that killed ≥99.9% of the starting inoculum was defined as the MBC endpoint. The double diluted inoculum suspension and 10 μL broth from 96-well with no visible growth above the MIC after 24 h incubation on MH agar, incubated for one or two nights and counted for colony, respectively, and calculated for the MBC further.

MICs of the facultative anaerobes tested under anaerobic conditions were determined according to the defined methodology of CLSI with little change in the anaerobic environement (80% N_2—10% CO_2—10% H_2). Bacteria for colony counting and MBC testing were cultured under aerobic condition.

All the experiments were performed in 3 replicates along with the quality control strains to ensure the accuracy of results.

2.3. Data Processing

For analytical purposes, the bacteria were grouped into species or genus groups. The calculation included in MIC_{50} (MBC at which 50% of the strains are inhibited), MBC_{90} (MBC at which 90% of the strains are inhibited), MBC_{50} (MBC at which 50% of the strains are killed), MBC_{90} (MBC at which 90% of the strains are killed), and the MBC/MIC ratios were calculated to determine the presence or absence of tolerance. MIC50, MBC50, MIC90, and MBC90 were calculated by using SPSS software. The breakpoint was set in present study as follow: susceptible, $MIC_{90} \leq 8$ μg/mL; intermediate, 16 μg/mL $\leq MIC_{90} \leq$ 32 μg/mL; resistant, $MIC_{90} \geq 64$ μg/mL. Tolerance was defined as an MBC/MIC ratio of $\geq$32 or an MBC/MIC ratio of $\geq$16 when the MBC was greater than or equal to the MIC resistance breakpoint.

3. Results

3.1. Susceptibility of Pig Pathogens to Cyadox

Under CLSI standard conditions, the MIC and MBC of cyadox against *Clostridium perfringen* were 0.5~1 μg/mL, which were more susceptible and stronger than that of other antibacterial agents. The cyadox was much more effective against *Pasteurella multocida, Salmonella choleraesui, Erysipelothrix,* and *Streptococcus* than olaquindox but weaker than chlortetracycline. *Streptococcus* were found to be resistant to chlortetracycline. Under anaerobic conditions for facultative anaerobes, the antibacterial activity of cyadox was enhanced by 4–6 times in *E. coli, Pasteurella multocida, Salmonella choleraesuis,* and *Erysipelothrix*. Compared with controls, the antibacterial activity of cyadox was stronger than that of other antibacterials against *Escherichia coli*; the actions of cyadox were stronger than or similar to that of olaquindox and weaker than that of chlortetracycline against other bacteria (Table 1).

3.2. Susceptibility of Poultry Pathogens to Cyadox

Following CLSI standards conditions, the most susceptible bacteria forcyadox were *C. jejuni* and *C. perfringen* with the MICs and MBCs were 0.25~1 μg/mL and 1 μg/mL, respectively. While *E. faecalis* and *E. faecium* were resistant against cyadox. Under anaerobic conditions for facultative anaerobes, the antibacterial activity of cyadox was enhanced by 4~16 times in *S. pullorum, E. coli,* and *Enterococcus* spp., which indicated an inclined effect of cyadox against these bacteria. Compared with controls, under the two incubating conditions, the antibacterial actions of cyadox were stronger than that of other antibacterial agents against *E. coli* and *C. perfringen*, and the action of cyadox was stronger than or similar to that of olaquindox but weaker than that of chlortetracycline against other bacteria (Table 2).

3.3. Susceptibility of Fish Pathogens to Cyadox

E. coli showed a susceptible effect to cyadox with the MIC and MBC was 1 μg/mL and 16 μg/mL, respectively. For *F. columnare*, cyadox and sulfadimidine showed only an inhibitory effect but not a bactericidal effect. Under anaerobic conditions for facultative anaerobes, the antibacterial activity was enhanced by 8~256 times in *Aeromonas* spp. (included *A. hydrophila, A. veronii, A. jandaei, A. caviae,* and *A. sobria*, excluding *A. punctata*), *V. fluvialis, A. baumannii,* and *Y. ruckeri*. MICs and MBCs of *Aeromonas* spp. (excluded *Aeromonas punctata*), *V. fluvialis,* and *Y. ruckeri* were declined to 0.5~2 μg/mL and 1~8 μg/mL. Compared with controls, the antibacterial activity of cyadox were stronger than that of other antibacterial agents against *E. coli*. For *Mycobacterium tuberculosis*, the action of cyadox was stronger or similar to sulfadimidine but weaker than that of chlortetracycline against other bacteria except for *A. baumannii* (Table 3).

Table 1. Antimicrobial susceptibility of cyadox and controls against pathogens isolated from pigs (unit: μg/mL).

Number	Serotype	Cyadox				Chlortetracycline				Olaquindox				Dimethyl Sulfoxide	
		MIC_S	MBC_S	MIC_N	MBC_N	MIC_S	MBC_S	MIC_N	MBC_N	MIC_S	MBC_S	MIC_N	MBC_N	MIC_S	MIC_N
	G $^-$ *E. coil*														
CVCC196	O8:K87,K88ac	32	64	2 (16)	8 (8)	4	32	0.5 (8)	8 (4)	16	128	4 (4)	8 (16)	128	128
CVCC220	O101:K32	32	128	2 (16)	8 (16)	64	128	16 (4)	32 (4)	16	128	4 (4)	8 (16)	128	128
CVCC216	O8:K87,K88ad	32	64	4 (8)	16 (4)	32	32–64	4 (8)	32 (1–2)	32	128	8 (4)	16 (8)	128	128
CVCC223	O141:K99	32	64	1 (32)	8 (8)	64	64	64 (1)	>64 (1)	16	>128	2 (8)	16 (>8)	>128	128
CVCC224	O149:K91,K88ac	32	64	2 (16)	16 (4)	64	64	64 (1)	>64 (1)	32	128	4 (8)	8 (16)	128	128
CVCC1500	O149:K88ac	32	128	2 (16)	16 (8)	64	128	64 (1)	64 (2)	32	128	8 (4)	16 (8)	128	64
CVCC1502	O9:K88	32	128	4 (8)	16 (8)	64–128	128	32 (2–4)	64 (2)	32	64	4 (8)	16 (4)	64	128
CVCC1513	O101:K99	32	>128	1 (32)	8(>16)	64	128	32 (2)	64 (2)	16	128	2 (8)	8 (16)	128	128
CVCC1519	O139	32	>128	2 (16)	32 (>4)	64	128	32 (2)	64 (2)	32	128	8 (4)	16 (8)	128	128
CVCC1514	O45:K99	32	128	0.5 (64)	16 (8)	64	128	8 (8)	64 (2)	8	16	2 (4)	8 (2)	128	128
		MIC_{50} = 32, MBC_{50} = 128		MIC_{N50} = 2, MBC_{N50} = 16		MIC_{50} = 64, MBC_{50} = 128		MIC_{50} = 32, MBC_{50} = 64		MIC_{50} = 16, MBC_{50} = 128		MIC_{50} = 4, MBC_{50} = 8			
		MIC_{90} = 32, MBC_{90} > 128		MIC_{90} = 4, MBC_{90} = 16		MIC_{90} = 64, MBC_{90} = 128		MIC_{90} = 64, MBC_{90} = 64		MIC_{90} = 32, MBCjhjhh$_{90}$ = 128		MIC_{90} = 8, MBC_{90} = 16			
		MBC_{50}/MIC_{50} = 4		MBC_{50}/MIC_{50} = 8		MBC_{50}/MIC_{50} = 2		MBC_{50}/MIC_{50} = 2		MBC_{50}/MIC_{50} = 8		MBC_{50}/MIC_{50} = 2			
	P. multocida														
CVCC430	B:2,5	16	16			0.5	2			32	64			128	
CVCC432	A:1	8	16			0.5	2			16	32			128	
CVCC433	D:7	2	4	0.13 (16)	0.5 (8)	0.5	2	0.06 (8)	0.5 (4)	4	8	0.5 (8)	4 (2)	64	128
CVCC435	A:1	16	32	0.25 (64)	1 (32)	0.5	2	0.03 (16)	0.25 (8)	16	64	2 (8)	4 (16)	128	64
CVCC436	A:1	8	64	0.25 (32)	1 (32)	0.5	2	0.03 (16)	0.25 (8)	16	64	1 (16)	4 (16)	128	64
CVCC437	A:6	4	8	1 (4)	2 (4)	0.5	4	0.03 (16)	0.25(16)	8–16	32	1(8–16)	4 (8)	128	128
CVCC438	A:1	4	8	0.25 (16)	1 (8)	1	4	0.03 (32)	0.5 (8)	2	8	1 (2)	4 (2)	128	128
CVCC439	D:3	8	16			0.5	2–4			8–16	32			128	
CVCC440	A:6	8	16	0.5 (16)	2 (8)	0.25–0.5	2	0.06(4–8)	0.25 (8)	8	32	2 (4)	8 (4)	128	128
CVCC441	B:2,5	4	8	0.5 (8)	2 (4)	0.5	4	0.03 (16)	0.25(16)	8–16	16	1(8–16)	4 (4)	128	64
CVCC443	A:1	8	16	0.5 (16)	2 (8)	0.5	2	0.03 (16)	0.25 (8)	8	16	1 (8)	4 (4)	128	64
CVCC444	A:1	8	16			0.5	4			16	32			128	
CVCC446	B:2,5	8	16	0.25 (32)	2 (8)	0.5	2	0.03 (16)	0.25 (8)	16	32	2 (8)	4 (8)	128	64
		MIC_{50} = 8, MBC_{50} = 16		MIC_{50} = 0.25, MBC_{50} = 2		MIC_{50} = 0.5, MBC_{50} = 2		MIC_{50} = 0.03, MBC_{50} = 0.25		MIC_{50} = 16, MBC_{50} = 32		MIC_{50} = 1, MBC_{50} = 4			
		MIC_{90} = 8, MBC_{90} = 32		MIC_{90} = 0.5, MBC_{90} = 2		MIC_{90} = 1, MBC_{90} = 4		MIC_{90} = 0.06, MBC_{90} = 0.25		MIC_{90} = 16, MBC_{90} = 64		MIC_{90} = 2, MBC_{90} = 4			
		MBC_{50}/MIC_{50} = 2		MBC_{50}/MIC_{50} = 8		MBC_{50}/MIC_{50} = 4		MBC_{50}/MIC_{50} = 8		MBC_{50}/MIC_{50} = 2		MBC_{50}/MIC_{50} = 4			

Table 1. *Cont.*

Number	Serotype	Cyadox				Chlortetracycline				Olaquindox				Dimethyl Sulfoxide	
		MIC_S	MBC_S	MIC_N	MBC_N	MIC_S	MBC_S	MIC_N	MBC_N	MIC_S	MBC_S	MIC_N	MBC_N	MIC_S	MIC_N
	S. choleraesuis														
CVCC503	6,7:C:1,5	8	>128	1 (8)	32 (>4)	4	64	1 (4)	64 (1)	32	>128	2 (16)	4 (>32)	>128	128
CVCC504	6,7:C:1,5	32	>128	4 (8)	64 (>2)	8	64	2 (4)	64 (1)	8	>128	2 (4)	8 (>16)	>128	128
		MBC/MIC > 16		MBC/MIC = 16–32		MBC/MIC = 8–16		MBC/MIC = 32–64		MBC/MIC > 16		MBC/MIC = 2–4			
	G^+														
	Erysipelothrix														
	1a	32	128	4 (8)	32 (4)	0.5	32	0.06 (8)	2 (16)	32	>128	32 (1)	64 (>2)	>128	128
	8	32	>128	4 (8)	64 (>2)	0.5	32	0.06 (8)	2 (16)	32	128	32 (1)	64 (2)	128	128
CVCC1293	5	32	>128	4 (8)	64 (>2)	0.5	16	0.06 (8)	2 (8)	32	128	32 (1)	64 (2)	128	128
		MIC_{50} = 32, MBC_{50} > 128		MIC_{50} = 4, MBC_{50} = 64		MIC_{50} = 0.5, MBC_{50} = 32		MIC_{50} = 0.06, MBC_{50} = 2		MIC_{50} = 32, MBC_{50} = 128		MIC_{50} = 32, MBC_{50} = 64			
		MBC_{50}/MIC_{50} > 4		MBC_{50}/MIC_{50} = 16		MBC_{50}/MIC_{50} = 64		MBC_{50}/MIC_{50} = 32		MBC_{50}/MIC_{50} = 4		MBC_{50}/MIC_{50} = 2			
	***Streptococcus* spp.**														
CVCC606	Gram-R group	32	64	16 (2)	64 (1)	8	128	0.25 (32)	8 (16)	>128	>128	64 (>2)	128 (>1)	128	128
CVCC607	Gram-R group	32	64	32 (1)	64 (1)	0.25	>128	0.06 (4)	1(>128)	>128	>128	64 (>2)	128 (>1)	>128	128
CVCC608	Gram-S group	32	64	32 (1)	64 (1)	0.25	>128	0.06 (4)	1(>128)	>128	>128	64 (>2)	128 (>1)	>128	128
CVCC609	Gram-S group	16	32	16 (1)	32 (1)	0.13	128	0.06 (2)	1 (128)	>128	>128	64 (>2)	128 (>1)	128	128
sc19	Capsule-IItype	64	>128	32 (2)	128 (>1)	64	128	16 (4)	16 (8)	>128	>128	64 (>2)	128 (>1)	128	128
sc109	Capsule-IItype	128	>128	64 (2)	128 (>1)	32	>128	0.25(128)	2 (>64)	>128	>128	64 (>2)	128 (>1)	>128	>128
		MIC_{50} = 32, MBC_{50} = 64		MIC_{50} = 32, MBC_{50} = 64		MIC_{50} = 0.25, MBC_{50} = 128		MIC_{50} = 0.06, MBC_{50} = 1		MIC_{50} > 128, MBC_{50} > 128		MIC_{50} = 64, MBC_{50} = 128			
		MBC_{50}/MIC_{50} = 2		MBC_{50}/MIC_{50} = 2		MBC_{50}/MIC_{50} = 512		MBC_{50}/MIC_{50} = 4				MBC_{50}/MIC_{50} = 2			
	C. perfringens														
CVCC1125	A	1	1			0.03	0.06			1	128			128	
CVCC1160	C	0.5–1	1			8	8			1	128			128	
		MBC/MIC = 1–2				MBC/MIC = 1–2				MBC/MIC = 128					

Note: (1) The lower symbol "$_S$" denotes the result was under CLSI condition, and "$_N$" denotes the result was under anaerobic condition. (2) Values in brackets are the multiple drop of MIC under anaerobic conditions from aerobic conditions. "+" denotes gram-positive and "−" denotes gram-negative.

Table 2. Antimicrobial susceptibility of cyadox and controls against pathogens isolated from poultry (unit: μg/mL).

Number	Serotype	Cyadox				Chlortetracycline				Bacitracin Zinc				Dimethyl Sulfoxide	
		MIC_S	MBC_S	MIC_N	MBC_N	MIC_S	MBC_S	MIC_N	MBC_N	MIC_S	MBC_S	MIC_N	MBC_N	MIC_S	MIC_N
	G^-														
	E. coil														
CVCC1496	O139:K^+	32	128	2 (16)	32 (4)	64	64	16 (4)	64 (1)	>128	>128	>128 (1)	>128 (1)	>128	>128
C84010	O1	16	64	1 (16)	8 (16)	32	64	8 (4)	64 (1)	128	>128	128 (1)	>128 (1)	>128	>128
E-O1	O1	16	64			32	128			>128	>128			>128	
E-O2	O2	32	64			32	128			>128	>128			>128	
E-O24	O24	64	>128			128	>128			>128	>128			>128	
E-O78	O78	32	64			64	64			>128	>128			>128	
W1		64	128			64	128			>128	>128			>128	
W2		32	64			16	32			>128	>128			>128	
W3		64	128			64	128			>128	>128			>128	
Ae1		32–64	128	4 (8–16)	32 (1–2)	32–64	32–64	16 (2–4)	64 (1)	>128	>128	>128 (1)	>128 (1)	>128	>128
		MIC_{50} = 32, MBC_{50} = 64		MIC_{50} = 2, MBC_{50} = 32		MIC_{50} = 32, MBC_{50} = 64		MIC_{50} = 16, MBC_{50} = 64		MIC_{50} > 128, MBC_{50} > 128		MIC_{50} > 128, MBC_{50} > 128			
		MIC_{90} = 64, MBC_{90} = 128		MBC_{50}/MIC_{50} = 16		MIC_{90} = 64, MBC_{90} = 128		MBC_{50}/MIC_{50} = 4		MIC_{90} > 128, MBC_{90} > 128 >128					
		MBC_{50}/MIC_{50} = 8				MBC_{50}/MIC_{50} = 2									
	P. multocida														
CVCC1729	A:1,3	2	32	2 (1)	16 (2)	0.25	0.5	0.03 (8)	0.5 (1)	64	>128	32 (2)	32 (>4)	128	>128
CVCC2083	A:1,4	2	32	2 (1)	32 (1)	0.25	8	0.03 (8)	0.5 (16)	>128	>128	64 (>2)	128 (>1)	>128	>128
Ap1		4	16	1 (4)	16 (1)	0.13	1	0.03 (4)	0.5 (2)	128	>128	32 (4)	64 (>2)	128	>128
		MIC_{50} = 2, MBC_{50} = 32		MIC_{50} = 2, MBC_{50} = 16		MIC_{50} = 0.25, MBC_{50} = 1		MIC_{50} = 0.03, MBC_{50} = 0.5		MIC_{50} = 128, MBC_{50} > 128		MIC_{50} = 32, MBC_{50} = 64			
		MBC_{50}/MIC_{50} = 16		MBC_{50}/MIC_{50} = 8		MBC_{50} /MIC_{50} = 4		MBC_{50}/MIC_{50} = 16				MBC_{50}/MIC_{50} = 2			
	S. pullorum														
Sa-s1		8	128	1 (8)	16 (8)	2	64	0.5 (4)	32 (2)	128	>128	128 (1)	>128 (1)	>128	>128
Sa-s2		8	128	1 (8)	16 (8)	2	64	0.5 (4)	32 (2)	64	>128	64 (1)	>128 (1)	>128	>128
Sa-h		8	128	1 (8)	16 (8)	128	>128	32 (4)	128 (2)	>128	>128	>128 (1)	>128 (1)	>128	>128
Sa-h2		8	128	1 (8)	16 (8)	2	64	0.5 (4)	64 (2)	128	>128	128 (1)	>128 (1)	>128	>128
Sa-x		16	128	2 (8)	32 (4)	2	64	0.5 (4)	32 (2)	128	>128	128 (1)	>128 (1)	>128	>128
Sa-p1		16	128	2 (8)	32 (4)	2	64	0.5 (4)	32 (2)	128	>128	64 (2)	>128 (1)	>128	>128
Sa-p2		32	128	2 (16)	32 (4)	2	32	0.5 (4)	32 (1)	128	>128	128 (1)	>128 (1)	>128	>128
X1		4	64			8	32			128	>128			>128	

Table 2. *Cont.*

Number	Serotype	Cyadox				Chlortetracycline				Bacitracin Zinc				Dimethyl Sulfoxide	
		MIC_S	MBC_S	MIC_N	MBC_N	MIC_S	MBC_S	MIC_N	MBC_N	MIC_S	MBC_S	MIC_N	MBC_N	MIC_S	MIC_N
		MIC_{50} = 8, MBC_{50} = 128		MIC_{50} = 1, MBC_{50} = 16		MIC_{50} = 2, MBC_{50} = 64		MIC_{50} = 0.5, MBC_{50} = 32		MIC_{50} = 128, MBC_{50} > 128		MIC_{50} = 128, MBC_{50} > 128			
		MIC_{90} = 16, MBC_{90} = 128		MIC_{90} = 2, MBC_{90} = 32		MIC_{90} = 8, MBC_{90} = 64		MIC_{90} = 0.5, MBC_{90} = 64		MIC_{90} = 128, MBC_{90} > 128		MIC_{90} = 128, MBC_{90} > 128			
		MBC_{50}/MIC_{50} = 16		MBC_{50}/MIC_{50} = 16		MBC_{50}/MIC_{50} = 32		MBC_{50}/MIC_{50} = 64							
	C. jejuni														
ATCC BAA-1062™		0.25	1			0.13	0.5			128	128			>128	
		MBC/MIC = 4				MBC/MIC = 4				MBC/MIC = 1					
	G^+														
	S. aureus														
As1		16–32	64			0.13	4			32	32			>128	
As2		32	64			16	32			16	32			>128	
Z1		64	>128			32	>128			16	>128			>128	
		MIC_{50} = 32, MBC_{50} = 64				MIC_{50} = 16, MBC_{50} = 32				MIC_{50} = 16, MBC_{50} = 32					
		MBC_{50}/MIC_{50} = 2				MBC_{50}/MIC_{50} = 2				MBC_{50}/MIC_{50} = 2					
	***Enterococcus* spp.**														
CVCC1297	Gram-D group	64	>128	8 (8)	64 (>2)	16	128	8 (2)	32 (4)	32	128	32 (1)	64 (2)	>128	>128
CVCC1298	Gram-D group	64	>128	16 (4)	64 (>2)	0.5	4	0.5 (1)	4 (1)	64	>128	32 (2)	64 (>2)	>128	>128
		MBC/MIC > 2		MBC/MIC = 4–8		MBC/MIC = 8		MBC/MIC = 4–8		MBC/MIC = 4		MBC/MIC = 2			
	C. perfringens														
CVCC2030	A	1	1			8	8			4	4			>128	
		MBC/MIC = 1				MBC/MIC = 1				MBC/MIC = 1					

Note: (1) The lower symbol "S" denotes the result was under CLSI condition, and "N" denotes the result was under anaerobic condition. (2) Values in brackets are the multiple drop of MIC under anaerobic conditions from aerobic conditions. (3) Includes *E. faecalis* (CVCC1297) and *E. faecium* (CVCC1298). "+" denotes gram-positive and "−" denotes gram-negative.

Table 3. Antimicrobial susceptibility of cyadox and controls against common pathogens isolated from fishes (unit: μg/mL).

Strains	Number	Cyadox				Chlortetracycline				Sulfadimidine				Dimethyl Sulfoxide	
		MIC_S	MBC_S	MIC_N	MBC_N	MIC_S	MBC_S	MIC_N	MBC_N	MIC_S	MBC_S	MIC_N	MBC_N	MIC_S	MIC_N
G^-															
E. coil	Se1	1	16			2	4			1	2			128	128
Y. ruckeri	SC90-2-4	32	128	2 (16)	8 (16)	2	16	0.25 (8)	1 (16)	128	>128	>128 (1)	>128 (1)	128	128
	XS91-4-1	64	128	1 (64)	2 (64)	0.5	0.5	0.13 (4)	0.25 (2)	>128	>128	64 (1)	>128 (1)	128	128
	Ah78	64	128	0.5 (128)	1 (128)	2	16	0.13 (16)	2 (32)	>128	>128	>128 (1)	>128 (1)	>128	128
A. hydrophila	Ah561	128	128	0.5 (256)	1 (128)	0.5	8	0.13 (4)	2 (4)	>128	>128	>128 (1)	>128 (1)	>128	64
	Ah563	128	128	1 (128)	2 (64)	0.5	2	0.13 (4)	0.5 (4)	64	128	64 (1)	128 (1)	>128	128
	A1	64	128	0.5 (128)	1 (128)	0.25	2	0.13 (2)	0.5 (4)	128	128	128 (1)	>128 (1)	128	128
		MIC_{50} = 64, MBC_{50} = 128		MIC_{50} = 0.5, MBC_{50} = 1		MIC_{50} = 0.5, MBC_{50} = 2		MIC_{50} = 0.13, MBC_{50} = 0.5		MIC_{50} > 128, MBC_{50} > 128		MIC_{50} = 128, MBC_{50} > 128			
		MBC_{50}/MIC_{50} = 2		MBC_{50}/MIC_{50} = 2		MBC_{50}/MIC_{50} = 4		MBC_{50}/MIC_{50} = 4							
A. veronii	ATCC9071	64	128	0.5 (128)	4 (32)	≤0.25	1	0.13 (≤2)	0.13 (8)	>128	>128	>128 (1)	>128 (1)	128	128
A. jandaei	F30-3	64	128	2 (32)	4 (32)	≤0.25	1	0.06 (≤4)	0.13 (8)	>128	>128	64 (>2)	>128 (1)	128	128
A. caviae	DMA1-A	64	128	1 (64)	4 (32)	≤0.25	1	0.25 (1)	0.5 (2)	>128	>128	>128 (1)	>128 (1)	128	128
A. punctata	58-20-9	128	128	128 (1)	128 (1)	128	128	64 (2)	128 (1)	>128	>128	>128 (1)	>128 (1)	128	128
	CR79-1-1	128	128	0.5 (256)	1 (128)	1	2	0.06 (16)	0.13 (16)	>128	>128	>128 (1)	>128 (1)	128	128
A. sobria	3-6	128	128			0.5	2			>128	>128			>128	
	3-7	64	128			4	8			>128	>128			>128	
	3-8	128	128			4	8			>128	>128			>128	
		MIC_{50} = 128, MBC_{50} = 128				MIC_{50} = 1, MBC_{50} = 2				MIC_{50} > 128, MBC_{50} > 128					
		MBC_{50}/MIC_{50} = 1				MBC_{50}/MIC_{50} = 2									
E. ictaluri	HSN-1	64	64	64 (1)	64 (1)	4	4	≤0.03 (≥128)	1 (4)	>128	>128	>128 (1)	>128 (1)	128	128
V. fluvialis	WY91-24-3	64	128	0.5 (128)	2 (32)	0.5	8	0.13 (4)	0.25 (32)	>128	>128	>128 (1)	>128 (1)	128	128

Table 3. *Cont.*

Strains	Number	Cyadox				Chlortetracycline				Sulfadimidine				Dimethyl Sulfoxide	
		MIC_S	MBC_S	MIC_N	MBC_N	MIC_S	MBC_S	MIC_N	MBC_N	MIC_S	MBC_S	MIC_N	MBC_N	MIC_S	MIC_N
F. columnare	G4	2	>128			0.5	16			8	128			64	
A. baumannii	Ab1	64	128	8 (8)	16 (8)	0.125	0.5	≤0.03 (≥4)	0.13 (4)	16	32	16 (1)	32 (1)	128	128
	W81-11	128	>128	128 (1)	>128 (1)	4	8	2 (2)	4 (2)	>128	>128	>128 (1)	>128 (1)	>128	128
	56-12-10	128	>128	128 (1)	128 (>1)	16	128	4 (4)	64 (2)	>128	>128	>128 (1)	>128 (1)	128	128
	1-1	128	>128			16	128			>128	>128			128	
	1-2	128	>128			16	128			>128	>128			128	
P. fluorescent	1-3	128	>128			32	128			>128	>128			128	
	1-4	128	>128			16	128			>128	>128			128	
	1-5	128	>128			16	128			>128	>128			128	
	1-6	128	>128			16	128			>128	>128			128	
	1-7	64	>128			16	128			>128	>128			128	
	1-8	64	>128			32	128			>128	>128			128	
		MIC_{50} = 128, MBC_{50}>128				MIC_{50} = 16, MBC_{50} = 128				MIC_{50} > 128, MBC_{50} > 128					
		MIC_{90} = 128, MBC_{90} > 128				MIC_{90} = 32, MBC_{90} = 128				MIC_{90} > 128, MBC_{90} > 128					
						MBC_{50}/MIC_{50} = 8									
G^+															
S. aureus	Fs1	64	128			0.125	0.5			16	128			128	
	Fs2	16	64			0.125	1			>128	>128			>128	
S. agalactiae	XQ-1	16	32	8 (2)	16 (2)	0.125	2	≤0.03 (2)	0.13 (16)	>128	>128	>128 (1)	>128 (1)	>128	128
	Asc-1.2II	16	32			8	32			>128	>128			>128	
M. tuberculosis	Asc-1.3II	32	64			32	64			>128	>128			>128	
	Asc-1.3V	32	64			32	128			>128	>128			>128	
	Cst-t-10	32	64			>128	>128			>128	>128			>128	
		MIC_{50} = 32, MBC_{50} = 64				MIC_{50} = 32, MBC_{50} = 64				MIC_{50}>128, MBC_{50}>128					
		MBC_{50}/MIC_{50} = 2				MBC_{50}/MIC_{50} = 2									

Note: (1) The lower symbol "$_S$" denotes the result was under CLSI condition, and "$_N$" denotes the result was under anaerobic condition. (2) Values in brackets are the multiple drop of MIC under anaerobic conditions from aerobic conditions. "+" denotes gram-positive and "−" denotes gram-negative.

Table 4. Antimicrobial susceptibility of cyadox and controls against pathogens isolated from others (unit: μg/mL).

Numbers of Strains	Serotype	Cyadox				Chlortetracycline				Olaquindox				Bacitracin zinc			Dimethyl Sulfoxide		
		MIC_S	MBC_S	MIC_N	MBC_N	MIC_S	MBC_S	MIC_N	MBC_N	MIC_S	MBC_S	MIC_N	MBC_N	MIC_S	MIC_N	MIC_S	MIC_N	MIC_S	MIC_N
	G⁻																		
	S. typhimurium																		
CVCC542	1,4,12:i:1,2	8	>128	8 (1)	64 (2)	8	128	0.5(16)	≥64 (1)	32	64	2 (16)	16 (4)	>128	>128	>128 (1)	>128 (1)	>128	>128
	Y. enterocolitica																		
ATCC 9610 TM	Group, O:8	32	128	16 (2)	64 (2)	1	4	0.5 (2)	8 (1)	8	16	4 (2)	16 (1)	-		>128 (1)	>128 (1)	>128	128
	P. mirabilis																		
ATCC 29245™		32	128	4 (8)	32 (4)	>128	>128	64 (>2)	128 (>1)	16	32	2 (8)	4 (8)	-		>128 (1)	128	>128	128
	P. pyocyanea																		
CVCC2087		128	>128	128 (1)	>128 (1)	32	128	8 (4)	32 (4)	>128	>128	64 (>2)	128 (>1)	>128	>128	128 (1)	>128 (1)	>128	>128

Note: (1) The lower symbol "S" denotes the result was under CLSI condition, and "N" denotes the result was under anaerobic condition. (2) Values in brackets are the multiple drop of MIC under anaerobic conditions from aerobic conditions. "+" denotes gram-positive and "−" denotes gram-negative.

3.4. Susceptibility of Other Pathogens to Cyadox

The results of antimicrobial susceptibility of cyadox against pathogenic bacteria isolated from humans and animals were listed in (Table 4). The antibacterial action of cyadox was stronger than that of other antibacterial agents against *S. typhimurium*, *Y. enterocolitica*, and *P. mirabilis* which was stronger than sulfonamide but weaker than chlortetracycline. Under anaerobic conditions, the antibacterial activity was enhanced by 8 times in *Proteus mirabilis*.

4. Discussion

Clinical breakpoints for quinoxalines have not been established by CLSI yet [15]. This study defines the clinical breakpoints for cyadox according to the antibacterial activities of cyadox and the antibiogram of olaquindox. Cyadox has a good effect against *E. coli* in vitro (MIC_{90} under anaerobic condition was 4 μg/mL in this test). The susceptible bacteria of olaquindox including gram-negative bacteria (*P. multocida, E. coli, S. choleraesui, Shigella* spp., and *Proteus* spp.) and gram-positive bacteria (*Staphylococci*), MIC_{90} of these bacteria under anaerobic condition were 8 μg/mL in this study. In addition, isolates were considered to be tolerant to antimicrobial agents that were known to be bactericidal but that do not show a killing effect.

The antimicrobial effect of cyadox against pathogens isolated from pigs and poultry was similar in vitro. Under standard conditions, susceptible bacteria for cyadox were *C. perfringen*, *C. jejuni*, and *P. multocida*. Intermediate bacteria were *Salmonella* spp. (including *S. choleraesui*, *S. typhimurium*, *S. pullorum*), *E. coli*, *Y. enterocolitica*, *P. mirabilis*, *Erysipelothrix*, *S. aureus*, and *Streptococcus* spp. The susceptibility of *C. perfringens* against cyadox was similar to previous studies conducted by [11]. Resistant bacteria were *P. pyocyanea*, *E. faecalis*, and *E. faecium*. Under anaerobic conditions, susceptible bacteria were *P. multocida*, *E. coli*, *Salmonella* spp., *P. mirabilis*, and *Erysipelothrix*, intermediate bacteria were *Y. enterocolitica*, *Streptococcus* spp, *E. faecalis*, and *E. faecium*, while *P. pyocyanea* was resistant bacterium against cyadox. However, cyadox showed growth inhibition with a ≥16-fold against *Salmonella* spp. and *Erysipelothrix* spp. While compared with other drugs, *Salmonella* spp., *Erysipelothrix* spp., and *Streptococcus* spp. have a high tolerance against chlortetracycline, and *C. perfringen* has a high tolerance against olaquindox.

Cyadox showed broad-spectrum activity against pathogens isolated from fish. Under standard conditions, susceptible bacteria for cyadox were *E. coli* and *F. columnare*, but for the later bacterium cyadox has no killing effect. Intermediate bacteria were *Yersinia ruckeri*, *Staphylococcus aureus*, *S. agalactiae*, and *Mycobacterium tuberculosis*. Nonsusceptible bacteria were *P. fluorescent*, *A. baumannii*, *Aeromonas* spp., *E. ictaluri*, and *V. fluvialis*. Under anaerobic conditions, susceptible bacteria were *Aeromonas* spp. (excluded *Aeromonas punctata)*, *V. fluvialis*, and *Y. ruckeri*, intermediate bacteria were *S. agalactiae* and *A. baumannii*, nonsusceptible bacteria were *P. fluorescent*, *A. punctata*, and *E. ictaluri*.

Compared with the source of pathogenic bacteria, the antimicrobial spectrum of cyadox against pigs and poultry in vitro was similar. The antimicrobial effect of cyadox against different serotypes or serogroup in the same species was almost similar, but the MICs of some *Streptococcus* isolated in recent years increased, which suggests no cross-resistance between quinoxalines except *Streptococcus*. The antimicrobial susceptibility of bacteria isolated from fish was different from that of bacteria from non-fish source, which mainly because the incubation temperature was different. Under aerobic conditions, the MICs and MBCs of cyadox in *E. coli* were the same as or higher than that of olaquindox, which means that the antibacterial effect of cyadox against *E. coli* is not as good as olaquindox in vitro. However, the effect of cyadox on the antibacterial activity in vitro was as good as that of olaquindox against *E. coli* infection demonstrated its activity under aerobic conditions [10]. Maybe it can turn to seek an answer from the bactericidal activity of cyadox and olaquindox under anaerobic conditions. The effect under anaerobic conditions is closer to that of the intestinal tract condition than that under the aerobic condition [16].

The antimicrobial activity of cyadox for most facultative anaerobes was significantly better in anaerobic conditions than in aerobic conditions, the sensitivity of control drug chlortetracycline and olaquindox were significantly improved as compared to Bacitracin-zinc and sulfadimidine. In this test, the MICs of *Escherichia coli* and *Salmonella* spp. under CLSI condition and anaerobic condition were in accordance with that reported previously [11]. The difference in antibacterial activity of some quinoxalines under anaerobic and aerobic conditions may be due to some free radicals [17]. The antibacterial mechanism may be similar to quindoxin. There was no evidence has been found for binding of quindoxin to DNA [18]. It suggested that some free radicals responsible for the lethal effect of quindoxin, and the free radicals were generated always accompanied by a reduction of the drug and occurred only under anaerobic conditions [18].

Usually, the treatment effect in vivo can be predicted by the results in vitro [19]. Cyadox exhibited excellent in vitro activity across an extended spectrum of bacteria, encompassing all major pathogens with clinical relevance of intestines infections in pigs, poultry, and fish [20]. Cyadox used as an antimicrobial growth promoter has good potential for disease resistance, which needs further clinical trials to validate especially in fish production. In addition, the better antimicrobial activity under anaerobic conditions provides a new aspect of investigation for further clinical studies.

In conclusion, this study has determined MICs of cyadox against pathogens from swine, chicken, and fish and established the antibacterial spectrum of activity of cyadox. It is shown that cyadox has a good antibacterial activity which is better than other quinoxaline derivatives. Under in vitro anaerobic conditions, the antibacterial activity of cyadox against most facultative anaerobes is considerably better which demonstrated that cyadox is an active compound in anaerobic conditions, which provides a reasonable theoretical foundation for the clinical application of cyadox. The overall in vitro results provide predictive evidence that cyadox has high antibacterial activity that can be used alone even though we are hunting appropriate medications for drug combinations.

Author Contributions: Data curation, Z.W., M.D. and G.C.; Formal analysis, Y.W.; Investigation, Z.W., M.D. and L.H.; Methodology, X.W. and L.H.; Project administration, L.H.; Supervision, Z.L., H.H. and X.W.; Writing—review & editing, M.K.M. All authors have read and agreed to the published version of the manuscript.

Funding: This work was partly supported by the National key research and development program (2018YFD0500301; 2016YFD0501310; 2017YFD0501400).

Conflicts of Interest: The authors have no conflicts of interest to declare.

References

1. Zhao, Y.; Cheng, G.; Hao, H.; Pan, Y.; Liu, Z.; Dai, M.; Yuan, Z. In vitro antimicrobial activities of animal-used quinoxaline 1,4-di-N-oxides against mycobacteria, mycoplasma and fungi. *BMC Vet. Res.* **2016**, *12*, 1–13. [CrossRef] [PubMed]
2. Huang, L.; Lin, Z.; Zhou, X.; Zhu, M.; Gehring, R.; Riviere, J.E.; Yuan, Z. Estimation of residue depletion of cyadox and its marker residue in edible tissues of pigs using physiologically based pharmacokinetic modelling. *Food Addit. Contam. Part A* **2015**, *49*, 1–16. [CrossRef] [PubMed]
3. Ding, M.X.; Yuan, Z.H.; Wang, Y.L.; Zhu, H.L.; Fan, S.X. Olaquindox and cyadox stimulate growth and decrease intestinal mucosal immunity of piglets orally inoculated with Escherichia coli. *J. Anim. Physiol. Anim. Nutr.* **2006**, *90*, 238–243. [CrossRef] [PubMed]
4. Wang, X.; He, Q.-H.; Wang, Y.-L.; Ihsan, A.; Huang, L.-L.; Zhou, W.; Su, S.-J.; Liu, Z.-L.; Yuan, Z.-H. A chronic toxicity study of cyadox in Wistar rats. *Regul. Toxicol. Pharmacol.* **2011**, *59*, 324–333. [CrossRef] [PubMed]
5. Wang, X.; Zhou, W.; Ihsan, A.; Chen, D.; Cheng, G.; Hao, H.; Liu, Z.; Wang, Y.; Yuan, Z. Assessment of thirteen-week subchronic oral toxicity of cyadox in Beagle dogs. *Regul. Toxicol. Pharmacol.* **2015**, *73*, 652–659. [CrossRef] [PubMed]
6. Li, Y.; Zhao, N.; Zeng, Z.; Gu, X.; Fang, B.; Yang, F.; Zhang, B.; Ding, H. Tissue deposition and residue depletion of cyadox and its three major metabolites in pigs after oral administration. *J. Agric. Food Chem.* **2013**, *61*, 9510–9515. [CrossRef] [PubMed]
7. Yan, D.; He, L.; Zhang, G.; Fang, B.; Yong, Y.; Li, Y. Simultaneous Determination of Cyadox and Its Metabolites in Chicken Tissues by LC-MS/MS. *Food Anal. Methods* **2012**, *5*, 1497–1505. [CrossRef]
8. He, Q.; Fang, G.; Wang, Y.; Wei, Z.; Wang, D.; Zhou, S.; Fan, S.; Yuan, Z.H. Experimental evaluation of cyadox phototoxicity to Balb/c mouse skin. *Photodermatol. Photoimmunol. Photomed.* **2006**, *22*, 100–104. [CrossRef] [PubMed]
9. Huang, L.; Maan, M.K.; Xu, D.; Bakr Shabbir, M.A.; Dai, M.; Yuan, Z. Pharmacokinetic-pharmacodynamic modeling of cyadox against *Escherichia coli* in swine. *Microb. Pathog.* **2019**, *135*, 103650. [CrossRef] [PubMed]

10. Xu, N.; Huang, L.; Liu, Z.; Pan, Y.; Wang, X.; Tao, Y.; Chen, D.; Wang, Y.; Peng, D.; Yuan, Z. Metabolism of cyadox by the intestinal mucosa microsomes and gut flora of swine, and identification of metabolites by high-performance liquid chromatography combined with ion trap/time-of-flight mass spectrometry. *Rapid Commun. Mass Spectrom.* **2011**, *25*, 2333–2344. [CrossRef] [PubMed]
11. Yan, L.; Xie, S.; Chen, D.; Pan, Y.; Tao, Y.; Qu, W.; Liu, Z.; Yuan, Z.; Huang, L. Pharmacokinetic and pharmacodynamic modeling of cyadox against *Clostridium perfringens* in swine. *Sci. Rep.* **2017**, *7*, 1–11. [CrossRef]
12. Huang, L.L. Effectiveness and Safety Studies of Cyadox In Broilers TT. Ph.D. Thesis, Huazhong Agricultural University, Wuhan, China, 2005.
13. Ihsan, A.; Wang, X.; Huang, X.; Liu, Y.; Liu, Q.; Zhou, W.; Yuan, Z. Acute and subchronic toxicological evaluation of Mequindox in Wistar rats. *Regul. Toxicol. Pharmacol.* **2010**, *57*, 307–314. [CrossRef]
14. Asmar, S.; Drancourt, M. Rapid culture-based diagnosis of pulmonary tuberculosis in developed and developing countries. *Front. Microbiol.* **2015**, *6*, 1184. [CrossRef] [PubMed]
15. Wayne, P.A. *Performance Standards for Antimicrobial Disk and Dilution Susceptibility Tests for Bacteria Isolated from Animals*; Approved Standard; Clinical and Laboratory Standards Institute: Wayne, PA, USA, 2009; ISBN 156238659X.
16. Zheng, M.; Jiang, J.; Wang, J.; Tang, X.; Ouyang, M.; Deng, Y. The mechanism of enzymatic and non-enzymatic N-oxide reductive metabolism of cyadox in pig liver. *Xenobiotica* **2011**, *41*, 964–971. [CrossRef] [PubMed]
17. Liu, Z.-Y.; Sun, Z.-L. The Metabolism of Carbadox, Olaquindox, Mequindox, Quinocetone and Cyadox: An Overview. *Med. Chem.* **2013**, *9*, 1017–1027. [CrossRef] [PubMed]
18. Suter, W.; Rosselet, A.; Knuesel, F. Mode of action of quindoxin and substituted quinoxaline-di-N-oxides on *Escherichia coli*. *Antimicrob. Agents Chemother.* **1978**, *13*, 770–783. [CrossRef]
19. Bulitta, J.B.; Ly, N.S.; Yang, J.C.; Forrest, A.; Jusko, W.J.; Tsuji, B.T. Development and qualification of a pharmacodynamic model for the pronounced inoculum effect of ceftazidime against *Pseudomonas aeruginosa*. *Antimicrob. Agents Chemother.* **2009**, *53*, 46–56. [CrossRef]
20. Nabuurs, M.J.A.; van der Molen, E.J.; de Graaf, G.J.; Jager, L.P. Clinical Signs and Performance of Pigs Treated with Different Doses of Carbadox, Cyadox and Olaquindox. *J. Vet. Med. Ser. A* **1990**, *37*, 68–76. [CrossRef] [PubMed]

antibiotics

MDPI

Article

Higher Prevalence of Extended-Spectrum Cephalosporin-Resistant *Enterobacterales* in Dogs Attended for Enteric Viruses in Brazil Before and After Treatment with Cephalosporins

Marília Salgado-Caxito [1,2,*], Andrea I. Moreno-Switt [2,3], Antonio Carlos Paes [1], Carlos Shiva [4], Jose M. Munita [2,5], Lina Rivas [2,5] and Julio A. Benavides [2,6,7,*]

1 Department of Animal Production and Preventive Veterinary Medicine, School of Veterinary Medicine and Animal Science, Sao Paulo State University, Botucatu 18618000, Brazil; ac.paes@unesp.br
2 Millennium Initiative for Collaborative Research on Bacterial Resistance (MICROB-R), Santiago 7550000, Chile; andrea.moreno@uc.cl (A.I.M.-S.); munita.jm@gmail.com (J.M.M.); linarivas@udd.cl (L.R.)
3 Escuela de Medicina Veterinaria, Pontificia Universidad Católica de Chile, Santiago 8940000, Chile
4 Faculty of Veterinary Medicine and Zootechnics, Universidad Cayetano Heredia of Peru, Lima 15102, Peru; carlos.shiva@upch.pe
5 Genomics and Resistant Microbes Group, Facultad de Medicina Clinica Alemana, Universidad del Desarrollo, Santiago 7550000, Chile
6 Departamento de Ecología y Biodiversidad, Facultad de Ciencias de la Vida, Universidad Andrés Bello, Santiago 8320000, Chile
7 Centro de Investigación para la Sustentabilidad, Facultad de Ciencias de la Vida, Universidad Andrés Bello, Santiago 8320000, Chile
* Correspondence: mariliasalgadovet@gmail.com (M.S.-C.); benavidesjulio@yahoo.fr (J.A.B.)

Citation: Salgado-Caxito, M.I.; Moreno-Switt, A.I; Paes, A.C.; Shiva, C.; Munita, J.M; Rivas, L.; Benavides, J.A Higher Prevalence of Extended-Spectrum Cephalosporin-Resistant *Enterobacterales* in Dogs Attended for Enteric Viruses in Brazil Before and After Treatment with Cephalosporins. *Antibiotics* **2021**, *10*, 122. https://doi.org/10.3390/antibiotics10020122

Academic Editors: Nikola Puvača, Chantal Britt and Jonathan Gómez-Raja
Received: 1 January 2021
Accepted: 22 January 2021
Published: 28 January 2021

Abstract: The extensive use of antibiotics is a leading cause for the emergence and spread of antimicrobial resistance (AMR) among dogs. However, the impact of using antibiotics to treat viral infections on AMR remains unknown. In this study, we compared the prevalence of extended-spectrum cephalosporin-resistant *Enterobacterales* (ESCR-E) between dogs with a suspected infection of canine parvovirus (CPV) and canine distemper (CDV) before and after treatment with third-generation cephalosporins. We found a higher prevalence of ESCR-E faecal carriage in dogs suspected of CPV (37%) and CDV (15%) compared to dogs with noninfectious pathologies (9%) even prior to the start of their treatment. A 7-day course of ceftriaxone or ceftiofur administrated to CPV and CDV-suspected dogs substantially increased their ESCR-E faecal carriage during treatment (85% for CPV and 57% for CDV), and 4 weeks after the treatment ended (89% for CPV and 60% for CDV) when dogs were back in their households. Most of the observed resistance was carried by ESCR-*E. coli* carrying *bla*$_{CTX-M}$ genes. Our results suggest the need to optimize prophylactic antibiotic therapy in dogs treated for a suspected viral infection to prevent ESCR-E emergence and spread in the community.

Keywords: antimicrobial resistance; antimicrobial prophylaxis; canine distemper; canine parvovirus; companion animals

1. Introduction

Antimicrobial resistance (AMR) in companion animals is one of the major challenges for the treatment of infections in veterinary practice [1]. Part of the burden of AMR is attributed to extended-spectrum cephalosporin-resistant *Enterobacterales* (ESCR-E), considered as "global priority pathogen" due to the limited options available for their effective treatment in both humans and animals [2,3]. ESCR-E are increasingly reported among dogs [4–8]. Although most studies identified ESCR-E in commensal *E. coli*, horizontal resistance gene transfer can spread resistance to other pathogenic microorganisms and result in severe bacterial infections with reduced treatment options [9]. However, the drivers for the acquisition and dissemination of ESCR-E in commensal bacteria in both clinical and community settings remain poorly understood in dogs.

The extensive use of antibiotics is the main driver for the emergence of ESCR-E faecal carriage in dogs [10–12]. Several antibiotics of critical importance to human health are commonly used to treat bacterial infections in dogs including extended-spectrum cephalosporins (third and fourth generation) and fluoroquinolones [13]. For example, these antibiotics are the most commonly prescribed by European veterinarians, although a few small animal veterinary centres have an antimicrobial stewardship policy [14]. The correlation between the frequency of antimicrobial use and AMR is well documented in livestock [15]. However, to our knowledge, no similar study has been conducted in dogs, limiting our understanding of how to optimize the use of antibiotics to reduce the emergence and spread of AMR in the veterinary practice.

Other than using antibiotics to treat bacterial infections, infections caused by other pathogens such as viruses can also require the use of antibiotics. Canine parvovirus (CPV) and canine *morbillivirus* (canine distemper, CDV) are often treated with third-generation cephalosporins due to the severe host immunosuppression and a risk of sepsis by bacterial translocation [16–22]. Despite been considered as an effective prophylactic treatment for these viruses, the use of third-generation cephalosporins in dogs could increase the selective pressure for ESCR-E [23]. CPV and CDV are one of the main causes of mortality in dogs, particularly puppies, with high prevalence estimated in several countries including Brazil [24–29]. However, despite the common circulation of these viruses, no study to our knowledge has evaluated the effects of prophylactic antibiotic therapy in CPV and CDV infections on the faecal carriage of antibiotic-resistant bacteria among dogs.

The spread of ESCR-E potentially emerging during the treatment into the community (e.g., to other household members) will depend on the duration of ESCR-E faecal carriage after treatment. The spread of ESCR-E will also depend on the supporting genetic material coding the ESCR. Resistance to broad-spectrum cephalosporins is often associated to the presence of extended-spectrum β-lactamases (ESBL) enzymes that can hydrolyse β-lactams antibiotics (i.e., penicillins, cephalosporins, and cephamycins), which is the main mechanism for ESCR-*E. coli* in dogs and cats [4,6,30–32]. Most ESBL genes spread by insertion on mobile genetic elements such as plasmids [32]. ESBL genes have been detected in isolates from dogs 3 days after administration of first-generation cephalosporins prior to surgical procedures [33]. In addition, faecal carriage of ESBL-*E. coli* has been detected for up to 3 months in dog faeces after intravenous treatment with cephalexin and cefovecin [12]. Thus, limited available evidence shows the potential for the spread of ESBL-*E. coli* after treatment. However, a few studies have monitored treated dogs for longer periods. In this study, we first compared the prevalence of ESCR-E faecal carriage in dogs with clinical signs of CPV or CDV infections with uninfected dogs before antibiotic therapy at the referral veterinary teaching hospital of the Sao Paulo State University (FMVZ-UNESP) of Botucatu, Brazil. Then, we tested whether the use of third-generation cephalosporins to treat dogs suspected with CPV and CDV infections increased the faecal carriage of ESCR-E in dogs returning to their household up to 14 weeks after treatment.

2. Results

2.1. Dogs' Characteristics

A total of 222 dogs were sampled from Botucatu (Southeast Brazil) (63%) and cities within a radius of approximately 350 Km (37%). CPV-suspected dogs were 5 months old on average (range: 1–30 months, median: 3), half (52%, 27/52) were male, and 56% were mixed breed. CDV-suspected dogs were 34 months old on average (range: 1–108 months, median: 24), half (50%, 20/40) were male, and 73% were mixed breed. Noninfected dogs were 58 months old on average (range: 1–120 months, median: 60); the majority were female (56.2%, 73/130) and 55% were purebred. The type of food provided to dogs by owners were majority kibble (noninfected dogs: 95%, 118/124; CPV-suspected dogs: 100%, 38/38; and CDV-suspected dogs: 94%, 30/32), but owners also provided raw (noninfected dogs: 8%, CPV-suspected dogs: 18%, CDV-suspected dogs: 16%,) and cooked meat/poultry (noninfected dogs: 63%; CPV-suspected dogs: 45%, CDV-suspected dogs: 66%).

2.2. Prevalence of Faecal Carriage and Characterization of ESCR-E Isolated from Dogs before Antibiotic Therapy

The prevalence of ESCR-E (i.e., *E. coli* and *K. pneumoniae*) faecal carriage in dogs prior to their admission at the referral veterinary teaching hospital FMVZ-UNESP was 16.7% (37/222) (95% CI: 12–22%). The prevalence of ESCR-E faecal carriage in CPV-suspected dogs (36.5% (95% CI: 25–50%) (19/52)) was higher than in CDV-suspected dogs (15% (95% CI: 7–29%) (6/40)) (Pearson's test, $p < 0.05$) and that in noninfected dogs (9.2% (95% CI: 5–16%) (12/130)) (Pearson's test, $p < 0.001$) (Table 1). No statistically significant difference was found between CDV-suspected dogs and noninfected dogs (Pearson's test, $p = 0.46$).

Table 1. Clinical signs, prevalence of extended-spectrum cephalosporin-resistant *Enterobacterales* (ESCR-*E*) and antimicrobial resistance profiles isolated from faeces of dogs clinically diagnosed with canine parvovirus (CPV) and canine distemper (CDV) infections before and after prophylactic antibiotic therapy with third-generation cephalosporin and from dogs with noninfectious diseases.

Variable	CPV-Suspected Dogs	CDV-Suspected Dogs	Noninfected Dogs
Main clinical signs	Haemorrhagic diarrhoea Vomiting Intense dehydration	Nonhaemorrhagic diarrhoea Respiratory disorders Neurological signs	Signs of noninfectious diseases
Prevalence BEFORE treatment	36.5% (19/52) [1] (95% CI: 25–50%)	15% (6/40) (95% CI: 7–29%)	9.2% (12/130) (95% CI: 5–16%)
AMR profiles BEFORE treatment	*E. coli* CroCpdCtx (n = 5) [2] CroCpdCtxAtm (n = 12) CroCpdCtxCazAtm (n = 1) CroCpdCtxCazFox (n = 2) CroCpdCtxCazFoxAtm (n = 4) *K. pneumoniae* CroCpdCtxAtm (n = 1) CroCpdCtxCazAtm (n = 2)	*E. coli* CroCpdCtx (n = 3) CroCpdCtxAtm (n = 1) CroCpdCtxCazAtm (n = 1) CroCpdCtxCazFox (n = 1) CroCpdCtxCazFoxAtm (n = 1)	*E. coli* CroCpdCtx (n = 8) CroCpdCtxAtm (n = 8) CroCpdCtxCazAtm (n = 2)
Prevalence DURING treatment	84.6% (11/13) (95% CI: 56–97%)	57.1% (4/7) (95% CI: 25–84%)	N/A
AMR profiles DURING treatment	*E. coli* CroCpdCtx (n = 2) CroCpdCtxAtm (n = 7) CroCpdCtxCazAtm (n = 2) *K. pneumoniae* CroCpdCtx (n = 1) CroCpdCtxCazAtm (n = 2)	*E. coli* CroCpdCtx (n = 1) CroCpdCtxAtm (n = 2) CroCpdCtxCazAtm (n = 1) CroCpdCtxCazFox (n = 1) CroCpdCtxCazFoxAtm (n = 1)	N/A
Prevalence 1–4 WEEKS after treatment	88.5% (23/26) (95% CI: 70–97%)	60% (6/10) (95% CI: 31–83%)	N/A
AMR profiles 1–4 WEEKS after treatment	*E. coli* CroCpdCtx (n = 17) CroCpdCtxAtm (n = 18) CroCpdCtxCazAtm (n = 5) CroCpdCtxCazFox (n = 5) CroCpdCtxCazFoxAtm (n = 4) CroCpdCtxFox (n = 2) * *K. pneumoniae* CroCpdCtx (n = 3) CroCpdCtxAtm (n = 2) CroCpdCtxCazAtm (n = 2) CroCpdCtxCazFoxAtm (n = 1)	*E. coli* CroCpdCtx (n = 2) CroCpdCtxAtm (n = 4) CroCpdCtxCazAtm (n = 2) CroCpdCtxCazFoxAtm (n = 1)	N/A
Prevalence 5-8 WEEKS after treatment	15.4% (2/13) (95% CI: 3–43.5%)	N/A	N/A
AMR profiles 5-8 WEEKS after treatment	*E. coli* CroCpdCtx (n = 1) CroCpdCtxAtm (n = 1)	N/A	
Prevalence over 9 WEEKS after treatment	0% (0/10)	N/A	N/A

[1] Number of positive dogs over the total number of sampled dogs. [2] Number of isolates. * Antimicrobial resistance phenotype only observed after treatment. Abbreviations: Cro—ceftriaxone, Cpd—cefpodoxime, Ctx—cefotaxime, Caz—ceftazidime, Fox—cefoxitin, Atm—aztreonam, N/A—data not available.

We recovered 49 ESCR-*E. coli* and 3 ESCR-*K. pneumoniae* isolates from 37 dogs sampled before antibiotic therapy (details on each isolate are given in Table S1). To avoid duplicating same strains, isolates from the same sample showing the same antimicrobial resistance pattern (antimicrobial resistance phenotype) and ESBL genes were excluded from further analysis. All isolates were resistant to ceftriaxone, cefpodoxime, and cefotaxime, 63.5% to aztreonam, 26.9% to ceftazidime, and 15.4% to cefoxitin (Table 1). No isolate was resistant to carbapenems. We found 5 antimicrobial resistance phenotypes among dogs suspected of CPV and CDV infection, and 3 of them were also observed in noninfected dogs. β-lactamases genes were detected in 67% (33/49) of ESCR-*E. coli* and in 100% of *K. pneumoniae* (3/3) isolates from 37 dogs (Table 2). $bla_{CTX\text{-}M}$ was detected in 60% (31/52) of isolates, bla_{TEM} in 21% (11/52), and bla_{SHV} in 6% (3/52). The ESBL $bla_{CTX\text{-}M}$ was predominately identified in isolates resistant to ceftriaxone, cefpodoxime, cefotaxime, and aztreonam.

2.3. *Effect of Prophylactic Antibiotic Treatment*

From the 92 dogs clinically diagnosed with CPV and CDV infections sampled and then treated with third generation of cephalosporins, we sampled 20 dogs during their 7-day treatment and 36 dogs 1–4 weeks after (Table 3). Half (52%) of the dogs followed died during the study period, 19 dogs could not be accessed either during or after treatment, and 5 dogs have subsequent negative results that discontinued their follow-up. Details of the follow-up are given in Table S2.

The prevalence of ESCR-E faecal carriage in dogs significantly increased during the 7-day course of treatment from 36.5% to 84.6% (95% CI: 56–97%) (11/13) in CPV-suspected dogs (Pearson's test, $p < 0.01$) and from 15% to 57.1% (95% CI: 25–84%) (4/7) in CDV-suspected dogs (Pearson's test, $p < 0.05$) (Figure 1). This prevalence remained high 1–4 weeks after the treatment in both CPV-suspected (88.5% (95% CI: 70–97%) (23/26)) and CDV-suspected dogs (60% (95% CI: 31–83%) (6/10)). Due to the high mortality of CDV-suspected dogs, only CPV-suspected dogs were monitored more than 9 weeks after treatment. The prevalence of ESCR-E faecal carriage in CPV-suspected dogs significantly decreased 5–8 weeks after treatment (15.4% (95% CI: 3–43.5%) (2/13)) (Pearson's test, $p<0.001$) compared to 1–4 weeks. No ESCR-*E. coli* was detected in the 10 dogs monitored more than 9 weeks after treatment.

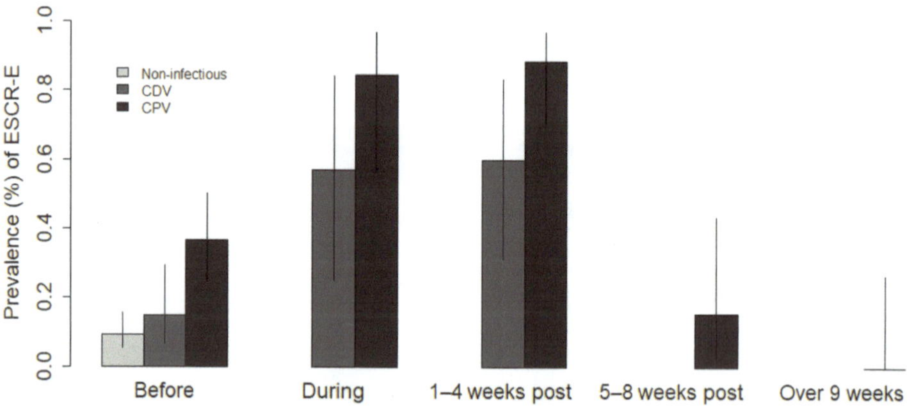

Figure 1. Prevalence of extended-spectrum cephalosporin-resistant *Enterobacterales* (ESCR-E) faecal carriage in dogs clinically diagnosed with canine parvovirus (CPV) and canine distemper (CDV) infections before, during, and after antibiotic therapy. The prevalence of dogs suspected of CPV and CDV infections was estimated at four periods after the start of antibiotic therapy with third-generation cephalosporin: "During" the 7-day course of ceftriaxone or ceftiofur, "1–4 weeks" post-treatment, "5–8 weeks" post-treatment, and "over 9 weeks" post-treatment. Before the treatment, the prevalence was compared to dogs without infectious diseases prior to their admission to the hospital for other health issues.

Table 2. Resistance profile and β-lactamases genes identified from ESCR-*E. coli* and ESCR-*K. pneumoniae* isolates of 19 CPV-suspected dogs, 6 CDV-suspected dogs, and 12 uninfected dogs before antibiotic therapy.

Dog ID	Bacteria Species	Strain	AMR Profile	CTX-M [1]	SHV	TEM
CPV-2	*E. coli*	MS1_001	CroCpdCtxCazFox	-	-	+
CPV-3	*E. coli*	MS1_018	CroCpdCtxCazFox	-	-	+
CPV-4	*E. coli*	MS1_022	CroCpdCtxCazFoxAtm	-	-	+
CPV-5	*E. coli*	MS1_034	CroCpdCtxCazFoxAtm	-	-	-
CPV-5	*E. coli*	MS1_035	CroCpdCtx	-	-	-
CPV-5	*K. pneumoniae*	MS1_036	CroCpdCtxCazAtm	+	+	+
CPV-5	*K. pneumoniae*	MS1_038	CroCpdCtxAtm	+	+	+
CPV-6	*E. coli*	MS1_052	CroCpdCtx	-	-	+
CPV-6	*E. coli*	MS1_053	CroCpdCtxCazFoxAtm	-	-	-
CPV-6	*E. coli*	MS1_054	CroCpdCtxAtm	-	-	-
CPV-7	*E. coli*	MS1_067	CroCpdCtx	-	-	+
CPV-7	*E. coli*	MS1_069	CroCpdCtxAtm	-	-	-
CPV-8	*E. coli*	MS1_083	CroCpdCtxCazFoxAtm	-	-	-
CPV-13	*E. coli*	MS1_111	CroCpdCtxAtm	+	-	-
CPV-14	*E. coli*	MS1_120	CroCpdCtxAtm	+	-	-
CPV-15	*E. coli*	MS1_123	CroCpdCtxAtm	+	-	-
CPV-16	*E. coli*	MS1_129	CroCpdCtxAtm	+	-	-
CPV-26	*E. coli*	MS1_152	CroCpdCtxAtm	+	-	-
CPV-41	*E. coli*	MS1_186	CroCpdCtx	+	-	-
CPV-42	*E. coli*	MS1_192	CroCpdCtxAtm	+	-	-
CPV-42	*E. coli*	MS1_194	CroCpdCtx	+	-	-
CPV-43	*E. coli*	MS1_198	CroCpdCtxCazAtm	+	-	-
CPV-43	*E. coli*	MS1_199	CroCpdCtxAtm	+	-	-
CPV-44	*E. coli*	MS1_204	CroCpdCtxAtm	+	-	-
CPV-45	*K. pneumoniae*	MS1_210	CroCpdCtxCazAtm	+	+	+
CPV-46	*E. coli*	MS1_213	CroCpdCtxAtm	+	-	-
CPV-50	*E. coli*	MS1_223	CroCpdCtxAtm	+	-	-
CDV-7	*E. coli*	MS1_234	CroCpdCtx	+	-	-
CDV-21	*E. coli*	MS1_249	CroCpdCtx	-	-	-
CDV-27	*E. coli*	MS1_252	CroCpdCtx	-	-	-
CDV-28	*E. coli*	MS1_258	CroCpdCtxAtm	+	-	-
CDV-29	*E. coli*	MS1_261	CroCpdCtxCazFox	-	-	-
CDV-29	*E. coli*	MS1_262	CroCpdCtxCazFoxAtm	-	-	-
CDV-37	*E. coli*	MS1_267	CroCpdCtxCazAtm	+	-	-
NI-11	*E. coli*	MS1_270	CroCpdCtxAtm	-	-	-
NI-11	*E. coli*	MS1_271	CroCpdCtx	-	-	-
NI-19	*E. coli*	MS1_273	CroCpdCtx	-	-	-
NI-29	*E. coli*	MS1_276	CroCpdCtxAtm	+	-	+
NI-29	*E. coli*	MS1_278	CroCpdCtxCazAtm	+	-	+
NI-43	*E. coli*	MS1_279	CroCpdCtx	-	-	-
NI-44	*E. coli*	MS1_282	CroCpdCtx	-	-	-
NI-44	*E. coli*	MS1_283	CroCpdCtxAtm	+	-	-
NI-59	*E. coli*	MS1_285	CroCpdCtxAtm	+	-	-
NI-72	*E. coli*	MS1_287	CroCpdCtx	+	-	-
NI-78	*E. coli*	MS1_290	CroCpdCtx	+	-	-
NI-78	*E. coli*	MS1_291	CroCpdCtxAtm	+	-	-
NI-93	*E. coli*	MS1_293	CroCpdCtxAtm	+	-	-
NI-94	*E. coli*	MS1_296	CroCpdCtxAtm	+	-	-
NI-94	*E. coli*	MS1_298	CroCpdCtx	+	-	+
NI-97	*E. coli*	MS1_299	CroCpdCtx	-	-	-
NI-106	*E. coli*	MS1_302	CroCpdCtxAtm	+	-	-
NI-106	*E. coli*	MS1_303	CroCpdCtxCazAtm	+	-	-

[1] Extended-spectrum β-lactamase, (+): detection of the gene, (-): no detection of the gene. Abbreviations: Cro—ceftriaxone, Cpd—cefpodoxime, Ctx—cefotaxime, Caz—ceftazidime, Fox—cefoxitin, Atm—aztreonam.

Table 3. Design and sample size of our longitudinal study tracking ESCR-E before and after antibiotic treatment.

Number of Dogs/Sampling Period	Before	During	1–4 Weeks after Treatment	5–8 Weeks after Treatment	Over 9 Weeks after Treatment
Number of CDV-suspected dogs	40	7	10	–	–
Number of CPV-suspected dogs	52	13	26	13	10
Median of sampling day resulting in ESCR-E isolates	–	4	14	50	–
Number of deaths	–	22	31	48	48
Number of dogs that were not accessed for sampling	–	49	21	22	3
Number of dogs sold	–	1	4	4	6
Number of dogs with subsequent negative results	–	–	–	5	5

We obtained 17 ESCR-*E. coli* and 3 ESCR-*K. pneumoniae* isolates from the 15 infected dogs sampled during antibiotic therapy, 60 ESCR-*E. coli* and 8 ESCR-*K. pneumoniae* isolates from the 29 infected dogs sampled 1–4 weeks after treatment, and 2 ESCR-*E. coli* from 2 infected dogs sampled 5–8 weeks after treatment (Table 1). All isolates obtained during and after the treatment were resistant to ceftriaxone, cefpodoxime, and cefotaxime, 61.1% to aztreonam, 30% to ceftazidime, and 16.7% to cefoxitin. No isolate was resistant to carbapenems. The five antimicrobial resistance phenotypes of isolates from dogs sampled before treatment were also found during and after treatment. Only one new antimicrobial resistance phenotype (resistance to ceftriaxone, cefpodoxime, cefotaxime, and cefoxitin) observed 1–4 weeks after treatment in 2 isolates of CPV-suspected dogs was not previously detected.

3. Discussion

Despite the common use of extended-spectrum cephalosporins to treat enteric viruses, their impact on the prevalence of ESCR-E faecal carriage in dogs has not been previously studied. We found that the faecal carriage of ESCR-E was higher in CPV-suspected dogs compared to CDV-suspected dogs or noninfected dogs prior to their admission at the veterinary university hospital in Botucatu, Brazil. During the 7-day course of third-generation cephalosporin, the prevalence of ESCR-E faecal carriage increased by more than 50% in both CPV-suspected and CDV-suspected dogs, remained high up to 4 weeks after treatment, and could still be detected in dogs for up to 7 weeks post-treatment. A diversity of antibiotic phenotypes was observed, and the majority of the observed in ESCR-E was associated with the presence of $bla_{\text{CTX-M}}$ genes.

Secondary bacterial infections frequently worsen the prognosis of enteric viruses such as CPV and CDV, requiring prophylactic antibiotic therapies including third-generation cephalosporins [16,21,22,34–37]. Our study showed that the use of ceftriaxone or ceftiofur increased faecal prevalence of ESCR-E in hospitalized dogs during the treatment and remained 4 weeks after hospital discharge. Ceftiofur and ceftriaxone are similar third-generation cephalosporins although ceftiofur has been developed exclusively for animal treatment [38]. Both cephalosporins contain an *oxyimino-aminothiazole* group (also found in other antimicrobials such as cefpodoxime, ceftazidime, cefotaxime, ceftizoxime, and aztreonam), which is hydrolysed by extended-spectrum β-lactamases conferring resistance to these β-lactams antibiotics [38,39]. Several studies have shown an increase in AMR *E. coli* in animals after selection pressure by use of β-lactams and fluoroquinolones [11,12,15,40–43]. For example, parenteral antibiotic therapy with extended-spectrum cephalosporins and hospitalization longer than 6 days increased the faecal carriage multidrug-resistant *E. coli* during hospitalization [44]. The presence of ESCR-E faecal carriage in the hospitalized dogs in our study suggests either independent circulation of these strains in the community or a selection in the hospital during treatment that is then spread in dogs of the community. Although we have not evaluated the clinical impact of the emergence of ESCR-E during treatment for enteric viruses, nosocomial infections by resistant bacteria in veterinary hospitals are been increasingly reported in small animal practices worldwide and several approaches should be used to reduce the risks [45–47]. Ensuring an appropriate use of third-generation cephalosporins may include de-escalation of antibiotic therapy or shorter duration of treatment when the clinical improvement of patients is observed [48]. However, the efficiency of these approaches should be first tested in veterinary practices. Optimizing antibiotic use without compromising its efficacy is particularly important when treating CPV-infected dogs because bacteremia and sepsis are commonly observed due to the loss of the intestinal barrier and translocation of Gram-negative bacteria [16,21,22].

Our results suggest that ESCR-*E. coli* faecal carriage in CPV-suspected dogs can last up to 7 weeks after treatment. Similar studies have shown that treatment with antibiotics increases the prevalence and persistence of AMR *Enterobacterales* [10,11]. For example, treatment with amoxicillin and clavulanic acid has been associated with ESCR-*E. coli* faecal carriage 1 month after treatment [12]. Alternatively to persistence, ESCR-*E. coli* may be reacquired after treatment from external sources, which could be evaluated in future molecular studies. Overall, our study calls for increasing awareness regarding the potential spread of ESCR-E in clinical and community settings caused by treatments of enteric viruses with antibiotics.

A total of six antimicrobial resistance profiles were obtained in our study. One profile was only detected after treatment. This new profile could reflect the emergence of new antibiotic resistance associated with the selection impose by the treatment or a low detection probability of all the resistant profiles before treatment given our limited sample size. Resistance to ceftriaxone, cefpodoxime, cefotaxime, and aztreonam was the main profile observed, which is often associated with ESBL production [32]. In fact, the majority (60%) of ESCR-E isolates (i.e., *E. coli* and *K. pneumoniae*) from CPV-suspected dogs and noninfected dogs (67%) carried $bla_{\text{CTX-M}}$ genes, followed by CDV-suspected dogs (43%). CTX-M genotype was the most prevalent genotype found among ESCR-E isolates, confirming the spread of ESBL in dogs [11,49–52]. Differences in the antimicrobial resistance phenotype between CTX-M-positive isolates might reflect the variety of CTX-M groups (i.e., CTX-M-1, CTX-M-2, CTX-M-8, CTX-M-9, and CTX-M-25) that may present different hydrolysing activities for cephalosporins [32,53]. In addition, the concomitant presence of AmpC genes (chromosomally encoded or plasmid-mediated) results in cefoxitin resistance and can mask the presence of ESBL [54,55]. Although our PCR protocol included primers specifically designed to detect common extended-spectrum β-lactamases genes, future molecular analyses including sequencing of these resistance genes (e.g., bla_{SHV} and bla_{TEM}) will confirm if they are ESBL genes and identify their variant. No β-lactamase genes were detected in 16 ESCR-E isolates but the phenotypic resistance observed may be due to other β-lactamases not tested in the current study (e.g., CMY, PER, and OXA), mutations in the chromosomal AmpC gene, efflux pumps, or pore deficiencies [56]. Therefore, further molecular studies such as whole-genome sequencing could help identifying all that antibiotic resistance mechanisms present among these bacteria.

To our knowledge, this is the first study showing a higher prevalence of faecal carriage of antibiotic-resistant bacteria in dogs presenting clinical signs of enteric viruses. Brazil has a high prevalence of CPV and CDV, and these viruses are the leading cause of mortality related to infectious diseases in dogs with an incidence above 45% in some areas with low vaccine coverage [57,58]. Thus, increase in ESCR-*E. coli* after treatment could have important implications for the spread of ESCR-*E. coli* among dogs in Brazil. CPV and CDV alter the host microbiota [16,17,34,59,60] and could be influencing the gut colonization by antibiotic-resistant bacteria such as ESCR-E. Since the immune system regulates the gut microbiota [61], host immunosuppression provoked by these viruses may favour mechanisms expressing different genes including ESBL genes. For instance, immunosuppressive treatments with a combination of prednisolone, mycophenolate mofetil, and tacrolimus increased the population of uropathogenic *E. coli* in treated humans [62]. CPV has a strong affinity of rapidly dividing cells causing destruction of crypt intestinal epithelial cells, which might generate a higher impact on the microbiota, including antimicrobial-resistant bacteria. Alternatively, other explanations for the observed outcome could include exposure to antibiotics by infected dogs prior to the period established in our inclusion criteria (3 months). However, this hypothesis is not supported by the observation that most infected dogs were puppies and thus, were probably not exposed directly to antibiotics' treatment. Thus, the mechanisms behind the higher prevalence of ESCR-E in CPV-suspected dogs remain unclear. Other explanations could include dogs been intensely exposed to antibiotic-resistant bacteria from other sources such as humans or livestock, and the puppies' mothers been a source of antibiotic-resistant bacteria. For example, adult dogs leaving in regions with low vaccine coverage favouring the acquisition of CPV [57] could be more likely to have concomitant diseases and/or a history of receiving antimicrobials, which could indirectly expose their puppies.

Several limitations of our study could encourage future research on the role of enteric viruses along with antimicrobial prophylaxis in the emergence of AMR. For examples, although most differences in prevalence between dog populations were statistically significant, the number of followed dogs after treatment was substantially reduced by the high mortality of infected dogs (52%) and difficulty to access dogs at their household. Therefore, the lack of detection of dogs with ESCR-E 50 days after treatment could be related to a low detection power due to our low sample size ($n = 5$) and could be further studied in future research. Furthermore, since the excretion of antibiotic-resistant bacteria hosted on the dog's intestinal microbiota can be shed intermittently on faeces, a lack of detection within a faecal sample does not necessarily indicate the absence of faecal carriage in the sampled dog. In addition, we were unable to follow uninfected dogs to confirm that the observed increased in ESCR-*E. coli* prevalence was associated with prophylactic treatment with antibiotics and no other factors such as colonization at the hospital after visit or unknown interactions between CPV or CDV and antibiotic-resistant bacteria. Further studies covering these limitations could explore in more detail both the effect of antibiotic prophylactic treatment and enteric viruses in relation to antimicrobial resistance. The potential misdiagnoses of a bacterial infection cannot be ruled out and require further studies using molecular detection of CPV and CDV to confirm the clinical diagnostics, which was not available at our hospital. However, pathognomonic clinical signs of CDV and CPV such as myoclonus (CDV) or acute haemorrhagic diarrhoea along with intense leukopenia on the peripheral blood (CPV) observed in these animals suggest that misdiagnosis should only represent a small percentage of our population. Furthermore, we cannot exclude the chances of coinfections with other enteropathogens; however, these clinical signs also suggest that illness severity was associated to the presence of these enteric viruses and not aggravated by another agent. Finally, molecular typing of resistant bacteria and detection of mobile genetic elements (e.g., plasmids) will help to understand whether the increase in ESCR-E after treatment is due to maintenance of the same ESCR-E strain, infection with new bacteria or transfer of genetic material across strains conferring antibiotic resistance.

4. Materials and Methods

4.1. Comparison of Prevalence of Dogs Carrying ESCR-E before Antibiotic Therapy

Between August and December 2018 at the referral veterinary teaching hospital of the Sao Paulo State University (FMVZ-UNESP) of Botucatu (Southeast Brazil), rectal swabs were collected from dogs suspected of CPV ($n = 52$) and CDV ($n = 40$). In addition, we also sampled 130 dogs classified as noninfected dogs by the veterinarian collecting the sample as a control group. Dogs were physically examined by a veterinarian and the owners were asked about the previous use of antibiotic in their dogs within the last 3 months. Two exclusion criteria were used: i) the use of antimicrobials within 3 months before sampling and ii) dogs more than 10 years old.

Dogs attended in the Animal Infectious Diseases sector presenting haemorrhagic diarrhoea, vomiting, dehydration, and intense leukopenia on peripheral blood [16] were diagnosed with CPV infection by the veterinarian attending while signals of nonhaemorrhagic diarrhoea, respiratory disorders, nasal and ocular discharges, hyperkeratosis, and neurological manifestation (i.e., myoclonus) were diagnosed as CDV infection [34]. To be included in this study, infected dogs had to present all the described clinical signs to guarantee homogeneity among CPV and CDV groups and to attest the severity of the illness. Noninfected dogs were attended in the sectors of Cardiology, Nephrology, Neurology, Surgery, or Ophthalmology and showed absence of clinical signs of infectious diseases and/or gastrointestinal disorders (dogs suspected of infection even without symptoms such as gastrointestinal alterations or respiratory disorders were not included).

The sample size required to estimate the prevalence of noninfected dogs was determined using Epi Info 7.2.2.6 TM [63]. Based on an expected prevalence of ESCR-*E. coli* of 9% estimated in a previous study conducted in Brazil [49], a dog population estimated in Botucatu of 27,735 dogs [64], an acceptable margin of error of 5% and confidence interval of 95%, the estimated sample size was 125 animals. A sampling of dogs suspected of viral infections was based on convenience, enrolling all suspected dogs with CPV and CDV admitted to the hospital in 5 months, considering that many dies before or during the treatment.

4.2. Faecal Prevalence of ESCR-E During and After Antibiotic Therapy With Third-Generation Cephalosporins in Dogs Suspected of CPV and CDV Infections

CPV and CDV suspected dogs were treated with parenteral ceftriaxone (30 mg/Kg) or ceftiofur (7.5 mg/Kg) every 24 h for 7 days. To test how the prevalence of ESCR-E in dogs changes after treatment, all treated dogs were sampled in the following periods: (1) before administration of third-generation cephalosporin, (2) during the 7-day course of treatment, and (3) after antibiotic therapy between the first and fourth week (1–4 weeks post-treatment). In dogs where ESCR-E was detected during or after treatment, subsequent sampling was done (4) between the fifth and eighth week (5–8 weeks post-treatment) and (5) above the ninth week (over 9 weeks post-treatment). The number of samples after antibiotic therapy varied from one to three per dog and sampling of dogs was not paired (Table S2). This study was approved by the Ethical Committee in Animal Use (CEUA) of the FMVZ-UNESP/Botucatu under protocol: 0090/2018 (registration number on CONCEA–National Council for Animal Control and Experimentation: CIAEP/CONCEA no. 01.0115.2014–05/06/2014), and all owners signed a consent form for inclusion of their dogs.

4.3. Microbiology Analysis

Rectal swabs were screened for ESCR-E using MacConkey agar supplemented with 2 μg/mL cefotaxime (Oxoid, Hampshire, England) and incubated at 37 °C for 48 h to select potential ESBL/AmpC-producing isolates [65]. *E. coli* strain containing the $bla_{\text{CTX-M15}}$ gene (provided by the Microbiology Laboratory of Institute of Biosciences-UNESP) and a non-resistant *E. coli* strain (donated by the Microbiology Laboratory of the Veterinary Teaching Hospital of FMVZ-UNESP) were used as positive and negative controls. Up to three isolates morphologic compatible with *E. coli* or *K. pneumoniae* were randomly selected in the plate and then confirmed by matrix-assisted laser desorption ionization-time of flight mass spectrometry (MALDI-TOF MS, BioMérieux, Marcy l'Etoile, France) at the Genomics and Resistant Microbes (GeRM) Group of the Millennium Initiative for Collaborative Research On Bacterial Resistance (MICROB-R), in Santiago, Chile. Other species identified were excluded from the further analysis (i.e., *Escherichia fergusonii*, *Raoultella ornithinolytica*, *Raoultella planticola*, and *Citrobacter freundii*).

According to the CLSI M100:28ED, cefpodoxime (10 μg) with inhibition zone $\leq$ 17 mm, ceftazidime (30 μg) with inhibition zone $\leq$ 22 mm, aztreonam (30 μg) with inhibition zone $\leq$27 mm, cefotaxime (30 μg) with inhibition zone $\leq$ 27 mm, and ceftriaxone (30 μg) with inhibition zone $\leq$25 mm of *E. coli* isolates may indicate ESBL production. To select extended-spectrum cephalosporins-resistant isolates, particularly the ESBL producers, we tested ceftriaxone (30 μg), cefpodoxime (10 μg), cefotaxime (30 μg), ceftazidime (30 μg), aztreonam (30 μg), and cefoxitin (30 μg) by the disk diffusion method according to the CLSI [65]. We preferred to include a combination of these antibiotics instead on only one of them, to improve the detection of ESBL production. To assess co-resistance to carbapenems, we also tested susceptibility to imipenem (10 μg), meropenem (10 μg), and ertapenem (10 μg). Breakpoints and a quality control *E. coli* ATCC25922 strain was used during each assay as recommended by CLSI [65]. A multiplex PCR protocol was performed to detect β-lactamases genes ($bla_{CTX\text{-}M}$, bla_{SHV}, and bla_{TEM}) in ESCR-*E. coli* and in ESCR-*K. pneumoniae* isolated before antibiotic therapy using primers previously published [66,67]. Primers sequence and PCR conditions are given in the additional data (Table S3). *E. coli* strain SCL-1290 of MICROB-R repository containing these three genes was used as a positive control.

4.4. Statistical Analysis

The prevalence of dogs colonized by ESCR-E, referred here as the number of individuals with at least one positive isolate of ESCR-*E. coli* or ESCR-*K. pneumoniae* over the total number of sampled animals, was reported with a 95% confidence interval using the *binom.confint* function (Agresti–Coull method) in the *binom* package in R 3.6.1 [68]. Differences in prevalence were tested using the Pearson test's chi-squared in R.

5. Conclusions

Our results show that prophylactic antibiotic therapy in dogs clinically diagnosed with enteric viruses (i.e., CPV and CDV) can play an important role in the dissemination of ESCR-E in clinical settings and the community. Although antimicrobial prophylaxis in these diseases is necessary, we highlight the importance of optimizing prophylactic antibiotic therapy in infected dogs by prioritizing first or second generation of cephalosporin in mild cases and third-generation cephalosporins only for life-threatening one. Even if new classes of antimicrobial agents are developed, they are unlikely to be available for veterinary medicine in the short term. Therefore, emergence and persistence of resistance to broad-spectrum cephalosporins observed in this study after treatment with third-generation of cephalosporins stress the need for widespread to veterinarians targeting the necessity to maintain the effectiveness of current antibiotic therapies. In addition, our findings suggest that the high prevalence of CPV and CDV may be aggravating the spread of ESCR-*E. coli* among dogs in Brazil, where vaccination against canine viruses with exception of rabies is not mandatory [57]. Therefore, reducing the circulation of CPV and CDV by improving vaccination coverage could help to reduce the dissemination of ESCR-E. Our results also call for further studies to identify the mechanisms behind the observed association between enteric viruses and faecal carriage of antimicrobial-resistant bacteria.

Supplementary Materials: The following are available online at https://www.mdpi.com/2079-6382/10/2/122/s1, Table S1: Characterization of isolates recovered from dogs clinically diagnosed with canine parvovirus (CPV) and canine distemper (CDV) infections and from dogs with noninfectious diseases before antibiotic therapy and of isolates recovered from dogs suspected of CPV and CDV infections after of antibiotic therapy with third-generation cephalosporin started; Table S2: Sampling details of the follow-up of the dogs suspected of CPV and CDV infections after of antibiotic therapy with third-generation cephalosporin; Table S3. Sequences, melting temperature, and amplicon size of primers used for detection of CTX-M-type, SHV-type, and TEM-type genes.

Author Contributions: Conceptualization, M.S.-C., A.C.P., C.S. and J.A.B.; data curation, J.A.B.; formal analysis, J.A.B.; funding acquisition, A.I.M.-S. and J.A.B.; investigation, M.S.-C. and J.A.B.; methodology, M.S.-C., J.M.M. and L.R.; project administration, A.I.M.-S., A.C.P. and J.A.B.; resources, M.S.-C., A.I.M.-S., A.C.P. and J.A.B.; supervision, A.I.M.-S., A.C.P. and J.A.B.; visualization, J.A.B.; writing—original draft, M.S.-C.; writing—review and editing, A.I.M.-S., A.C.P., C.S. and J.A.B. All authors have read and agreed to the published version of the manuscript.

Funding: This study was financed by the Coordenação de Aperfeiçoamento de Pessoal de Nível Superior-Brasil (CAPES)-Finance Code 001, supported by FONDECYT 1181167 awarded to AMS. This work was funded by the National Agency for Research and Development (ANID) FONDECYT Iniciación 11181017, awarded to J.B., and by the ANID Millennium Science Initiative/Millennium Initiative for Collaborative Research on Bacterial Resistance, MICROB-R, NCN17_081.

Institutional Review Board Statement: This study was approved by the Ethical Committee in Animal Use (CEUA) of the FMVZ-UNESP/Botucatu under protocol: 0090/2018 (registration number on CONCEA–National Council for Animal Control and Experimentation: CIAEP/CONCEA no. 01.0115.2014–05/06/2014).

Informed Consent Statement: All owners signed a consent form for inclusion of their dogs.

Acknowledgments: We would like to thank dog owners and their families for their willingness, kindness, and patience to participate in this study, particularly with dogs that were very ill. This work is dedicated to all the dogs that unfortunately died during this study from CPV and CDV, two preventable diseases. We would continue fighting to avoid these painful deaths. We thank veterinary teaching hospital of FMVZ-UNESP and the Laboratory of Microbiology of FMVZ-UNESP. We thank members of the MonkeyLab at Universidad Andrés Bello, Patricia Poeta, Ana Gales, José Carlos Pantoja, and Marcio Garcia Ribeiro for their useful comments and suggestions with the manuscripts.

Conflicts of Interest: The authors declare no conflict of interest.

References

1. Bengtsson, B.; Greko, C. Antibiotic Resistance—Consequences for Animal Health, Welfare, and Food Production. *Ups. J. Med. Sci.* **2014**, *119*, 96–102. [CrossRef]
2. Ventola, C.L. The Antibiotic Resistance Crisis—Part 1. *P T* **2015**, *40*, 277–283. [PubMed]
3. WHO. *Global Priority List of Antibiotic-Resistant Bacteria to Guide Research, Discovery, and Development of New Antibiotics*; WHO: Geneva, Switzerland, 2017.
4. Rocha-Gracia, R.C.; Cortés-Cortés, G.; Lozano-Zarain, P.; Bello, F.; Martínez-Laguna, Y.; Torres, C. Faecal *Escherichia Coli* Isolates from Healthy Dogs Harbour CTX-M-15 and CMY-2 β-Lactamases. *Vet. J.* **2015**, *203*, 315–319. [CrossRef] [PubMed]
5. Ortega-Paredes, D.; Haro, M.; Leoro-Garzón, P.; Barba, P.; Loaiza, K.; Mora, F.; Fors, M.; Vinueza-Burgos, C.; Fernández-Moreira, E. Multidrug-Resistant *Escherichia Coli* Isolated from Canine Faeces in a Public Park in Quito, Ecuador. *J. Glob. Antimicrob. Resist.* **2019**, *18*, 263–268. [CrossRef] [PubMed]
6. Dupouy, V.; Abdelli, M.; Moyano, G.; Arpaillange, N.; Bibbal, D.; Cadiergues, M.-C.; Lopez-Pulin, D.; Sayah-Jeanne, S.; de Gunzburg, J.; Saint-Lu, N.; et al. Prevalence of Beta-Lactam and Quinolone/Fluoroquinolone Resistance in *Enterobacteriaceae* from Dogs in France and Spain—Characterization of ESBL/PAmpC Isolates, Genes, and Conjugative Plasmids. *Front. Vet. Sci.* **2019**, 6. [CrossRef]
7. Abbas, G.; Khan, I.; Mohsin, M.; Sajjad-ur-Rahman, S.-R.; Younas, T.; Ali, S. High Rates of CTX-M Group-1 Extended-Spectrum Beta-Lactamases Producing *Escherichia Coli* from Pets and Their Owners in Faisalabad, Pakistan. *IDR* **2019**, *12*, 571–578. [CrossRef]
8. Albrechtova, K.; Kubelova, M.; Mazancova, J.; Dolejska, M.; Literak, I.; Cizek, A. High Prevalence and Variability of CTX-M-15-Producing and Fluoroquinolone-Resistant *Escherichia Coli* Observed in Stray Dogs in Rural Angola. *Microb. Drug Resist.* **2014**, *20*, 372–375. [CrossRef]
9. Loayza, F.; Graham, J.P.; Trueba, G. Factors Obscuring the Role of *E. Coli* from Domestic Animals in the Global Antimicrobial Resistance Crisis: An Evidence-Based Review. *Int J. Environ. Res. Public Health* **2020**, *17*, 3061. [CrossRef]
10. Van den Bunt, G.; Fluit, A.C.; Spaninks, M.P.; Timmerman, A.J.; Geurts, Y.; Kant, A.; Scharringa, J.; Mevius, D.; Wagenaar, J.A.; Bonten, M.J.M.; et al. Faecal Carriage, Risk Factors, Acquisition and Persistence of ESBL-Producing *Enterobacteriaceae* in Dogs and Cats and Co-Carriage with Humans Belonging to the Same Household. *J. Antimicrob. Chemother.* **2020**, *75*, 342–350. [CrossRef]
11. Wedley, A.L.; Dawson, S.; Maddox, T.W.; Coyne, K.P.; Pinchbeck, G.L.; Clegg, P.; Nuttall, T.; Kirchner, M.; Williams, N.J. Carriage of Antimicrobial Resistant *Escherichia Coli* in Dogs: Prevalence, Associated Risk Factors and Molecular Characteristics. *Vet. Microbiol.* **2017**, *199*, 23–30. [CrossRef]
12. Schmidt, V.M.; Pinchbeck, G.; McIntyre, K.M.; Nuttall, T.; McEwan, N.; Dawson, S.; Williams, N.J. Routine Antibiotic Therapy in Dogs Increases the Detection of Antimicrobial-Resistant Faecal *Escherichia Coli*. *J. Antimicrob. Chemother.* **2018**, *73*, 3305–3316. [CrossRef] [PubMed]
13. WHO. Critically Important Antimicrobials for Human Medicine, 6th Revision. Available online: http://www.who.int/foodsafety/publications/antimicrobials-sixth/en/ (accessed on 23 November 2020).
14. De Briyne, N.; Atkinson, J.; Borriello, S.P.; Pokludová, L. Antibiotics Used Most Commonly to Treat Animals in Europe. *Vet. Rec.* **2014**, *175*, 325. [CrossRef] [PubMed]
15. Chantziaras, I.; Boyen, F.; Callens, B.; Dewulf, J. Correlation between Veterinary Antimicrobial Use and Antimicrobial Resistance in Food-Producing Animals: A Report on Seven Countries. *J. Antimicrob. Chemother.* **2014**, *69*, 827–834. [CrossRef] [PubMed]
16. Mylonakis, M.E.; Kalli, I.; Rallis, T.S. Canine Parvoviral Enteritis: An Update on the Clinical Diagnosis, Treatment, and Prevention. *Vet. Med.* **2016**, *7*, 91–100. [CrossRef] [PubMed]
17. Zhao, N.; Li, M.; Luo, J.; Wang, S.; Liu, S.; Wang, S.; Lyu, W.; Chen, L.; Su, W.; Ding, H.; et al. Impacts of Canine Distemper Virus Infection on the Giant Panda Population from the Perspective of Gut Microbiota. *Sci. Rep.* **2017**, *7*, 39954. [CrossRef] [PubMed]
18. Kilian, E.; Suchodolski, J.S.; Hartmann, K.; Mueller, R.S.; Wess, G.; Unterer, S. Long-Term Effects of Canine Parvovirus Infection in Dogs. *PLoS ONE* **2018**, 13. [CrossRef]

19. Mangia, S.; Paes, A. Cinomose. In *Doenças Infecciosas em Animais de Produção e de Companhia*, 1st ed.; Megid, J., Ribeiro, M.G., Paes, A.C., Eds.; Roca: Rio de Janeiro, Brazil, 2016; pp. 560–579.
20. Paes, A. Parvovirose Canina. In *Doenças Infecciosas em Animais de Produção e de Companhia*, 1st ed.; Megid, J., Ribeiro, M.G., Paes, A.C., Eds.; Roca: Rio de Janeiro, Brazil, 2016; pp. 768–785.
21. Sunghan, J.; Akatvipat, A.; Granick, J.; Chuammitri, P.; Boonyayatra, S. Clinical Factors Associated with Death during Hospitalization in Parvovirus Infection Dogs. *Vet. Integr. Sci.* **2019**, *17*, 171–180.
22. Sunghan, J.; Pichpol, D.; Chuammitri, P.; Akatvipat, A. Bacteremia and Multidrug Resistance in Naturally Parvovirus Infection Dogs. *Thai J. Vet. Med.* **2019**, *49*, 193–196.
23. Burdet, C.; Grall, N.; Linard, M.; Bridier-Nahmias, A.; Benhayoun, M.; Bourabha, K.; Magnan, M.; Clermont, O.; d'Humières, C.; Tenaillon, O.; et al. Ceftriaxone and Cefotaxime Have Similar Effects on the Intestinal Microbiota in Human Volunteers Treated by Standard-Dose Regimens. *Antimicrob. Agents Chemother.* **2019**, 63. [CrossRef]
24. DiGangi, B.A.; Dingman, P.A.; Grijalva, C.J.; Belyeu, M.; Tucker, S.; Isaza, R. Prevalence and Risk Factors for the Presence of Serum Antibodies against Canine Distemper, Canine Parvovirus, and Canine Adenovirus in Communities in Mainland Ecuador. *Vet. Immunol. Immunopathol.* **2019**, *218*, 109933. [CrossRef]
25. Kelman, M.; Ward, M.P.; Barrs, V.R.; Norris, J.M. The Geographic Distribution and Financial Impact of Canine Parvovirus in Australia. *Transbound. Emerg. Dis.* **2019**, *66*, 299–311. [CrossRef] [PubMed]
26. Kulkarni, M.B.; Deshpande, A.R.; Gaikwad, S.S.; Majee, S.B.; Suryawanshi, P.R.; Awandkar, S.P. Molecular Epidemiology of Canine Parvovirus Shows CPV-2a Genotype Circulating in Dogs from Western India. *Infect. Genet. Evol.* **2019**, *75*, 103987. [CrossRef] [PubMed]
27. Da Costa, V.G.; Saivish, M.V.; Rodrigues, R.L.; de Lima Silva, R.F.; Moreli, M.L.; Krüger, R.H. Molecular and Serological Surveys of Canine Distemper Virus: A Meta-Analysis of Cross-Sectional Studies. *PLoS ONE* **2019**, 14. [CrossRef] [PubMed]
28. Litster, A.; Nichols, J.; Volpe, A. Prevalence of Positive Antibody Test Results for Canine Parvovirus (CPV) and Canine Distemper Virus (CDV) and Response to Modified Live Vaccination against CPV and CDV in Dogs Entering Animal Shelters. *Vet. Microbiol.* **2012**, *157*, 86–90. [CrossRef]
29. Decaro, N.; Buonavoglia, C.; Barrs, V.R. Canine Parvovirus Vaccination and Immunisation Failures: Are We Far from Disease Eradication? *Vet. Microbiol.* **2020**, *247*, 108760. [CrossRef] [PubMed]
30. Yousfi, M.; Mairi, A.; Touati, A.; Hassissene, L.; Brasme, L.; Guillard, T.; De Champs, C. Extended Spectrum β-Lactamase and Plasmid Mediated Quinolone Resistance in *Escherichia Coli* Fecal Isolates from Healthy Companion Animals in Algeria. *J. Infect. Chemother.* **2016**, *22*, 431–435. [CrossRef]
31. Bevan, E.R.; Jones, A.M.; Hawkey, P.M. Global Epidemiology of CTX-M β-Lactamases: Temporal and Geographical Shifts in Genotype. *J. Antimicrob. Chemother.* **2017**, *72*, 2145–2155. [CrossRef]
32. Bush, K.; Jacoby, G.A. Updated Functional Classification of β-Lactamases. *AAC* **2010**, *54*, 969–976. [CrossRef]
33. Kimura, A.; Yossapol, M.; Shibata, S.; Asai, T. Selection of Broad-Spectrum Cephalosporin-Resistant *Escherichia Coli* in the Feces of Healthy Dogs after Administration of First-Generation Cephalosporins: Cephalosporin-Resistant *E. Coli* in Dog Feces. *Microbiol. Immunol.* **2017**, *61*, 34–41. [CrossRef]
34. Rendon-Marin, S.; da Fontoura Budaszewski, R.; Canal, C.W.; Ruiz-Saenz, J. Tropism and Molecular Pathogenesis of Canine Distemper Virus. *Virol. J.* **2019**, *16*, 30. [CrossRef]
35. Dash, S.; Das, M.; Senapati, S.; Patra, R.; Behera, P.; Sathapathy, S. Effect of Therapeutic Regimen on the Survivility and Mortality Rates in Canine Parvovirus Infection. *J. Entomol. Zool. Stud.* **2020**, *8*, 392–395.
36. Eregowda, C.G.; De, U.K.; Singh, M.; Prasad, H.; Akhilesh; Sarma, K.; Roychoudhury, P.; Rajesh, J.B.; Patra, M.K.; Behera, S.K. Assessment of Certain Biomarkers for Predicting Survival in Response to Treatment in Dogs Naturally Infected with Canine Parvovirus. *Microb. Pathog.* **2020**, *149*, 104485. [CrossRef]
37. Kataria, D.; Agnihotri, D.; Jain, V.; Charaya, G.; Singh, Y. Molecular Occurrence and Therapeutic Management of Canine Parvovirus Infection in Dogs. *Int. J. Curr. Microbiol. Appl. Sci.* **2020**, *9*, 1770–1779. [CrossRef]
38. Hornish, R.; Katarski, S. Cephalosporins in Veterinary Medicine—Ceftiofur Use in Food Animals. *CTMC* **2002**, *2*, 717–731. [CrossRef]
39. Bush, K. The ABCD's of β-Lactamase Nomenclature. *J. Infect. Chemother.* **2013**, *19*, 549–559. [CrossRef] [PubMed]
40. Buckland, E.L.; O'Neill, D.; Summers, J.; Mateus, A.; Church, D.; Redmond, L.; Brodbelt, D. Characterisation of Antimicrobial Usage in Cats and Dogs Attending UK Primary Care Companion Animal Veterinary Practices. *Vet. Rec.* **2016**, *179*, 489. [CrossRef] [PubMed]
41. Burow, E.; Simoneit, C.; Tenhagen, B.-A.; Käsbohrer, A. Oral Antimicrobials Increase Antimicrobial Resistance in Porcine *E. Coli*—A Systematic Review. *Prev. Vet. Med.* **2014**, *113*, 364–375. [CrossRef] [PubMed]
42. Chang, S.-K.; Lo, D.-Y.; Wei, H.-W.; Kuo, H.-C. Antimicrobial Resistance of *Escherichia Coli* Isolates from Canine Urinary Tract Infections. *J. Vet. Med. Sci.* **2015**, *77*, 59–65. [CrossRef]
43. Okpara, E.O.; Ojo, O.E.; Awoyomi, O.J.; Dipeolu, M.A.; Oyekunle, M.A.; Schwarz, S. Antimicrobial Usage and Presence of Extended-Spectrum β-Lactamase-Producing *Enterobacteriaceae* in Animal-Rearing Households of Selected Rural and Peri-Urban Communities. *Vet. Microbiol.* **2018**, *218*, 31–39. [CrossRef]
44. Gibson, J.S.; Morton, J.M.; Cobbold, R.N.; Filippich, L.J.; Trott, D.J. Risk Factors for Dogs Becoming Rectal Carriers of Multidrug-Resistant *Escherichia Coli* during Hospitalization. *Epidemiol. Infect.* **2011**, *139*, 1511–1521. [CrossRef]

45. Hamilton, E.; Kruger, J.M.; Schall, W.; Beal, M.; Manning, S.D.; Kaneene, J.B. Acquisition and Persistence of Antimicrobial-Resistant Bacteria Isolated from Dogs and Cats Admitted to a Veterinary Teaching Hospital. *J. Am. Vet. Med. Assoc.* **2013**, *243*, 990–1000. [CrossRef] [PubMed]
46. Grönthal, T.; Moodley, A.; Nykäsenoja, S.; Junnila, J.; Guardabassi, L.; Thomson, K.; Rantala, M. Large Outbreak Caused by Methicillin Resistant *Staphylococcus Pseudintermedius* ST71 in a Finnish Veterinary Teaching Hospital—From Outbreak Control to Outbreak Prevention. *PLoS ONE* **2014**, *9*, e110084. [CrossRef] [PubMed]
47. Keck, N.; Dunie-merigot, A.; Dazas, M.; Hirchaud, E.; Laurence, S.; Gervais, B.; Madec, J.-Y.; Haenni, M. Long-Lasting Nosocomial Persistence of Chlorhexidine-Resistant Serratia Marcescens in a Veterinary Hospital. *Vet. Microbiol.* **2020**, *245*, 108686. [CrossRef] [PubMed]
48. De Waele, J.J.; Schouten, J.; Beovic, B.; Tabah, A.; Leone, M. Antimicrobial De-Escalation as Part of Antimicrobial Stewardship in Intensive Care: No Simple Answers to Simple Questions—A Viewpoint of Experts. *Intensive Care Med.* **2020**, *46*, 236–244. [CrossRef]
49. Carvalho, A.C.; Barbosa, A.V.; Arais, L.R.; Ribeiro, P.F.; Carneiro, V.C.; Cerqueira, A.M.F. Resistance Patterns, ESBL Genes, and Genetic Relatedness of *Escherichia Coli* from Dogs and Owners. *Braz. J. Microbiol.* **2016**, *47*, 150–158. [CrossRef]
50. Aslantaş, Ö.; Yilmaz, E.Ş. Prevalence and Molecular Characterization of Extended-Spectrum β-Lactamase (ESBL) and Plasmidic AmpC β-Lactamase (PAmpC) Producing *Escherichia Coli* in Dogs. *J. Vet. Med. Sci.* **2017**, *79*, 1024–1030. [CrossRef]
51. Melo, L.C.; Oresco, C.; Leigue, L.; Netto, H.M.; Melville, P.A.; Benites, N.R.; Saras, E.; Haenni, M.; Lincopan, N.; Madec, J.-Y. Prevalence and Molecular Features of ESBL/PAmpC-Producing *Enterobacteriaceae* in Healthy and Diseased Companion Animals in Brazil. *Vet. Microbiol.* **2018**, *221*, 59–66. [CrossRef]
52. Moreno, A.; Bello, H.; Guggiana, D.; Domínguez, M.; González, G. Extended-Spectrum β-Lactamases Belonging to CTX-M Group Produced by *Escherichia Coli* Strains Isolated from Companion Animals Treated with Enrofloxacin. *Vet. Microbiol.* **2008**, *129*, 203–208. [CrossRef]
53. Doi, Y.; Iovleva, A.; Bonomo, R.A. The Ecology of Extended-Spectrum β-Lactamases (ESBLs) in the Developed World. *J. Travel Med.* **2017**, *24*, S44–S51. [CrossRef]
54. Baudry, P.J.; Nichol, K.; DeCorby, M.; Mataseje, L.; Mulvey, M.R.; Hoban, D.J.; Zhanel, G.G. Comparison of Antimicrobial Resistance Profiles among Extended-Spectrum-β-Lactamase-Producing and Acquired AmpC β-Lactamase-Producing *Escherichia Coli* Isolates from Canadian Intensive Care Units. *Antimicrob. Agents Chemother.* **2008**, *52*, 1846–1849. [CrossRef]
55. Song, W.; Bae, I.K.; Lee, Y.-N.; Lee, C.-H.; Lee, S.H.; Jeong, S.H. Detection of Extended-Spectrum β-Lactamases by Using Boronic Acid as an AmpC β-Lactamase Inhibitor in Clinical Isolates of *Klebsiella* Spp. and *Escherichia Coli*. *J. Clin. Microbiol.* **2007**, *45*, 1180–1184. [CrossRef]
56. Baede, V.O.; Wagenaar, J.A.; Broens, E.M.; Duim, B.; Dohmen, W.; Nijsse, R.; Timmerman, A.J.; Hordijk, J. Longitudinal Study of Extended-Spectrum-β-Lactamase- and AmpC-Producing *Enterobacteriaceae* in Household Dogs. *Antimicrob. Agents Chemother.* **2015**, *59*, 3117–3124. [CrossRef] [PubMed]
57. Alves, C.D.B.T.; Granados, O.F.O.; Budaszewski, R.D.F.; Streck, A.F.; Weber, M.N.; Cibulski, S.P.; Pinto, L.D.; Ikuta, N.; Canal, C.W.; Alves, C.D.B.T.; et al. Identification of Enteric Viruses Circulating in a Dog Population with Low Vaccine Coverage. *Braz. J. Microbiol.* **2018**, *49*, 790–794. [CrossRef] [PubMed]
58. Budaszewski, R.D.F.; Pinto, L.D.; Weber, M.N.; Caldart, E.T.; Alves, C.D.B.T.; Martella, V.; Ikuta, N.; Lunge, V.R.; Canal, C.W. Genotyping of Canine Distemper Virus Strains Circulating in Brazil from 2008 to 2012. *Virus Res.* **2014**, *180*, 76–83. [CrossRef] [PubMed]
59. Wang, B.; Wang, X.-L. Species Diversity of Fecal Microbial Flora *in Canis Lupus Familiaris* Infected with Canine Parvovirus. *Vet. Microbiol.* **2019**, *237*, 108390. [CrossRef] [PubMed]
60. Zheng, Y.; Hao, X.; Lin, X.; Zheng, Q.; Zhang, W.; Zhou, P.; Li, S. Bacterial Diversity in the Feces of Dogs with CPV Infection. *Microb. Pathog.* **2018**, *121*, 70–76. [CrossRef]
61. Willing, B.P.; Gill, N.; Finlay, B.B. The Role of the Immune System in Regulating the Microbiota. *Gut Microbes* **2010**, *1*, 213–223. [CrossRef]
62. Tourret, J.; Willing, B.P.; Dion, S.; MacPherson, J.; Denamur, E.; Finlay, B.B. Immunosuppressive Treatment Alters Secretion of Ileal Antimicrobial Peptides and Gut Microbiota, and Favors Subsequent Colonization by Uropathogenic *Escherichia Coli*. *Transplantation* **2017**, *101*, 74–82. [CrossRef]
63. Centers for Disease Control and Prevention (CDC). Epi Info^{TM}. Available online: https://www.cdc.gov/epiinfo/support/downloads.html (accessed on 18 June 2020).
64. Instituto Pasteur Campanhas de Vacinação—Secretaria Da Saúde—Governo Do Estado de São Paulo. Available online: http://www.saude.sp.gov.br/instituto-pasteur/paginas-internas/vacinacao/campanhas-de-vacinacao (accessed on 18 June 2020).
65. CLSI. *Performance Standards for Antimicrobial Susceptibility Testing*, 28th ed.; CLSI supplement M100; Clinical and Laboratory Standards Institute: Wayne, PA, USA, 2018; ISBN 978-1-56238-838-6.
66. Taşli, H.; Bahar, I.H. Molecular Characterization of TEM- and SHV-Derived Extended-Spectrum Beta-Lactamases in Hospital-Based *Enterobacteriaceae* in Turkey. *Jpn. J. Infect. Dis.* **2005**, *58*, 162–167.
67. Jena, J.; Sahoo, R.K.; Debata, N.K.; Subudhi, E. Prevalence of TEM, SHV, and CTX-M Genes of Extended-Spectrum β-Lactamase-Producing *Escherichia Coli* Strains Isolated from Urinary Tract Infections in Adults. *3 Biotech.* **2017**, *7*, 244. [CrossRef]
68. R. Core Team. *R: A Language and Evironmetnt for Stastical Computing*; R Foundation for Stastical Computing: Vienna, Austria, 2015.

antibiotics

MDPI

Article

A Pilot Study in Sweden on Efficacy of Benzylpenicillin, Oxytetracycline, and Florfenicol in Treatment of Acute Undifferentiated Respiratory Disease in Calves

Virpi Welling [1], Nils Lundeheim [2] and Björn Bengtsson [3,*]

[1] Farm and Animal Health, Kungsängens Gård, SE-753 23 Uppsala, Sweden; virpi.welling@gardochdjurhalsan.se

[2] Department of Animal Breeding and Genetics, Swedish University of Agricultural Sciences, Box 7023, SE-750 07 Uppsala, Sweden; nils.lundeheim@slu.se

[3] Department of Animal Health and Antimicrobial Strategies, National Veterinary Institute, SE-751 89 Uppsala, Sweden

* Correspondence: bjorn.bengtsson@sva.se

Received: 29 September 2020; Accepted: 25 October 2020; Published: 26 October 2020

Abstract: Bovine respiratory disease (BRD) is a major indication for antibiotic treatment of cattle worldwide and some of the antibiotics used belong to classes of highest priority among those listed by WHO as critically important for human medicine. To preserve the efficacy of "newer" antibiotics, it has been suggested that "older" drugs should be revisited and used when possible. In this pilot study, we evaluated the efficacy of benzylpenicillin (PEN), oxytetracycline (OTC), and florfenicol (FLO) for treatment of naturally occurring BRD on two farms raising calves for slaughter. Farm personnel selected calves for enrolment, assigned calves to one of the three regimens in a systematically random manner, treated the calves, and registered the results. Overall, 117 calves were enrolled in the study. Nineteen calves relapsed in BRD before slaughter and were retreated (16.2%) and three died (2.6%). For PEN, treatment response rates after 30 days, 60 days, and until slaughter were 90.2%, 87.8%, and 80.5%, respectively; for OTC, 90.0%, 85.0%, and 85.0%, respectively; and for FLO, 86.1%, 83.3%, and 77.8%, respectively. There were no statistically significant differences in relapse, mortality, or response rates between the three treatment regimens. This indicates that PEN, OTC, and FLO were equally effective for treatment of BRD but the results need to be confirmed in a more elaborate study with a higher statistical power. The findings support the current recommendations from the Swedish Veterinary Association and the Medical Products Agency to use benzylpenicillin as a first line antibiotic for treatment of calves with undifferentiated respiratory disease in Sweden. Due to differences in the panorama of infectious agents and presence of acquired antibiotic resistance, the findings might not be applicable in other geographical areas.

Keywords: cattle; respiratory disease; treatment; benzylpenicillin; oxytetracycline; florfenicol

1. Introduction

Bovine respiratory disease (BRD) is recognized worldwide as a common and persistent problem in cattle raised intensively for meat production [1–4]. BRD has a multifactorial background that includes infectious agents and environmental factors but also the immunological and general status of the animals [5,6]. The pathogenesis and clinical presentation of BRD varies depending on which infectious agents and predisposing factors are present in a herd, but in general, viral infections of the respiratory tract precede secondary bacterial infections [7]. The bacteria commonly involved often reside in the upper airways of healthy calves and include *Pasteurella multocida*, *Mannheimia haemolytica*, *Histophilus somni*, and *Mycoplasma bovis* [7,8]. Due to the complex background of BRD, morbidity and mortality vary between herds, but both can be very high [9,10] leading to animal welfare problems and economic losses for the farmers [6,11].

There is no curative therapy for viral respiratory infections available for use in cattle and treatment of manifest BRD therefore relies on antibiotics to control secondary bacterial infections of the lower respiratory tract and NSAIDs to alleviate the inflammatory response. Worldwide, antibiotics are also used extensively for prophylactic or metaphylactic medication to prevent or curb outbreaks of BRD in groups of calves or growing cattle [9,12]. Thus, BRD is the major indication for antibiotic treatment of cattle [9,13] and the risk of emerging antibiotic resistance from this has been emphasized [14]. Some of the antibiotics used to control BRD, for example, fluoroquinolones, third generation cephalosporins, and macrolides, belong to antibiotic classes of highest priority among those listed by WHO as critically important for human medicine (CIA) [15].

Due to concerns for human and animal health from emerging resistance, WHO recently suggested that CIAs should not be used for treatment of food-producing animals if alternatives are available [16]. It has also been suggested that to preserve the efficacy of "newer" antibiotics "older" drugs should be re-investigated and used when possible [17]. In Sweden, benzylpenicillin is recommended by the Swedish Veterinary Association [18] and by the Medical products agency [19] as first line treatment of cattle with lower respiratory tract infections. The rationale for using this "old" antibiotic is a lower risk for emergence of resistance from the use of the narrow-spectrum benzylpenicillin than the broad-spectrum antibiotics available for treatment of BRD in Sweden, i.e., oxytetracycline, florfenicol, enrofloxacin, amoxicillin, tulathromycin, gamithromycin, trimethoprim-sulphonamide, and ceftiofur.

Penicillin resistance in respiratory pathogens from calves is uncommon in Sweden [20] and *M. bovis* has hitherto been found only rarely [21]. In most herds, the efficacy of benzylpenicillin should therefore not be compromised by these factors. The efficacy of benzylpenicillin for the treatment of BRD has, however, never been evaluated in Swedish cattle herds and studies are also scarce in the scientific literature [10,22]. Information on performance of benzylpenicillin in Swedish herds would be valuable to uphold, or reevaluate, the current recommendation. The aim of this pilot study was therefore to evaluate the efficacy of benzylpenicillin (PEN) for treatment of calves with naturally occurring BRD in comparison with two other antibiotics used in Sweden, i.e., oxytetracycline (OTC) and florfenicol (FLO).

2. Results

2.1. Descriptive Data

The study was designed to include three farms and 180 calves in total, but one farm dropped out at an early stage. On the remaining two farms (H and S), 120 calves were enrolled in the study. Due to uncertainties in farm records, three calves were excluded, one calf on farm S and two calves on farm H, leaving 117 calves for final evaluation (Table 1). Of these, 59 calves were from farm S treated between February and April 2016 and 58 from farm H treated between February 2016 and May 2017. The stipulated order of assignment to treatment regime (PEN, OTC, FLO) at enrolment was upheld throughout the study but with minor deviations on both farms.

Table 1. Descriptive data for 117 calves treated with procaine benzylpenicillin (PEN), oxytetracycline (OTC), or florfenicol (FLO) for respiratory disease on farm S and H.

		PEN			OTC			FLO			PEN & OTC & FLO		
Farm		**S**	**H**	**S & H**	**S**	**H**	**S & H**	**S**	**H**	**S & H**	**S**	**H**	**S & H**
No. of calves		20	21	**41**	21	19	**40**	18	18	**36**	59	58	**117**
Age when treated (days) [a]	Mean (range)	42.6 (16–81)	51.2 (29–121)	**47.2** (16–121)	43.5 (10–88)	55.6 (25–107)	**49.6** (10–107)	40.7 (9–77)	53.6 (29–121)	**47.9** (9–121)	42.4 ** (9–88)	53.4 ** (25–121)	**48.2** (9–121)
Rectal temp. 0 h (°C)	Mean (range)	39.8 (38.4–41.5)	39.8 (38.4–41.3)	**39.8** (38.4–41.3)	40.1 (38.8–41.4)	39.6 (38.1–41.1)	**39.9** (38.1–41.4)	39.9 (37.1–41.3)	39.6 (37.5–41.0)	**39.8** (37.1–41.3)	39.9 (37.1–41.5)	39.7 (37.5–41.3)	**39.8** (37.1–41.5)
Rectal temp. 48 h (°C)	Mean (range)	38.4 (37.4–40.1)	38.4 (37.7–39.1)	**38.4** (37.4–40.1)	38.3 (36.3–40.4)	38.6 (37.5–39.9)	**38.4** (36.3–40.4)	38.2 (37.0–39.1)	38.3 (37.2–40.0)	**38.3** (37.0–40.0)	38.3 (36.3–40.4)	38.5 (37.2–40.0)	**38.4** (36.3–40.4)
Retreatment:													
<30 days	No.	0	2	**2**	2 [c]	0	**2**	5 [d]	0	**5**	7	2	**9**
30–60 days	No.	1	0	**1**	2	0	**2**	1 [e]	0	**1**	4	0	**4**
>60 days	No.	3	0	**3**	1	0	**1**	2	0	**2**	6	0	**6**
Total	No.	4	2	**6**	4	0	**5**	6	0	**8**	17 **	2 **	**19**
Case fatality:													
<30 days	No.	1	1	**2**	0	0	**0**	0	0	**0**	1	1	**2**
30–60 days	No.	0	0	**0**	0	0	**0**	0	0	**0**	0	0	**0**
>60 days	No.	1 (day 90)	0	**1**	0	0	**0**	0	0	**0**	1	0	**1**
Total Case fatality	No	2	1	**3**	0	0	**0**	0	0	**0**	2	1	**3**
Age at slaughter (days) [b]	Mean (range)	540 (450–597)	533 (482–574)	**536** (450–597)	544 (453–612)	526 (476–569	**535** (453–612)	552 (474–648)	539 (479–588)	**545** (474–648)	545 (450–648)	532 (476–588)	**539** (450–648)
Carcass weight (kg)	Mean (range)	311.8 (230–369)	326.8 (286–358)	**319.3** (230–369)	320.7 (260–364)	317.7 (287–356)	**319.2** (260–364)	315.0 (276–341)	318.1 (257–384)	**316.5** (257–384)	316.0 (230–369)	321.0 (257–384)	**318.4** (230–384)

[a] Data for 8 calves missing (farm S: 2 PEN, 2 OTC, 4 FLO); [b] data for 22 calves missing (farm S: 4 PEN, 4 OTC, 5 FLO; Farm H: 4 PEN, 1 OTC, 4 FLO); [c] 1 calf retreated 66 days after first retreatment; [d] 1 calf retreated 99 days after first retreatment; [e] 1 calf retreated 59 days after first retreatment. Statistically significant differences between mean values indicated by ** ($p < 0.01$).

The mean age of the calves at enrollment was 48.2 days and did not differ significantly between treatment regimens, but calves on farm H were significantly older (53.4 days) at enrollment than calves on farm S (42.4 days) ($p = 0.004$) (Table 1). The mean rectal temperature at enrolment was 39.8 °C, the mean age at slaughter 539 days, and the mean carcass weight at slaughter 318.4 kg (Table 1). None of these parameters differed significantly ($p > 0.05$) between treatment regimens or between the two farms (Table 1).

Of the 117 calves, 19 (16.2%) relapsed in respiratory disease after first treatment and were retreated (Table 1, Supplementary Material S1). The relapse rate, from first treatment up to slaughter, was 14.6% for PEN, 12.5% for OTC, and 22.2% for FLO. The relapse rate did not differ between regimens ($p > 0.05$) but was significantly higher on farm S (28.8%) than on farm H (3.5%) ($p = 0.0002$) (Table 1). Three calves relapsed twice, one of these was first treated with OTC and two with FLO (Table 1). Three calves died (2.6%), two on farm S and one on farm H (Table 1, Supplementary Material S1). All three calves were first treated with PEN and two died during the first treatment and one during retreatment with PEN 88 days after the first treatment. There was no statistically significant difference in mortality between treatment regimens or between farms ($p > 0.05$).

2.2. Efficacy Parameters

Most calves, 115 (98.3%), fulfilled the criteria for a positive temperature reaction (TEMP) (Table 2, Supplementary Material S1). Response rates for the three treatment regimens at 30 days ($RESP_{30}$), 60 days ($RESP_{60}$), and until slaughter ($RESP_{tot}$) were 90.2%, 87.8%, and 80.5%, respectively, for PEN; 90.0%, 85.0%, and 85.0%, respectively, for OTC; and 86.1%, 83.3%, and 77.8%, respectively, for FLO (Table 2). There were no statistically significant differences in response rates between treatment regimens ($p > 0.05$) (Table 2). There was also no difference in mean $RESP_{30}$ between farms ($p > 0.05$), but mean $RESP_{60}$ was significantly lower on farm S (76.3%) than on farm H (94.8%) ($p = 0.0044$) and the mean $RESP_{to}t$ was also significantly lower on farm S (67.8%) than on farm H (94.8%) ($p = 0.0002$) (Table 2). The perceived treatment effect at five days (PTE) was scored as "Good" for 91.2% of the calves and as "Poor" for 8.8% and did not differ between treatment regimens or between farms (Table 2). The mean average daily live weight gain from birth to slaughter (ADG) was 1006 grams/day and did not differ significantly between treatment regimens or between farms ($p > 0.05$) Table 2).

Table 2. Efficacy parameters for the treatment regimens procaine benzylpenicillin (PEN), oxytetracycline (OTC), and florfenicol (FLO) in 117 calves treated for respiratory disease on two farms, S and H. Percentage of calves fulfilling the criteria for the parameters: TEMP, $RESP_{30}$, $RESP_{60}$ and $RESP_{tot}$; percentage of calves scored in the categories "Poor" or "Good" of parameter PTE; mean average daily live weight gain (ADG).

Farm			PEN			OTC			FLO			PEN & OTC & FLO		
			S	H	S & H	S	H	S & H	S	H	S & H	S	H	S & H
No. of calves			20	21	**41**	21	19	**40**	18	18	**36**	59	58	**117**
TEMP		%	100	100	**100**	90.5	100	**95.0**	100	100	**100**	96.6	100	**98.3**
		(no./total)	(20/20)	(21/21)	(41/41)	(19/21)	(19/19)	(38/40)	(18/18)	(18/18)	(36/36)	(57/59)	(58/58)	(115/117)
$RESP_{30}$		%	95.0	85.7	**90.2**	81.0	100	**90.0**	72.2	100	**86.1**	83.1	94.8	**88.9**
(n = 117)		(no./total)	(19/20)	(18/21)	(37/41)	(17/21)	(19/19)	(36/40)	(13/18)	(18/18)	(31/36)	(49/59)	(55/58)	(104/117)
$RESP_{60}$		%	90.0	85.7	**87.8**	71.4	100	**85.0**	66.7	100	**83.3**	76.3 **	94.8 **	**85.5**
(n = 117)		(no./total)	(18/20)	(18/21)	(36/41)	(15/21)	(19/19)	(34/40)	(12/18)	(18/18)	(30/36)	(45/59)	(55/58)	(100/117)
$RESP_{tot}$		%	75.0	85.7	**80.5**	71.4	100	**85.0**	55.6	100	**77.8**	67.8 ***	94.8 ***	**81.2**
(n = 117)		(no./total)	(15/20)	(18/21)	(33/41)	(15/21)	(19/19)	(34/40)	(10/18)	(18/18)	(28/36)	(40/59)	(55/58)	(95/117)
PTE	Poor	%	11.1	10.0	**10.5**	5.0	5.3	**5.3**	5.5	16.7	**11.1**	7.1	10.5	**8.8**
(n = 113) [a]		(no./total)	(2/18)	(2/20)	(4/38)	(1/20)	(1/19)	(2/39)	(1/18)	(3/18)	(4/36)	(4/56)	(6/57)	(10/113)
	Good	%	88.8	90.0	**89.5**	95.0	94.7	**94.9**	94.4	83.3	**88.9**	92.9	89.5	**91.2**
		(no./total)	(16/18)	(18/20)	(34/38)	(19/20)	(18/19)	(37/39)	(17/18)	(15/18)	(32/36)	(52/56)	(51/57)	(103/113)
ADG		grams/day	1039	1104	**1072**	1063	1185	**1074**	1033	1063	**1048**	1046	1086	**1066**
(n = 99) [b]		(range)	(835–1266)	(925–1204)	(835–1266)	(887–1243)	(936–1239)	(887–1243)	(784–1210)	(804–1189)	(784–1210)	(784–1266)	(804–1239)	(784–1266)

[a] Data for 4 calves missing (farm S: 2 PEN, 1 OTC; farm H: 1 PEN); [b] data for 18 calves missing (farm S: 3 PEN, 2 OTC, 4 FLO; farm H: 4 PEN, 1 OTC, 4 FLO). Statistically significant differences between mean values indicated by ** ($p < 0.01$) and *** ($p < 0.001$).

3. Discussion

Benzylpenicillin is one of the oldest antibiotics used for treatment of BRD and has to a great extent been replaced by newer substances with a broader antibacterial spectrum [23]. However, in this study, we observed no difference in efficacy of benzylpenicillin, oxytetracycline, or florfenicol for treatment of naturally occurring BRD in Swedish calves raised for meat production. The response rates (RESP) at 30 days, 60 days, and until slaughter were 90.2%, 87.8%, and 80.5%, respectively, for PEN; 90.0%, 85.0%, and 85.0%, respectively, for OTC; and 86.1%, 83.3%, and 77.8%, respectively, for FLO and did not differ between the three regimens ($p > 0.05$). Moreover, the perceived treatment effects (PTE) scored by farmers at five days were high. In 91.2% of the calves, the effect was scored as good and did not differ between treatment regimens. A response rate of 80–85% after the first treatment is considered acceptable for BRD in feedlot cattle [23], and all three regimens evaluated in this study can therefore be considered adequate.

The overall response rates at 30 days and 60 days after first treatment in the present study are similar to response rates of about 85% at 28 days observed after treatment of weaned feedlot cattle with benzylpenicillin, oxytetracycline, or trimethoprim/sulphonamide reported by Bateman et al. [10] and higher than rates of about 50–60% at 60 days after treatment with these antibiotics reported by Mechor et al. [22]. Furthermore, the overall response rate up until slaughter in the present study (81.2%) was higher than reported for treatment of feedlot cattle with enrofloxacin, about 60–70% [24], or tilmicosin (34–67%) [25–27], and within the interval of success rates reported for florfenicol (23–97%) [25–27], tulathromycin (53–88%) [24,26,27], trimethoprim/sulphonamide (77%) [28], and ceftiofur (90%) [28]. Moreover, in a review of randomized control trials on BRD treatment with various antibiotics, the median success rate was 71% in treated animals and 24% in untreated controls [29]. Notably, in mixed treatment comparison meta-analyses of results from BRD-treatment studies performed in North American feedlots, tulathromycin ranked the highest and oxytetracycline the lowest with florfenicol ranking as number four on the list of 12 antibiotics evaluated; penicillin was not included in the analysis [30].

To compare success rates between BRD treatments studies should, however, be made cautiously due to possible differences in study design, e.g., study populations, dosing regimens, case definition, and the criteria used for evaluation of success or failure [29]. Additionally, the outcome of antimicrobial therapy for BRD is most likely influenced by the disease challenge in a herd [31], and extrapolation of results between different settings should be made cautiously. In Sweden, some infectious agents of importance in BRD elsewhere are not present, for example, BVDV and BHV-1 [32] and *M. haemolytica*, *H. somni*, and *M. bovis* are less often diagnosed [19,21]. The bacterial pathogen mainly isolated from calves with BRD in Sweden is *P. multocida*, and antimicrobial resistance to benzylpenicillin, oxytetracycline, or florfenicol in this bacterial species is uncommon [19,20]. The good performance of the antibiotics studied was therefore probably to some extent due to a relatively low disease challenge. The results of this study might therefore not be relevant in other settings where, for example, *M. bovis* is more common, such as North American feedlots [2], or where the occurrence of acquired antibiotic resistance is higher.

The total mortality in the study (2.6%) was lower than the overall mortality, including fatalities unrelated to BRD, on farm S (3.3%) and farm H (4.5%) in 2016. Notably, the three calves that died in the study were all treated with benzylpenicillin but there were no statistically significant differences in mortality between treatment regimens. Since no post-mortem examinations were performed, it is not known if these calves had comorbidities unrelated to BRD, for example, the calf that died about three months after the first treatment. Still, this finding is intriguing and warrants clarification in a more elaborate study.

The frequency of BRD treatment was similar on the two farms, at about 20%, but the overall response rates $RESP_{60}$ and $RESP_{tot}$ were significantly lower on farm S (76.3% and 67.8%, respectively) than on farm H (94.8% and 94.8%, respectively). The reasons for the difference are unclear, but farm S yearly purchases and raises about ten times more animals than farm H, and a greater flow of animals likely influences the spectrum of infectious agents present. The immunological and general status of the animals is also possibly more diverse on a larger farm and the supervision and management of diseased animals more complicated. This has probably an impact on the outcome of BRD treatments.

All calves in the present study were treated with NSAID (meloxicam) in conjunction with antibiotic therapy because this is recommended in the treatment of BRD in Sweden [33]. The initial drop in rectal temperature in all but 2 of the 117 calves was probably to some extent due to the antipyretic effect of meloxicam in agreement with the conclusions of a review on ancillary treatment of BRD by Francoz et al. [34]. These authors also concluded that NSAIDs may be beneficial from an animal welfare perspective and possibly also reduce lung lesions at slaughter whereas beneficial effects on clinical signs at the end of treatment and on productivity are not documented. To what extent the ancillary treatment influenced the overall response in the present study cannot be evaluated, but since all calves were treated with meloxicam, any impact on the conclusions regarding relative efficacy of the three regimens is likely to be small.

Respiratory infections in calves are known to negatively impact the productivity [5,35] but this aspect was not directly evaluated in the current study. However, the mean age at slaughter (539 days), the mean carcass weight (318.4 kg), and the average daily live weight gain (1066 grams/day) of the treated calves were higher than the national average for dairy breed bull calves in Sweden, 615 days, 334 kg, and 980 grams/day, respectively [36], and did not differ between the three treatment regimens or the two farms. This indicates a successful management on the two farms but also that all the three treatment regimens restored the long-term productivity of the calves.

A main limitation of this study is the small number of animals and farms included. The study was originally designed to include three farms, but the drop-out of one farm led to a loss of statistical power in the evaluation of the study. With the current number of observations, using a significance level of 0.05 and a statistical power of 80%, only a difference of about 20% between treatment regimens could be detected. Other limitations are that calves were selected for treatment by farm personnel based on visual inspection and rectal temperature. Selection in this manner inevitably leads to underdiagnosis of calves needing antibiotic therapy [6,9] but also to a selection of calves that would have recovered spontaneously [29]. Inclusion of calves that would have recovered spontaneously would overestimate the efficacy of the treatment regimens studied. However, the proportion of calves that would have recovered spontaneously is probably similar for the three regimens and the comparison of efficacy between regimes would remain unaffected. More concerning is that farm personnel, also on visual inspection and temperature recordings, decided which calves should be retreated and thereby considered relapses which directly impacts response rates. Furthermore, farm personnel were not blinded with respect to treatment regimen in individual calves and their perception of the efficacy of the antibiotics used could have biased the likelihood of selecting calves for retreatment. Another limitation is that calves that died not were submitted for post-mortem investigation and the causes of the fatalities are not known and could be unrelated to BRD. Moreover, isolation of respiratory tract pathogens or susceptibility testing of relevant isolates were not performed.

Despite these limitations, we consider it valuable to share the results obtained in this pilot study, although the conclusions should be confirmed in studies accounting for these constraints and with a higher statistical power.

4. Materials and Methods

4.1. Study Design

The study was designed to evaluate the efficacy of benzylpenicillin, oxytetracycline, and florfenicol in treatment of naturally occurring BRD in Swedish herds raising calves for slaughter (for an overview see Supplementary Material S2). The intention was to perform a non-inferiority pilot study using three herds selected by convenience and with a minimum of intervention in farm routines and extra work for farm personnel. Initially, three farms were enrolled in the study and a total of 60 calves were to be treated with each of the three regimens. At an expected treatment success rate of 85%, this would have given the study a power of 80% to detect a true difference in success rates between regimens of about 15% at a significance level of 5% (Sealed Envelope LTD. 2012). This was considered sufficient for a preliminary evaluation of the performance of the studied antibiotics, but, unfortunately, one of the herds dropped out of the study which reduced the non-inferiority limit to 20%.

4.2. *Farms and Animals*

The study was conducted in 2016 and 2017 on two farms (S and H) that purchased unweaned calves from dairy farms and raised them for slaughter at an age of about 18 months. Calves were purchased and received to both farms in batches over the whole year and kept in groups of 10–15 animals. Calves were fed milk substitutes, and gradually concentrates and silage, until weaned at a bodyweight of 90–100 kg and an age of about 8–12 weeks. After weaning, calves were mixed on both farms in larger groups of 20–30 animals and raised to slaughter on a mixed ration of concentrates and silage. On both farms, calves commonly contracted respiratory disease 1–2 weeks after arrival. During 2016, farm S received 2528 calves emanating from 59 different farms. Of these calves, 530 (20.9%) were treated for BRD, 43 (1.7%) died or were euthanized before reaching a bodyweight of 100 kg, and 40 calves (1.6%) died or were euthanized in the period thereafter and up until slaughter. The same year, farm H received 268 calves emanating from one single dairy farm, and of these, 64 (23.9%) were treated for BRD, 4 (1.5%) died or were euthanized before reaching a bodyweight of 100 kg, and 8 (3.0%) calves died or were euthanized in the period thereafter. Prophylactic antibiotic treatment, or use of antibiotics for growth promotion, is not allowed in Sweden and accordingly not practiced on the farms.

4.3. *Inclusion Criteria*

On both farms, calves were visually inspected daily by farm personnel for signs of disease and rectal temperature was recorded for calves showing clinical symptoms. For this study, farm personnel were instructed to identify calves with signs of respiratory disease, including (I) forced breathing and/or cough, (II) purulent nasal and/or ocular discharge, (III) depressed attitude, and (IV) a rectal temperature of >39.5 °C. Calves fulfilling at least three of the criteria I–IV were enrolled in the study. These criteria for starting antibiotic treatment of calves with suspected respiratory infection were the same as those used on both farms also before the start of the study. Calves with comorbidities or calves older than 6 months were not eligible for enrollment.

4.4. *Treatment Regimens*

Calves enrolled in the study were treated according to one of the following three regimens according to the manufacturers recommendations—PEN: procaine benzylpenicillin 40 mg/kg BW IM, 5 doses 24 H apart (Penovet® vet, Boehringer Ingelheim Animal Health, Copenhagen, Denmark); OTC: oxytetracycline 20 mg/kg BW IM, 2 doses 48 H apart (Engemycin® vet, Intervet AB, Stockholm, Sweden); FLO: florfenicol 20 mg/kg BW, 2 doses 48 H apart (Florselect® vet, Nordvacc Läkemedel AB, Hägersten, Sweden). Calves were assigned to a regimen in order of enrollment, where the first calf identified for treatment on a farm received PEN, the second OTC, and the third FLO. This order of treatments was to be repeated until a total of 60 calves had been treated on each farm. If farm personnel considered that the clinical response of a calf was unsatisfactory, they could change the treatment to one of the other two regimens. Calves relapsing in respiratory disease after completed initial treatment were again treated with one of the three regimens at the discretion of the farm personnel.

At the start of antibiotic therapy, all calves were treated with an NSAID given as a single subcutaneous dose of meloxicam at 0.5 mg/kg BW, (Metacam®, Boehringer Ingelheim Vetmedica, Malmö, Sweden).

4.5. Data Registered on Farm

On enrollment (0 h), farm personnel registered calf identity, date, assigned treatment regimen, and rectal temperature. At 48 h, rectal temperature was again registered and at 120 h the perceived treatment effect (PTE) was scored by farm personnel (see below). Changes of an assigned treatment, relapse in respiratory disease after completed treatment, and case fatality up until slaughter were also registered. Due to practical constraints, the study could not be performed in a blinded manner at the farm level. Data on birth date of calves, live weight on arrival to the farm, and age at slaughter were available from farm records.

4.6. Data Registered at Slaughter

At slaughter, carcass weights of the calves were recorded by slaughterhouse personnel unaware of the treatment of individual calves.

4.7. Efficacy Parameters

Treatment efficacy was evaluated by the following parameters:

- TEMP (temperature): A positive reaction was a rectal temperature ≤39.5 °C and/or a drop by ≥1 °C 48 h after first treatment.
- RESP (response to treatment): A positive RESP was a positive reaction for the TEMP parameter (see above), no change of initial treatment and no relapse or fatality within 30 days ($RESP_{30}$), 60 days ($RESP_{60}$), or until slaughter ($RESP_{tot}$).
- PTE (perceived treatment effect): Scored by farm personnel five days after first treatment as "Good" for a calf with noticeable improvements regarding clinical signs and general attitude, or "Poor" for a calf without noticeable improvements.
- ADG (average daily live weight gain from birth to slaughter).

4.8. Statistical Analyses

Possible differences in age and rectal temperatures at enrollment between calves enrolled in the three treatment regimen groups were evaluated by analysis of variance (PROC GLM) according to a statistical model including the fixed effects of treatment regimen (n = 3) and farm (n = 2).

To evaluate differences in efficacy between the three treatment regimens, the binary efficacy parameters TEMP, PTE, $RESP_{30}$, $RESP_{60}$, and $RESP_{tot}$ were analyzed by logistic regression (PROC GLIMMIX) with a statistical model including the fixed effects of treatment regimen (n = 3) and farm (n = 2). Differences in total relapse and case fatality rates were analyzed with the same model. Differences between treatment regimens in age at slaughter, carcass weight, and average daily gain from birth to slaughter (ADG) were evaluated by analysis of variance (PROC GLM), with a statistical model that included the fixed effects of treatment (n = 3) and farm (n = 2).

Descriptive statistics was obtained using EXCEL, and statistical analyses were performed using the SAS software (SAS Inst. Inc., Cary, NC). A 5% level of significance was used to assess statistical differences.

4.9. Ethics Approval

This study was approved by the regional ethical committee in Uppsala (DNR C 147/15).

5. Conclusions

The findings of this study indicate that PEN, OTC, and FLO were equally effective for treatment of undifferentiated BRD in calves, but the results need to be confirmed in a more elaborate study with a higher statistical power.

Supplementary Materials: The following are available online at http://www.mdpi.com/2079-6382/9/11/736/s1, S1: Flow chart for the outcome of 117 calves enrolled in the study. S2: Overview of the design and elaboration of the study.

Author Contributions: V.W., N.L., and B.B. designed the study, V.W. coordinated fieldwork and collection of data, V.W., N.L., and B.B. analyzed the data, N.L. performed statistical calculations, and B.B. drafted the manuscript. All authors have read and agreed to the published version of the manuscript.

Funding: This study was performed as part of the SvarmPat project, a cooperation between the National Veterinary Institute and Farm & Animal Health, financed by the Swedish Board of Agriculture and supported by Cost Action CA18217: European Network for Optimization of Veterinary Antimicrobial Treatment.

Acknowledgments: The authors express their profound gratitude for all the voluntary work put into this study by the farm personnel on the two participating farms.

Conflicts of Interest: The authors declare no conflict of interest.

References

1. Gay, E.; Barnouin, J. A nation-wide epidemiological study of acute bovine respiratory disease in France. *Prev. Vet. Med.* **2009**, *89*, 265–271. [CrossRef] [PubMed]
2. Griffin, D. Bovine pasteurellosis and other bacterial infections of the respiratory tract. *Vet Clin North Am Food Anim. Pract.* **2010**, *26*, 57–71. [CrossRef] [PubMed]
3. Hay, K.E.; Morton, J.M.; Mahony, T.J.; Clements, A.C.; Barnes, T.S. Associations between animal characteristic and environmental risk factors and bovine respiratory disease in Australian feedlot cattle. *Prev. Vet. Med.* **2016**, *125*, 66–74. [CrossRef] [PubMed]
4. Murray, G.M.; O'Neill, R.G.; More, S.J.; McElroy, M.C.; Earley, B.; Cassidy, J.P. Evolving views on bovine respiratory disease: An appraisal of selected key pathogens—Part 1. *Vet. J.* **2016**, *217*, 95–102. [CrossRef] [PubMed]
5. Delabouglise, A.; James, A.; Valarcher, J.F.; Hagglund, S.; Raboisson, D.; Rushton, J. Linking disease epidemiology and livestock productivity: The case of bovine respiratory disease in France. *PLoS ONE* **2017**, *12*, e0189090. [CrossRef] [PubMed]
6. Edwards, T.A. Control methods for bovine respiratory disease for feedlot cattle. *Vet. Clin. North. Am. Food Anim. Pract.* **2010**, *26*, 273–284. [CrossRef] [PubMed]
7. Caswell, J.L. Failure of respiratory defenses in the pathogenesis of bacterial pneumonia of cattle. *Vet. Pathol.* **2014**, *51*, 393–409. [CrossRef] [PubMed]
8. Taylor, J.D.; Fulton, R.W.; Lehenbauer, T.W.; Step, D.L.; Confer, A.W. The epidemiology of bovine respiratory disease: What is the evidence for predisposing factors? *Can. Vet. J.* **2010**, *51*, 1095–1102.
9. Baptiste, K.E.; Kyvsgaard, N.C. Do antimicrobial mass medications work? A systematic review and meta-analysis of randomised clinical trials investigating antimicrobial prophylaxis or metaphylaxis against naturally occurring bovine respiratory disease. *Pathog. Dis.* **2017**, *75*, ftx083. [CrossRef]
10. Bateman, K.G.; Martin, S.W.; Shewen, P.E.; Menzies, P.I. An evaluation of antimicrobial therapy for undifferentiated bovine respiratory disease. *Can. Vet. J.* **1990**, *31*, 689–696.
11. Barrett, D.C. Cost-effective antimicrobial drug selection for the management and control of respiratory disease in European cattle. *Vet. Rec.* **2000**, *146*, 545–550. [CrossRef] [PubMed]
12. Abell, K.M.; Theurer, M.E.; Larson, R.L.; White, B.J.; Apley, M. A mixed treatment comparison meta-analysis of metaphylaxis treatments for bovine respiratory disease in beef cattle. *J. Anim. Sci.* **2017**, *95*, 626–635. [CrossRef] [PubMed]
13. Pagel, S.W.; Gautier, P. Use of antimicrobial agents in livestock. *Rev. Sci. Tech.* **2012**, *31*, 145–188. [CrossRef] [PubMed]
14. Murray, G.M.; O'Neill, R.G.; More, S.J.; McElroy, M.C.; Earley, B.; Cassidy, J.P. Evolving views on bovine respiratory disease: An appraisal of selected control measures—Part 2. *Vet. J.* **2016**, *217*, 78–82. [CrossRef]
15. WHO. *Critically Important Antimicrobials for Human Medicine, 5th Revision*; World Health Organisation: Geneva, Switzerland, 2016.
16. WHO. *WHO Guidelines on Use of Medically Important Antimicrobials in Food-Producing Animals*; World Health Organization: Geneva, Switzerland, 2017; Licence: CC BY-NC-SA 3.0 IGO.
17. Bush, K.; Courvalin, P.; Dantas, G.; Davies, J.; Eisenstein, B.; Huovinen, P.; Jacoby, G.A.; Kishony, R.; Kreiswirth, B.N.; Kutter, E.; et al. Tackling antibiotic resistance. *Nat. Rev. Microbiol.* **2011**, *9*, 894–896. [CrossRef]

18. Swedish Veterinary Association. *Guidelines for the Use of Antibiotics in Production Animals—Cattle, Pigs, Sheep and Goats*; Swedish Veterinary Association: Stockholm, Sweden, 2017; pp. 1–55.
19. Medical Products Agency. *Information från Läkemedelsverket: Dosering av antibiotika till nötkreatur och får—ny rekommendation*; Medical Products Agency: Uppsala, Sweden, 2013; Volume 24, pp. 1–50.
20. Swedres-Svarm. *Consumption of Antibiotics and Occurrence of Resistance in Sweden*; Public Health Agency of Sweden: Solna, Sweden; National Veterinary Institute: Uppsala, Sweden, 2018; ISSN 1650-6332.
21. Ericsson Unnerstad, H.; Fungbrant, K.; Persson Waller, K.; Persson, Y. *Mycoplasma bovis* hos kor och kalvar i Sverige. *Svensk veterinärtidning* **2012**, *13*, 17–20.
22. Mechor, G.D.; Jim, G.K.; Janzen, E.D. Comparison of penicillin, oxytetracycline, and trimethoprim-sulfadoxine in the treatment of acute undifferentiated bovine respiratory disease. *Can. Vet. J.* **1988**, *29*, 438–443. [PubMed]
23. Apley, M. Antimicrobial therapy of bovine respiratory disease. *Vet. Clin. North. Am. Food Anim. Pract.* **1997**, *13*, 549–574. [CrossRef]
24. Robb, E.J.; Tucker, C.M.; Corley, L.; Bryson, W.L.; Rogers, K.C.; Sturgess, K.; Bade, D.J.; Brodersen, B. Efficacy of tulathromycin or enrofloxacin for initial treatment of naturally occurring bovine respiratory disease in feeder calves. *Vet. Ther.* **2007**, *8*, 127–135.
25. Hoar, B.R.; Jelinski, M.D.; Ribble, C.S.; Janzen, E.D.; Johnson, J.C. A comparison of the clinical field efficacy and safety of florfenicol and tilmicosin for the treatment of undifferentiated bovine respiratory disease of cattle in western Canada. *Can. Vet. J.* **1998**, *39*, 161–166.
26. Nutsch, R.G.; Skogerboe, T.L.; Rooney, K.A.; Weigel, D.J.; Gajewski, K.; Lechtenberg, K.F. Comparative efficacy of tulathromycin, tilmicosin, and florfenicol in the treatment of bovine respiratory disease in stocker cattle. *Vet. Ther.* **2005**, *6*, 167–179. [PubMed]
27. Skogerboe, T.L.; Rooney, K.A.; Nutsch, R.G.; Weigel, D.J.; Gajewski, K.; Kilgore, W.R. Comparative efficacy of tulathromycin versus florfenicol and tilmicosin against undifferentiated bovine respiratory disease in feedlot cattle. *Vet. Ther.* **2005**, *6*, 180–196. [PubMed]
28. Jim, G.K.; Booker, C.W.; Guichon, P.T. A comparison of trimethoprim-sulfadoxine and ceftiofur sodium for the treatment of respiratory disease in feedlot calves. *Can. Vet. J.* **1992**, *33*, 245–250. [PubMed]
29. DeDonder, K.D.; Apley, M.D. A review of the expected effects of antimicrobials in bovine respiratory disease treatment and control using outcomes from published randomized clinical trials with negative controls. *Vet. Clin. North. Am. Food Anim. Pract.* **2015**, *31*, 97–111. [CrossRef]
30. O'Connor, A.M.; Yuan, C.; Cullen, J.N.; Coetzee, J.F.; da Silva, N.; Wang, C. A mixed treatment meta-analysis of antibiotic treatment options for bovine respiratory disease—An update. *Prev. Vet. Med.* **2016**, *132*, 130–139. [CrossRef]
31. Hendrick, S.H.; Bateman, K.G.; Rosengren, L.B. The effect of antimicrobial treatment and preventive strategies on bovine respiratory disease and genetic relatedness and antimicrobial resistance of *Mycoplasma bovis* isolates in a western Canadian feedlot. *Can. Vet. J.* **2013**, *54*, 1146–1156.
32. National Veterinary Institute. *Surveillance of Infectious Diseases in Animals and Humans in Sweden 2017*; National Veterinary Institute: Uppsala, Sweden, 2018.
33. Medical Products Agency. *Information från Läkemedelsverket: Behandling med NSAID till Nötkreatur, får, get och Gris—Ny Rekommendation*; Medical Products Agency: Uppsala, Sweden, 2009; Volume 20, pp. 1–40.
34. Francoz, D.; Buczinski, S.; Apley, M. Evidence related to the use of ancillary drugs in bovine respiratory disease (anti-inflammatory and others): Are they justified or not? *Vet. Clin. North Am. Food Anim. Pract.* **2012**, *28*, 23–38. [CrossRef]
35. Griffin, D. The monster we don't see: Subclinical BRD in beef cattle. *Anim Health Res. Rev.* **2014**, *15*, 138–141. [CrossRef]
36. Växa Statistik KAP Kokontroll 2004–2018. 2019. Available online: www.vxa.se (accessed on 25 August 2020).

Publisher's Note: MDPI stays neutral with regard to jurisdictional claims in published maps and institutional affiliations.

antibiotics

MDPI

Article

Comparative Evaluation of *qnrA*, *qnrB*, and *qnrS* Genes in *Enterobacteriaceae* Ciprofloxacin-Resistant Cases, in Swine Units and a Hospital from Western Romania

Alexandru O. Doma [1], Roxana Popescu [2], Mihai Mitulețu [2], Delia Muntean [2], János Dégi [1], Marius V. Boldea [1], Isidora Radulov [1], Eugenia Dumitrescu [1], Florin Muselin [1], Nikola Puvača [3,*] and Romeo T. Cristina [1,*]

1 Faculty of Veterinary Medicine, Banat's University of Agricultural Sciences and Veterinary Medicine Timișoara, Calea Aradului 119, 300645 Timișoara, Romania; dao_west@yahoo.com (A.O.D.); janosdegi@usab-tm.ro (J.D.); marius_boldea@usab-tm.ro (M.V.B.); isidoraradulov@yahoo.com (I.R.); eugeniadumitrescu@usab-tm.ro (E.D.); florinmuselin@usab-tm.ro (F.M.)

2 Department of Cellular and Molecular Biology, University of Medicine and Pharmacy Timișoara, Piaţa Eftimie Murgu, 2, 300041 Timişoara, Romania; popescu.roxana@umft.ro (R.P.); mihai.mituletu@umft.ro (M.M.); muntean.delia@umft.ro (D.M.)

3 Department of Engineering Management in Biotechnology, Faculty of Economics and Engineering Management in Novi Sad, University Business Academy in Novi Sad, Cvećarska 2, 21000 Novi Sad, Serbia

* Correspondence: nikola.puvaca@fimek.edu.rs (N.P.); romeocristina@usab-tm.ro (R.T.C.); Tel.: +381-65-219-1284 (N.P.); Tel./Fax: +40-246-277140 (R.T.C.)

Received: 18 August 2020; Accepted: 13 October 2020; Published: 14 October 2020

check for updates

Abstract: Excessive use of antimicrobials and inadequate infection control practices has turned antimicrobial resistance (AMR) into a global, public health peril. We studied the expression of *qnrA*, *qnrB*, and *qnrS* plasmid in ciprofloxacin (CIP)-resistant strains of *Escherichia coli* in swine and humans from Romania, using the Polymerase Chain Reaction (PCR) technique. Antibiotic Susceptibility Testing (AST) for human subjects (H) on 147 samples and 53 swine (S) was ascertained as well as the isolation of bacterial DNA (*E. coli*) as follows: bacteriolysis, DNA-binding, rinsing, elution, amplification, and nucleic acids' migration and U.V. visualization stages. From 24 samples of *E. coli* resistant to CIP collected from H subjects and 15 from S, for PCR analysis, 15 H and 12 S were used, with DNA purity of 1.8. The statistically analyzed results using the *Crosstabs* function (IBM SPSS Statistics-Ver. 2.1.), revealed the *qnrS* (417 bp) gene in 13 human subjects (52.0%), as well as in all swine samples studied. The *qnrB* (526 bp) gene was exposed in 9 of the human patients (36.0%) and in all swine isolates, and the *qnrA* (516 bp) gene was observed only in 3 of the isolates obtained from human subjects (12.0%) and was not discovered in pigs ($p > 0.05$). The presence of plasmids *qnrA*, *qnrB*, and *qnrS* in the human samples and of *qnrB* and *qnrS* in swine, facilitates the survival of pathogens despite the CIP action. The long-term use of CIP could cause a boost in the prevalence of *qnr* resistance genes, and resistance in the pigs destined for slaughter, a perturbing fact for public health and the human consumer.

Keywords: *Enterobacteiaceae*; ciprofloxacin-resistant; *qnrA*; *qnrB*; *qnrS*; genes

1. Introduction

Antimicrobial resistance (AMR) is the capacity of microorganisms to adjust to antimicrobials, particularly antibiotics. Excessive and improper uses of antimicrobial drugs and inadequate infection control practices have turned AMR into a severe global public health peril [1,2].

According to the European Commission (EC), the influence of the imprudent use of anti-infectives is substantial. Thus, more than 70% of bacteria, accountable for intra-hospital infectivity, were found to be resistant to at least one antibiotic structure. AMR is also responsible for more than 25,000 human deaths/year in the EU, and 700,000 worldwide, and might lead to more deaths than cancer by 2050 [3,4].

In this respect, databases and surveillance systems, from both the human health and veterinary sector, are becoming increasingly ample in data, since resistance was reported for nearly all antibiotic structures. In Romania, the main indicator for antimicrobial consumption in the veterinary sector is the Population Correction Unit (PCU), who revealed that the consumed amount of antibiotics was 100.5 mg $\times$ PCU^{-1}, an almost identical value with the EU average (100.6 mg $\times$ PCU^{-1}) in 2015 [2,5]. Between 2010 and 2030, global antimicrobial consumption in the livestock sector is expected to increase by approximately 70%, however, only a quarter of countries have implemented a national policy to combat AMR [5].

Though the antimicrobials have greatly modernized current medical practices, today, this advantage is particularly at risk due to intense or improper use of antimicrobials. The irresponsible use of antibiotics has amplified the occurrence and spread of multidrug-resistant bacteria, making optimization of veterinary antimicrobial treatment a priority [6].

Along with antibiotics used in human medicine, their use for treatment or prophylaxis practices used in animal breeding have led to selective pressure, favoring the emergence and rapid spread of resistant bacterial strains [7–9]. In this aim, animals can serve as mediators, reservoirs, and disseminators of resistant bacterial strains and/or resistance genes. Multiple studies have reported that excessive or inadequate use of antimicrobial substances in animals destined for production in the food industry can have a negative impact on the health of hired farm workers, of employees from meat processing units, as well as the on the final consumer [7–9].

The link between antibiotic and antimicrobial resistance has already been statistically demonstrated for *Escherichia coli* resistant to fluoroquinolones in humans [10,11] or animals [12–14], and also, *E. coli* resistant to cephalosporins from third and fourth generation in humans, *E. coli* resistant to tetracyclines and polymyxins in animals, *Klebsiella pneumoniae* resistant to carbapenems and polymyxins in humans, and *Campylobacter* spp. strains that are resistant to macrolides from animals associated with cross-resistance in animals and humans. Multiple resistances have also been reported in *Salmonella typhimurium* strains to antibiotics such as ampicillin, chloramphenicol, streptomycin, sulfonamides, and tetracycline [3,4,9,12,15].

The quick identification and antimicrobial susceptibility testing have considerable effects on the clinical outcome of severe infections in humans and animals. The frequent emergence of resistance to quinolones occurring in common infections with *Campylobacter* spp. and *E. coli* in humans, as a result of their massive use in animal feed, as well as the transmission of human-resistant bacteria through meat and animal products, causes great awareness [8,13,14].

Fluoroquinolones impede DNA gyrase and topoisomerase IV enzymes, both with crucial roles in bacterial DNA replication, and resistance to quinolones is regularly associated to amino-acid substitutions of *gyrA* and *gyrB* gyrases, DNA topoisomerase IV subunits, the quinolone-resistance-determining regions, followed by target modification [16,17].

Quinolones group have been used for prophylaxis against Gram-negative infections both in humans and animals, but the impact on the resistance mechanisms of this important group nonetheless require additional exploration [18,19].

The *qnr* genes provide low resistance level to quinolones in *Enterobacteriaceae*, but the multi-resistance dimension is of great importance, and studies about the resistance of *E. coli* to ciprofloxacin (CIP) and the specific *qnrA*, *qnrB*, and *qnrS* genes' detection and expression have been published in the last years [20–22].

In these cases, the use of Polymerase Chain Reaction (PCR) offers a simple, rapid, and accurate detection of the antibiotic resistance profiles, becoming a regularly used method of antibio-resistance diagnosis and surveillance in the epidemiological and ecological studies [23–25].

Since we were concerned with the quinolone group's resistance, emergent in Western Romania, to humans and animals, the present study tried to identify CIP-resistant cases and monitored the *qnrA*, *qnrB*, and *qnrS* plasmids in *E. coli*, using the molecular technique. The aim was to analyze the extent to which these ciprofloxacin resistance genes are present, and to examine their clone relatedness in pigs and human samples from our region.

2. Results

2.1. Antibiotic Susceptibility Testing (AST)

The results obtained from AST and the evolution of the resistance tendency showed the considerable presence of the multi-resistant strains in swine isolates where, from 53 samples analyzed, 15 isolates were presenting resistance to CIP and also multi-resistance to other antibiotics, including other quinolone representatives like, enrofloxacin, in the majority of cases, and norfloxacin (Table 1).

Table 1. Swine strains found with multiple resistances to CIP, 15 isolates from a total of 53.

No.	CIP-Resistant Sample No.	Antibiotics Where Resistance Was Identified	Total Antibiotics
1.	S.2.	CIP; NOR; FLO; AMX; CEF; SPCM; TC	7
2.	S.6.	CIP; ENR; AMX; CEF; OXA; FLO; SPCM	7
3.	S.7.	CIP; AMX; OXA; CEF; SPCM; TC	6
4.	S.13.	CIP; ENR; NOR; AMX; FLO; CEF; SPCM; TC	8
5.	S.14.	CIP; AMX; FLO; CEF; TC	5
6.	S.16.	CIP; NOR; AMX; FLO; CEF; SPCM; TC	7
7.	S.22.	CIP; ENR	2
8.	S.28.	CIP ENR; AMX; PSTR; NEO; CST; TC	7
9.	S.35.	CIP; ENR AMX; FLO; LCM; NEO; TC	7
10.	S.36.	CIP; ENR; FLO; AMX; LCM; NEO; TC	7
11.	S.38.	CIP; ENR; AMP; AMX; FLO; LCM; NEO; TC	8
12.	S.46.	CIP; ENR; AMP; GEN; NEO; FLO; LCM; TC; POS	9
13.	S.47.	CIP; ENR; AMP; GEN; NEO; FLO; LCM; TC; POS	9
14.	S.49.	CIP; ENR; AMP; AMX; NEO; STR; GEN; FLO; LCM; TC; POS	11
15.	S.50.	CIP; ENR; AMP; AMX; NEO; STR; FLO; LCM; TC; POS	10

Legend: S—Swine sample; Amoxicillin—AMX; Ampicillin—AMP; Cefalothin—CEF; Ciprofloxacin—CIP; Colistin—CST; Enrofloxacin—ENR; Florfenicol—FLO; Gentamicin—GEN; Lincomycin—LCM; Neomycin—NEO; Norfloxacin—NOR; Oxacillin—OXA; Penicillin-streptomycin—PSTR; Potentiated sulfonamides—POS; Spectinomycin—SPCM; Streptomycin—STR; Tetracycline—TC.

The AST results obtained from 147 human samples also presented high CIP resistance levels, but proportionally lower compared to swine, with 38 isolates presenting resistance, and among these, 17 were found with resistance for more than two antibiotics (Table 2).

Table 2. Human strains found with multiple resistances to CIP, 38 isolates from a total of 147.

No.	CIP -Resistant Sample No.	Antibiotics Where Resistance Was Identified	Total Antibiotics	No.	CIP -Resistant Sample No.	Antibiotics Where Resistance Was Identified	Total Antibiotics
1.	H.6.	CIP; LVX; PIP; SAM; GEN	5	20.	H.78.	CIP; PIP; SAM; CAZ; CTX; CFPM; TZP	7
2.	H.13.	CIP; LVX; TPM	3	21.	H.79.	CIP, PIP	2
3.	H.15.	CIP; LVX; PIP	3	22.	H.80.	CIP, LVX; PIP	3
4.	H.16.	CIP; LVX; PIP; TPM	4	23.	H.85.	CIP; PIP; CTX; CXM	4
5.	H.19.	CIP	1	24.	H.88.	CIP; LVX; PIP; CXM; TPM	5
6.	H.20.	CIP, LVX	2	25.	H.90.	CIP; LVX; GEN; PIP	4
7.	H.21.	CIP, LVX; PIP	3	26.	H.94.	CIP; PIP; CAZ; CTX; CXM; TPM	6
8.	H.22.	CIP; PIP; CAP; CTX; CXM; GEN	6	27.	H.97.	CIP; PIP; SAM; TPM	4
9.	H.24.	CIP; PIP; CTX; TPM	4	28.	H.102.	CIP; PIP; CAZ; CXM	4
10.	H.26.	CIP, LVX	2	29.	H.104.	CIP; PIP; CAZ. CTX; CFPM; TPM	6
11.	H.32.	CIP; PIP; SAM; CTX; CXM	5	30.	H.106.	CIP; PIP.	2
12.	H.35	CIP; PIP; CXM; TPM	4	31.	H.110.	CIP; PIP; TPM	3
13.	H.49.	CIP; LVX; PIP; CTX; CXM	5	32.	H.116.	CIP; LVX; PIP; CXM; TPM	5
14.	H.50.	CIP; LV	2	33.	H.119.	CIP; PIP; SAM; TPM	4
15.	H.60.	CIP; PIP; TPM	3	34.	H.130.	CIP; LVX; SAM; CAZ; CTX; CFPM; GEN; TZP	8
16.	H.65.	CIP; LVX; PIP; SAM; CAZ; CTX; CFPM; GEN	8	35.	H.134.	CIP; TPM.	2
17.	H.68.	CIP; LVX	2	36.	H.142.	CIP; CXM.	2
18	H.70.	CIP; LVX; PIP; CTX; CXM	5	37.	H.144.	CIP; TPM	2
19	H.71.	CIP; PIP; CTX; CXM; TPM	5	38.	H.147.	CIP; PIP; SAM; TPM.	4

Legend: Human sample—H; Ampicillin-sulbactam—SAM; Cefepime—CFPM; Ceftazidime—CAZ; Ceftriaxone—CTX; Cefuroxime—CXM; Ciprofloxacin—CIP; Gentamicin—GEN; Levofloxacin—LVX; Piperacillin—PIP; Piperacillin-tazobactam—TZP; Trimethoprim—TPM.

Crosstabs function and statistics for human and swine samples are presented in Tables 3 and 4.

Table 3. Antibiotic Susceptibility Testing (AST) results for human subjects (H) and swine (S).

Cross-Tabulation Results											
Humans (H)						**Swine (S)**					
Antibacterial		**Results**			**Total**	**Antibacterial**		**Results**			**Total**
		N	**R**	**S**				**N**	**R**	**S**	
Amikacin	count	4	1	142	147	Amoxicillin	count	6	43	4	53
	%	2.7	0.7	96.6	100.0		%	11.32	81.13	7.55	100.0
Ampicillin-sulbctam	count	20	14	113	147	Ampicillin	count	44	9	0	53
	%	13.6	9.5	76.9	100.0		%	83.02	16.98	0.0	100.0
Aztreonam	count	145	0	2	147	Sulfadoxin	count	49	0	4	53
	%	98.6	0.0	1.4	100.0		%	92.45	0.0	7.55	100.0
Cefepime	count	5	5	137	147	Cefalotin	count	36	17	0	53
	%	3.4	3.4	93.2	100.0		%	67.92	32.08	0.0	100.0
Cefoperazona-sulbactam	count	146	0	1	147	Ceftiofur	count	41	0	12	53
	%	99.3	0.0	0.7	100.0		%	77.35	0.0	22.65	100.0
Ceftazidime	count	6	9	132	147	Ciprofloxacin	count	22	15	16	53
	%	4.1	6.1	89.8	100.0		%	41.51	28.30	30.19	100.0
Ceftriaxone	count	11	15	121	147	Cefquinome	count	46	0	7	53
	%	7.5	10.2	82.3	100.0		%	86.79	0.0	13.21	100.0
Cefuroxime	count	11	21	115	147	Colistin	count	22	14	17	53
	%	7.5	14.3	78.2	100.0		%	41.51	26.42	32.07	100.0
Ciprofloxacin	count	4	39	104	147	Doxycycline	count	37	10	6	53
	%	2.7	26.5	70.7	100.0		%	68.81	18.87	11.32	100.0
Colistin sulphate	count	36	0	111	147	Enrofloxacin	count	16	13	24	53
	%	24.5	0.0	75.5	100.0		%	30.19	24.53	45.28	100.0
Gentamicin	count	10	6	131	147	Erythromycin	count	39	12	2	53
	%	6.8	4.1	89.1	100.0		%	73.58	22.65	3.77	100.0
Imipenem	count	0	0	147	147	Florfenicol	count	5	27	21	53
	%	0.0	0.0	100.0	100.0		%	9.43	50.95	39.62	100.0
Levofloxacin	count	10	19	118	147	Gentamycin	count	4	8	41	53
	%	6.8	12.9	80.3	100.0		%	7.55	15.09	77.36	100.0
Meropeneme	count	3	0	144	147	Lincomycin	count	27	15	11	53
	%	2.0	0.0	98.0	100.0		%	50.95	28.30	20.75	100.0
Minocycline	count	145	0	2	147	Neomycin	count	19	30	4	53
	%	98.6	0.0	1.4	100.0		%	35.85	56.60	7.55	100.0
Ofloxacime	count	145	0	2	147	Norfloxacin	count	36	6	11	53
	%	98.6	0.0	1.4	100.0		%	67.92	11.32	20.75	100.0
Piperacillin-tazobactam	count	16	4	127	147	Oxacillin	count	36	4	13	53
	%	10.9	2.7	86.4	100.0		%	67.92	7.55	24.53	100.0
Piperacillin	count	9	71	67	147	Penicillin-Streptomycin	count	49	3	1	53
	%	6.1	48.3	45.6	100.0		%	92.45	5.66	1.89	100.0
Ticarcillin	count	145	0	2	147	Spectinomycin	count	36	13	4	53
	%	98.6	0.0	1.4	100.0		%	67.92	24.53	7.55	100.0
Tobramycin	count	145	0	2	147	Streptomycin	count	44	7	2	53
	%	98.6	0.0	1.4	100.0		%	83.02	13.21	3.77	100.0
Trimethoprim	count	28	42	77	147	Sulfonamides	count	44	8	1	53
	%	19.0	28.6	52.4	100.0		%	83.02	15.09	1.89	100.0
						Tetracycline	count	16	31	6	53
							%	30.19	58.49	11.32	100.0
Total		1044	246	1497	3087	Tiamulin	count	36	3	14	53
							%	67.92	5.66	26.42	100.0
						Total		710	288	221	1219

Legend: N = Non-aligned (Intermediary sensitive), R = Resistant, S = Susceptible.

Table 4. Statistical results of *E. coli* resistance to CIP.

	Humans (H)			**Swine (S)**		
Chi-Square Tests	Value	*df*	Asymp. Sig. (2-sided)	Value	*df*	Asymp. Sig. (2-sided)
Pearson Chi-Square	2925.127 [a]	40	0.000	574.795 [a]	44	0.000
Likelihood Ratio	3113.083	40	0.000	588.576	44	0.000
0 cells (0.0%) have expected count less than 5.0. The minimum expected count is 11.71.				0 cells (0.0%) have expected count less than 5.0. The minimum expected count is 9.61.		

Case Processing Summary	Valid		Missing		Total		Valid		Missing		Total	
	3087	100.0%	0	0.0%	3087	100.0%	1219	100.0%	0	0.0%	1219	100.0%

Legend: *df*—degree of freedom; Asymp. Sig.—Asymptotic Significance; [a]—with statistical significance ($p > 0.05$).

From a statistical point of view and according to the obtained results, percentage 0.0% should be less than 20% and 0.000 less than $p > 0.05$, so the null hypothesis is rejected, meaning there are significant differences between antibiotics with an error of $p > 0.05$.

2.2. PCR Techniques—Isolation of Bacterial DNA (E. coli) in Humans and Swine

For PCR analysis, only samples with DNA purity of approximately 1.8 were processed, with the values recorded below this level signifying the samples' contamination. Thus, from the *E. coli* cultures collected for PCR analysis from humans (H), we used 15 DNA samples from a total of 24 taken from the culture media, and of 15 swine (S) samples studied, only 12 had quantitatively and qualitatively appropriate genetic material.

Following the isolation, we carried on with the migration of the DNA in agarose gel for the additional verification of the genetic material's integrity.

The extent to which CIP resistance genes (*qnrA*, *qnrB*, and *qnrS*) were present in the bacterial genome isolated from pigs and human subjects is presented in Table 5.

Table 5. Presentation of CIP-resistant genes in human subjects and swine *E. coli* isolates.

Humans (H)	Gene	Swine (S)	Gene
H.1.	*qnrS* + *qnrB* + *qnrA*	S.1.	*qnrS* + *qnrB*
H.2.	*qnrS* + *qnrB*	S.2.	*qnrS* + *qnrB*
H.3.	*qnrS* + *qnrB* + *qnrA*	S.3.	*qnrS* + *qnrB*
H.4.	*qnrS*	S.4.	*qnrS* + *qnrB*
H.5.	-	S.5.	*qnrS* + *qnrB*
H.6.	*qnrS*	S.6.	*qnrS* + *qnrB*
H.7.	*qnrS*	S.7.	*qnrS* + *qnrB*
H.8.	*qnrS* + *qnrB*	S.8.	*qnrS* + *qnrB*
H.9.	*qnrS*	S.9.	*qnrS* + *qnrB*
H.10.	*qnrS* + *qnrB* +*qnrA*	S.10.	*qnrS* + *qnrB*
H.11.	-	S.11.	*qnrS* + *qnrB*
H.12.	*qnrS* + *qnrB*	S.12.	*qnrS* + *qnrB*
H.13.	*qnrS* + *qnrB*	-	-
H.14.	*qnrS* + *qnrB*	-	-
H.15.	*qnrS* + *qnrB*	-	-

The presence of the *qnrS* gene (417 base pairs—bp) was identified in 13 of the human subjects and in all pigs registered in our study.

PCR amplification for the *qnrB* gene (526 bp) showed its presence in 9 of the human patients and in all cases of isolates obtained from pigs.

The *qnrA* gene (516 bp) was observed only in 3 of the isolates obtained from human subjects, but it was absent in pig isolates.

Accordingly, in cultures of *E. coli* isolated from human samples, *qnrS* was detected in 52%, *qnrB* in 36%, and *qnrA* in 12% of cases, respectively. Similarly, in swine samples, *qnrS* and *qnrB* were reported in 100% of swine samples but no *qnrA* genes were reported. The obtained results point out an increased prevalence of *qnr* resistance genes in CIP-resistant *E. coli.* A differentiation between the two situations studied is the presence of *qnrA* genes only in humans. This leads to the assumption of direct or indirect contact of these subjects with low concentrations of CIP, which may increase resistance through the presence of plasmid *qnrA*, a mechanism that facilitates the survival of pathogenic *E. coli* germs.

3. Discussion

The introduction of ciprofloxacin in the therapeutic protocols of the 80's represented a real progress for the medicine of those times. After only a decade of use, unfortunately, the first cases of resistance appeared, with much lower incidence compared to current times [26–28].

The expansion of this phenomenon over time may coincide with the massive detection of *qnr* genes. This has been a suspicion of various researchers due to the close links between *qnr* genes and diverse quinolones resistance. It has been demonstrated through "in vitro" procedures on *qnrA* plasmid, which facilitated the development of this phenomenon in *Enterobacteriaceae*, at the chromosomal level [29–32].

The present study confirmed an increased prevalence of *qnrA*, *qnrB*, and *qnrS* resistance genes in quinolones in both human and swine subjects, and the presence of *qnrA* genes at a 12% rate in humans only stands as a differentiation between the two situations analyzed. This leads to the hypothesis regarding direct or indirect contact of these subjects with low concentrations of ciprofloxacin, which may increase resistance through the presence of plasmid *qnrA*—a mechanism that facilitates the survival of pathogenic *E. coli* [31,32].

After testing the pigs, however, some significant differences of the resistance phenomenon can be observed and confirmed through statistical interpretation of the results using the Crosstabs function. The presence of these differences can be based on the following assumptions:

- Dissimilar evolution of bacterial diseases on farms,
- Diverse treatment protocols between units,
- Organization of antimicrobial products through treatment rotation.

A simple comparison between the values obtained by us in the hospital in Timișoara and the clinical units in other areas of the world, show the increased incidence of quinolone-resistant *Enterobacteriaceae*: at a 32% rate in UK—Liverpool [12], and at an overwhelming rate of 78% genes encoded by *qnrA* in the Netherlands [10].

In the USA, the presence of the *qnrA* and *qnrB* genes only, was also reported [15]. In Taiwan and Korea, the presence of these genes was around 17% (*qnrA* 0.6%, *qnrB* 10%, and *qnrS* 6.5%) [11,32].

After analyzing this situation in other hospitals, from the first discovery of a quinolone resistance gene in 1998, until now, we can state that the evolution of this phenomenon differs greatly, depending on the area and the therapeutic protocols. From a genotypic and structural point of view, it is known that the composition of the two genes includes 218 amino acids with a variety lower than 10% between *qnrA* and *qnrS*. Similarities between *qnrB* and *qnrA* are of only 40%, with the first being composed of 214 amino acids [25,32].

The situation of the Romanian farms studied does not differ much from those in China, in terms of gene type presence. In both cases, the *qnrA* gene is missing, and as a differentiation, the incidence of *qnrB* plasmids is lower in Chinese farms. In the case of pigs from Chinese households, the presence of resistance genes is around 6%. Furthermore, in swine farms from Taiwan, the presence of the *qnrS* gene was reported to be around 3.33% [31].

It is general knowledge today that the long-term use of quinolones was followed by an increase in prevalence of *qnr* resistance genes, and cases of resistance have also been reported in pigs. Also, in our study, we ascertained an associated antibio-resistance of CIP with enrofloxacin and norfloxacin, which confirmed the multi-resistance high tendency for the quinolones group. Thus, some alarm signals were raised about the zoonotic transmission of this phenomenon through the food chain [3,5,7–9,24,25].

Healthcare organizations, as well as recent research, have focused on the global assessment of this phenomenon of resistance. The impact of much more restrictive protocols on the handling and use of antimicrobials has already led to a trend of significant percentage decrease in resistance—between 9% and 30%. In order to avoid the propagation of this phenomenon, the precautionary principle is recommended. The legislative revision of used therapeutic protocols, by establishing new limitations on the handling and use of antimicrobials, has become an absolute priority [33].

4. Materials and Methods

4.1. Location and Samples Collecting for AST

The study was conducted over one year (from Jan 2019–Jan 2020).

The experiment took place in the Western part of Romania, in Timiș and Arad Counties, areas well developed from the perspective of swine breeding, with an annual population of over one million pigs, in the intensive system only. A big part of this production is destined for meat consumption, as well as meat-derived products. For the purpose of this research, we included large capacity swine exploiting units, where clinical cases were diverse, and the incidence of colibacillary infections was high.

4.1.1. Samples

The examination was performed on biological material, from pure *E. coli* cultures (of maximum 20 mg), collected directly from the fresh intestinal contents of swine.

The samples from humans were provided for the lab processing from a large hospital from Timișoara city, Romania, with the blood samples being gathered in blood collection K3-EDTA vacutainer tubes (13 × 100 mm) (Kima, Bucharest, Romania).

4.1.2. Microbial Testing

Subsequently, bacterial resistance of 147 isolated *E. coli* strains from humans and 53 for swine were tested for susceptibility to twenty-one commonly used antibiotics in human medicine and fifteen frequently utilized antibiotics and associations, through the Kirby–Bauer standardized disk diffusion technique.

Interpretation of antibiotic resistance was performed through measuring the diameter of the growth inhibition zone and the strains were categorized as Non-aligned (Intermediary sensitive), Resistant, or Sensitive to the drug according to manufacturer's instructions and according with the current interpretation standards, which can be found in the Clinical Laboratory Standards Institute (CLSI), Performance Standards for Antimicrobial Disk Susceptibility Tests.

4.2. PCR Techniques—Isolation of Bacterial DNA (E. coli) in Humans and Swine Samples

Samples were taken in Phosphate Buffered Saline (PBS) solution (Sigma-Aldrich, Darmstadt, Germany) to culture plates and cultivation of *E. coli* strains was on McKonkey (Oxoid Ltd., Basingstoke, UK) selective media, then *E. coli* was sampled in tubes for PCR analysis.

Bacterial DNA isolation was performed using the PureLink® Genomic DNA Mini Kit (Invitrogen, Carlsbad, CA, USA) according to the manufacturer's protocol.

Analysis of the quality and quantification of DNA extracted from bacterial cultures was performed using UV spectroscopy. For appreciating DNA purity, we analyzed the Optical Density (OD) at 260/280 on a ScanDrop nano-volume spectrophotometer (Analitik Jena, Jena, Germany).

For PCR analysis, we took into account only samples with DNA purity of approximately 1.8, with the values recorded below this level indicating the contamination of samples.

DNA amplification was performed in PCR on a thermo-cycler (BiometraTM, Analitik Jena, Jena, Germany), for 35 cycles, using FIRESol® Master Mix (Solis BioDyne, Tartu, Estonia) and specific primers for *qnrS*, *qnrA*, and *qnrB* genes.

Work protocol used 500 µL tubes to obtain a 50 µL reaction volume, by adding 45 µL PCR mix and 5 µL primers and 1:1 DNA sample. Multiplex reagents were performed for *qnr* analysis, and sequence of primers used, genes, and fragment size are shown in Table 6.

Table 6. Sequence primers used genes and fragments size.

Gene	Primer Used	Fragment Size
qnrS	F: ACGACATTCGTCAACTGGAA R: TTAATTGGCACCCTGTAGGC	417 bp
qnrA	F: ATTTCTCACGCCAGGATTTG R:GATCGGCAAAGGTTAGGTCA	516 bp
qnrB	F: GTTGGCGAAAAAATTGACAGAA R: ACTCCGAATTGGTCAGATCG	526 bp

4.3. Statistical and Data Analysis

Statistical analysis of data obtained in the experiment regarding the use of antibiotics in the swine units was performed using the IBM SSPS Statistics (Version 2.1.) and Crosstabs function, where 0.000 was less than $p > 0.05$, so the null hypothesis is rejected, i.e., there are significant differences between antibiotics with an error of $p > 0.05$.

5. Conclusions

After evaluating this case, we can state that the main *qnrA* gene (516 bp) was not found in swine. Moreover, the presence of *qnrA* (12%), *qnrB* (36%), and *qnrS* (52%) genes in human samples and of *qnrB* and *qnrS* in swine can facilitate the survival of pathogens under the action of antimicrobials from the quinolone group, in our case, CIP alone, or CIP-associated multiple-resistance, both in veterinary practice and in human hospitals' therapeutic protocol.

Thus, the hypothesis of transmitting resistance on the human-animal-human food chain is demonstrated. The long-term use of CIP could lead to an increase in the prevalence of *qnr* resistance genes, and resistance emergence in the healthy pigs destined for slaughter.

Author Contributions: Conceptualization, R.T.C. and A.O.D.; methodology, R.P., D.M., M.M., and J.D.; software, M.V.B. and F.M. validation, R.T.C.; formal analysis, N.P. and S.D.; investigation I.R., R.P., D.M., M.M., and J.D.; resources, R.T.C. and I.R.; data curation, E.D.; writing—original draft preparation, R.T.C. and A.O.D.; writing—review and editing, R.T.C. and S.D.; visualization and supervision, S.D. and N.P.; project administration and funding acquisition, R.T.C. and E.D. All authors have read and agreed to the published version of the manuscript.

Funding: This work was supported by USAMVBT—Institutional development projects—Projects for financing excellence in CDI under the Grant 35SFE.

Acknowledgments: The present research was carried out within the Project 7 PCCDI/2018/Subprogram 1.2-Institutional performance/Complex Projects accomplished in CDI consortia, Romania/2018-2020. One part of this research was supported by COST Action CA18217—European Network for Optimization of Veterinary Antimicrobial Treatment.

Conflicts of Interest: The authors declare no conflict of interest.

Abbreviations

Antimicrobial Resistance—AMR; Polymerase Chain Reaction—PCR; Ultraviolet radiation—UV; European Commission—EC; Population Correction Unit—PCU; ciprofloxacin—CIP; Antibiotic Susceptibility Testing—AST; base pairs—bp; human subjects—H; swine—S; Phosphate Buffered Saline—PBS; Optical Density—OD; Electrophoresis Buffer-Acetic Acid Buffer—EDTA-TAE; proteinase K—pk; quinolone resistant—qnr; Amoxicillin—AMX; Ampicillin—AMP; Cefalothin—CEF; Ciprofloxacin—CIP; Colistin—CST; Enrofloxacin—ENR; Florfenicol—FLO; Gentamicin—GEN; Lincomycin—LCM; Neomycin—NEO; Norfloxacin—NOR; Oxacillin—OXA; Potentiated sulfonamides—POS; Spectinomycin—SPCM; Tetracycline—TC; Human sample—H; Ampicillin-sulbactam—SAM; Cefepime—CFPM; Ceftazidime—CAZ; Ceftriaxone—CTX; Cefuroxime—CXM; Ciprofloxacin—CIP; Levofloxacin—LVX; Piperacillin—PIP; Piperacillin-tazobactam—TZP; Trimethoprim—TPM; Clinical Laboratory Standards Institute—CLSI.

References

1. Aslam, B.; Wang, W.; Arshad, M.I.; Khurshid, M.; Muzammil, S.; Rasool, M.H.; Nisar, M.A.; Alvi, R.F.; Aslam, M.A.; Qamar, M.U.; et al. Antibiotic resistance: A rundown of a global crisis. *Infect. Drug Resist.* **2018**, *11*, 1645–1658. [CrossRef] [PubMed]
2. Cristina, R.T.; Doma, A.O.; Dumitrescu, E.; Muselin, F.; Chirilă, B.A. About the Development and Implications of the Drug Resistance Phenomenon of Veterinary Antinfectious and Parasitic Drugs and the Evolution of this Phenomenon in Romania. *Med. Vet./Vet. Drug* **2018**, *12*, 4–49. Available online: http://www.veterinarypharmacon.com/docs/1948-2018_VD_12(1)_ART2.RO.pdf (accessed on 20 March 2020).
3. European Centre for Disease Prevention and Control (ECDC); European Food Safety Authority (EFSA); European Medicines Agency (EMA). ECDC/EFSA/EMA second joint report on the integrated analysis of the consumption of antimicrobial agents and occurrence of antimicrobial resistance in bacteria from humans and food-producing animals. *EFSA J.* **2017**, *15*, e04872. [CrossRef]
4. Frieri, M.; Kumar, K.; Boutin, A. Antibiotic Resistance. *J. Inf. Public Health* **2017**, *10*, 369–378. [CrossRef]
5. Moruzi, R.F.; Tîrziu, E.; Muselin, F.; Dumitrescu, E.; Huțu, I.; Mircu, C.; Tulcan, C.; Doma, A.O.; Degi, J.; Degi, D.M.; et al. The Importance of Databases to Manage the Phenomenon of Resistance to Antimicrobials for Veterinary Use. *Rev. Rom. Med. Vet.* **2019**, *29*, 40–57.
6. Khameneh, B.; Diab, R.; Ghazvini, K.; Bazzaz, B.S.F. Breakthroughs in bacterial resistance mechanisms and the potential ways to combat them. *Microb. Pathog.* **2016**, *95*, 32–42. [CrossRef]
7. Marshall, B.M.; Levy, S.B. Food Animals and Antimicrobials: Impacts on Human Health. *Clin. Microbiol. Rev.* **2011**, *24*, 718–733. [CrossRef]
8. Muloi, D.; Ward, M.J.; Pedersen, A.B.; Fèvre, E.M.; Woolhouse, M.E.J.; van Bunnik, B.A.D. Are Food Animals Responsible for Transfer of Antimicrobial Resistant Escherichia coli or their Resistance Determinants to Human Populations? A Systematic Review. *Foodborne Pathog. Dis.* **2018**, *15*, 464–474. [CrossRef]
9. Tang, K.L.; Caffrey, N.P.; Nóbrega, D.B.; Cork, S.C.; Ronksley, P.E.; Barkema, H.W.; Polachek, A.J.; Ganshorn, H.; Sharma, N.; Kellner, J.D.; et al. Restricting the use of antibiotics in food-producing animals and its associations with antibiotic resistance in food-producing animals and human beings: A systematic review and meta-analysis. *Lancet Planet. Health* **2017**, *1*, e316–e327. [CrossRef]
10. Paauw, A.; Fluit, A.C.; Verhoef, J.; Hall, M.A.L.-V. Enterobacter cloacae Outbreak and Emergence of Quinolone Resistance Gene in Dutch Hospital. *Emerg. Infect. Dis.* **2006**, *12*, 807–812. [CrossRef]
11. Tamang, M.D.; Seol, S.Y.; Oh, J.-Y.; Kang, H.Y.; Lee, J.C.; Lee, Y.C.; Cho, D.T.; Kim, J. Plasmid-Mediated Quinolone Resistance Determinants qnrA, qnrB, and qnrS among Clinical Isolates of Enterobacteriaceae in a Korean Hospital. *Antimicrob. Agents Chemother.* **2008**, *52*, 4159–4162. [CrossRef]
12. Corkill, J.E.; Anson, J.J.; Hart, C.A. High prevalence of the plasmid-mediated quinolone resistance determinant qnrA in multidrug-resistant Enterobacteriaceae from blood cultures in Liverpool, UK. *J. Antimicrob. Chemother.* **2005**, *56*, 1115–1117. [CrossRef]
13. Cristina, R.T.; Doma, A.O.; Moșneang, C.L. Use of antibiotics and about quinolones in veterinary therapy. *Med. Vet./Vet. Drug* **2012**, *6*, 4–67. Available online: http://www.veterinarypharmacon.com/docs/1116-2012-6(2)-ART.2-ro.pdf (accessed on 20 March 2020).
14. Du, X.D.; Lian, M.X.; LI, D.X.; Zhang, S.M.; Liu, J.H.; Pan, Y.S.; Li, X.S. Detection of Plasmid-mediated Quinolone Resistant Genes among Escherichia coli Strains Isolated from Healthy Pigs. *Jiangxi J. Agric. Sci.* **2009**, *21*, 9–11.

15. Robicsek, A.; Strahilevitz, J.; Sahm, D.F.; Jacoby, G.A.; Hooper, D.C. qnr Prevalence in Ceftazidime-Resistant Enterobacteriaceae Isolates from the United States. *Antimicrob. Agents Chemother.* **2006**, *50*, 2872–2874. [CrossRef]
16. Martínez-Martínez, L.; Pascual, A.; Jacoby, G.A. Quinolone resistance from a transferable plasmid. *Lancet* **1998**, *351*, 797–799. [CrossRef]
17. Azargun, R.; Barhaghi, M.H.S.; Kafil, H.S.; Oskouee, M.A.; Sadeghi, V.; Memar, M.Y.; Ghotaslou, R. Frequency of DNA gyrase and topoisomerase IV mutations and plasmid-mediated quinolone resistance genes among Escherichia coli and Klebsiella pneumoniae isolated from urinary tract infections in Azerbaijan, Iran. *J. Glob. Antimicrob. Resist.* **2019**, *17*, 39–43. [CrossRef]
18. Yanat, B.; Rodríguez-Martínez, J.M.; Touati, A. Plasmid-mediated quinolone resistance in Enterobacteriaceae: A systematic review with a focus on Mediterranean countries. *Eur. J. Clin. Microbiol. Infect. Dis.* **2016**, *36*, 421–435. [CrossRef]
19. Vieira, D.C.; Lima, W.G.; Paiva, M.C. Plasmid-mediated quinolone resistance (PMQR) among Enterobacteriales in Latin America: A systematic review. *Mol. Biol. Rep.* **2019**, *47*, 1471–1483. [CrossRef]
20. Mahmoud, A.T.; Salim, M.T.; Ibrahem, R.A.; Gabr, A.; Halby, H.M. Multiple Drug Resistance Patterns in Various Phylogenetic Groups of Hospital-Acquired Uropathogenic *E. coli* Isolated from Cancer Patients. *Antibiotics* **2020**, *9*, 108. [CrossRef]
21. Salah, F.D.; Soubeiga, S.T.; Ouattara, A.K.; Sadji, A.Y.; Metuor-Dabire, A.; Obiri-Yeboah, D.; Kere, A.B.; Karou, S.D.; Simpore, J. Distribution of quinolone resistance gene (qnr) in ESBL-producing Escherichia coli and Klebsiella spp. in Lomé, Togo. *Antimicrob. Resist. Infect. Control* **2019**, *8*, 1–8. [CrossRef]
22. Hamed, S.M.; Elkhatib, W.F.; El-Mahallawy, H.A.; Helmy, M.M.; Ashour, M.S.; Aboshanab, K. Multiple mechanisms contributing to ciprofloxacin resistance among Gram negative bacteria causing infections to cancer patients. *Sci. Rep.* **2018**, *8*, 12268. [CrossRef]
23. Kindle, P.; Zurfluh, K.; Nüesch-Inderbinen, M.; Von Ah, S.; Sidler, X.; Stephan, R.; Kümmerlen, D. Phenotypic and genotypic characteristics of Escherichia coli with non-susceptibility to quinolones isolated from environmental samples on pig farms. *Porc. Health Manag.* **2019**, *5*, 9. [CrossRef]
24. Kuo, H.-C.; Chou, C.-C.; Tu, C.; Gong, S.-R.; Han, C.-L.; Liao, J.-W.; Chang, S.-K. Characterization of plasmid-mediated quinolone resistance by the qnrS gene in Escherichia coli isolated from healthy chickens and pigs. *Vet. Med.* **2009**, *54*, 473–482. [CrossRef]
25. Yue, L.; Jiang, H.-X.; Liao, X.-P.; Liu, J.-H.; Li, S.-J.; Chen, X.-Y.; Chen, C.-X.; Lü, D.-H.; Liu, Y.-H. Prevalence of plasmid-mediated quinolone resistance qnr genes in poultry and swine clinical isolates of Escherichia coli. *Vet. Microbiol.* **2008**, *132*, 414–420. [CrossRef]
26. Jacoby, G.A.; Strahilevitz, J.; Hooper, D.C. Plasmid-mediated Quinolone Resistance: A multifaceted threat. *Clin. Microbiol. Rev.* **2009**, *22*, 664–689. [CrossRef]
27. Jacoby, G.; Cattoir, V.; Hooper, D.; Martínez-Martínez, L.; Nordmann, P.; Pascual, A.; Poirel, L.; Wang, M. qnr Gene Nomenclature. *Antimicrob. Agents Chemother.* **2008**, *52*, 2297–2299. [CrossRef]
28. Jacoby, G.A.; Walsh, K.E.; Mills, D.M.; Walker, V.J.; Oh, H.; Robicsek, A.; Hooper, D.C. qnrB, Another Plasmid-Mediated Gene for Quinolone Resistance. *Antimicrob. Agents Chemother.* **2006**, *50*, 1178–1182. [CrossRef]
29. Liu, J.H.; Deng, Y.T.; Zeng, Z.L.; Gao, J.H. Coprevalence of Plasmid-Mediated Quinolone Resistance Determinants qepA, qnr, and AAC(6′)-Ib-cr among 16S rRNA Methylase RmtB-Producing Escherichia coli Isolates from Pigs. *Antimicrob. Agents Chemother.* **2008**, *52*, 2992–2993. [CrossRef]
30. Poirel, L.; Nguyen, T.V.; Weintraub, A.; Leviandier, C.; Nordmann, P. Plasmid-mediated quinolone resistance determinant qnrS in Enterobacter cloacae. *Clin. Microbiol. Infect.* **2006**, *12*, 1021–1023. [CrossRef]
31. Wang, M.; Tran, J.H.; Jacoby, G.A.; Zhang, Y.; Wang, F.; Hooper, D.C. Plasmid-Mediated Quinolone Resistance in Clinical Isolates of Escherichia coli from Shanghai, China. *Antimicrob. Agents Chemother.* **2003**, *47*, 2242–2248. [CrossRef]

32. Wu, J.-J.; Ko, W.-C.; Tsai, S.-H.; Yan, J.-J. Prevalence of Plasmid-Mediated Quinolone Resistance Determinants QnrA, QnrB, and QnrS among Clinical Isolates of Enterobacter cloacae in a Taiwanese Hospital. *Antimicrob. Agents Chemother.* **2007**, *51*, 1223–1227. [CrossRef]
33. Commission Staff Document. EU Action on Antimicrobial Resistance. 2019. Available online: https://ec.europa.eu/health/amr/antimicrobial-resistance_en (accessed on 15 February 2020).

Publisher's Note: MDPI stays neutral with regard to jurisdictional claims in published maps and institutional affiliations.

antibiotics

Article

Antimicrobial Resistance Genes in Porcine *Pasteurella multocida* Are Not Associated with Its Antimicrobial Susceptibility Pattern

Máximo Petrocchi-Rilo [1], César-B. Gutiérrez-Martín [1,*], Esther Pérez-Fernández [1], Anna Vilaró [2], Lorenzo Fraile [3] and Sonia Martínez-Martínez [1]

1 Departamento de Sanidad Animal, Unidad de Microbiología e Inmunología, Universidad de León, s/n, 24071 León, Spain; mpetr@unileon.es (M.P.-R.); eperf@unileon.es (E.P.-F.); smarm@unileon.es (S.M.-M.)
2 Grup de Sanejament Porcí, 25192 Lleida, Spain; micro@gsplleida.net
3 Departament de Ciència Animal, ETSEA, Universitat de Lleida-Agrotecnio, 25198 Lleida, Spain; Lorenzo.fraile@udl.cat
* Correspondence: cbgutm@unileon.es; Tel.: +34-98729-1203

Received: 2 September 2020; Accepted: 16 September 2020; Published: 17 September 2020

Abstract: Forty-eight *Pasteurella multocida* isolates were recovered from porcine pneumonic lungs collected from farms in "Castilla y León" (north-western Spain) in 2017–2019. These isolates were characterized for their minimal inhibition concentrations to twelve antimicrobial agents and for the appearance of eight resistance genes: *tetA*, *tetB*, bla_{ROB1}, bla_{TEM}, *ermA*, *ermC*, *mphE* and *msrE*. Relevant resistance percentages were shown against tetracyclines (52.1% for doxycycline, 68.7% for oxytetracycline), sulphamethoxazole/trimethoprim (43.7%) and tiamulin (25.0%), thus suggesting that *P. multocida* isolates were mostly susceptible to amoxicillin, ceftiofur, enrofloxacin, florfenicol, marbofloxacin and macrolides. Overall, 29.2% of isolates were resistant to more than two antimicrobials. The tetracycline resistance genes (*tetA* and *tetB*) were detected in 22.9% of the isolates, but none were positive to both simultaneously; bla_{ROB1} and bla_{TEM} genes were found in one third of isolates but both genes were detected simultaneously in only one isolate. The *ermC* gene was observed in 41.7% of isolates, a percentage that decreased to 22.9% for *msrE*; finally, *ermA* was harbored by 16.7% and *mph*E was not found in any of them. Six clusters were established based on hierarchical clustering analysis on antimicrobial susceptibility for the twelve antimicrobials. Generally, it was unable to foresee the antimicrobial susceptibility pattern for each family and the association of each particular isolate inside the clusters established from the presence or absence of the resistance genes analyzed.

Keywords: *Pasteurella multocida*; antimicrobial resistance genes; antimicrobial susceptibility patterns; swine

1. Introduction

The Porcine Respiratory Disease Complex (PRDC) is a syndrome that results from a combination of infectious and non-infectious factors. *Pasteurella multocida* is one of the most common bacterial agents isolated from respiratory clinical cases [1]. It belongs to the commensal organisms in the upper portion of the porcine respiratory tract that can also cause pneumonia in growing and finishing pigs worldwide. *P. multocida* is normally considered as a secondary agent but it has also been described as a primary agent of haemorrhagic septicaemia in pigs, mainly caused by B:2 [2] or E:5 serotypes [3]. Moreover, the prevalence of *P. multocida* serotypes can vary considerably from region to region and over time in a given region [4].

The use of antimicrobials could be necessary to control bacteria entailed in PRDC with a therapeutic or a metaphylactic goal [5], but their use may be one of the factors involved in the emergence and spread of bacterial resistance from pig origin across the world [6,7]. Although *P. multocida* had been generally susceptible to the majority of antimicrobials, the emergence of multidrug-resistant pathogenic bacteria has been widely reported in recent times probably associated with the abusive use of antimicrobials [4]. Tetracyclines have been used for prophylaxis, in such a way that the effects of long-term consumption of these drugs probably resulted in increased levels of resistance [8,9], with global problems for public health [10]. Some of these resistance genes are often located on mobile genetic elements, frequently transmissible plasmids and transposons [11]; in addition, exchanges of resistance genes are common not only in the genus *Pasteurella*, but also in the family *Pasteurellaceae* [12].

The term of antimicrobial resistome has been proposed for describing the collection of all known antimicrobial resistance genes in the microbial ecosystem [13]. This concept supports the theory that resistant organisms and their antimicrobial resistome are settled after birth in living beings and are gained from the mother or by direct contact with resistant bacteria in the adjoining environment [14].

In this study, the antimicrobial susceptibility patterns observed in *P. multocida* strains isolated from pigs in Spain between 2017 and 2019 was linked with the presence or absence of antimicrobial resistance genes in order to decipher whether it is possible to determine the feasibility of selecting antimicrobials from the identification of resistance genes by molecular biology.

2. Results

2.1. Antimicrobial Resistance

The MIC (minimum inhibitory concentration) range, MIC_{50}, MIC_{90} and antimicrobial resistance of the 48 *P. multocida* isolated from porcine pneumonic lungs in Spain from 2017 to 2019 are shown in Table 1. All isolates were susceptible to ceftiofur, florfenicol, tildipirosin and tulathromycin, while most of them (>95%) were susceptible to amoxicillin, the two quinolones tested (enrofloxacin and marbofloxacin), and tilmicosin. In addition, 25% of isolates showed resistance to tiamulin and 31.2% or 43.7% to sulphamethoxazole/trimethoprim depending on the selected breakpoint (*Staphylococcus aureus* and *Escherichia coli*, or *Streptococcus suis*, respectively). On the other hand, doxycycline and oxytetracycline cannot be used to treat 52.1% and 68.7% of the cases, respectively. In addition, the distribution of the MIC range of amoxicillin, doxycycline, tiamulin, tilmicosin and tulathromycin was clearly unimodal, whereas *P. multocida* isolates seemed to show a bimodal distribution to enrofloxacin, and a multimodal bend to sulphamethoxazole/trimethoprim. Tailing of isolates over the MIC range was found for ceftiofur, marbofloxacin, oxytetracycline and tildipirosin (Table 1).

Table 1. MIC (minimum inhibitory concentration) range, MIC_{50}, MIC_{90} and percentage of resistant *Pasteurella multocida* isolates recovered in Spain between 2017 and 2019.

Antimicrobial Agent	Range (µg/mL)	MIC_{50} (µg/mL)	MIC_{90} (µg/mL)	Breakpoint (µg/mL) *	Antimicrobial Resistance (%)
Amoxicillin	1–8	0.25	8	0.5 $	2.1
Ceftiofur	0.06–0.25	0.06	0.12	2	0
Doxycycline	0.25–2	1	>2	0.5 $$	52.1
Enrofloxacin	0.03–0.5	0.03	0.12	0.25	2.1
Florfenicol	0.5	0.5	0.5	2	0
Marbofloxacin	0.03–0.5	0.03	0.12	0.25 &	4.2
Oxytetracycline	0.5–8	2	>8	0.5	68.7
Sulphamethoxazole/trimethoprim (19/1 ratio) §	0.06–4	0.25	>4	0.5 && 2 §§	43.7 31.2
Tiamulin	2–32	16	>32	16	25
Tildipirosin	0.5–4	1	4	4	0

Table 1. *Cont.*

Antimicrobial Agent	Range (µg/mL)	MIC_{50} (µg/mL)	MIC_{90} (µg/mL)	Breakpoint (µg/mL) *	Antimicrobial Resistance (%)
Tilmicosin	2–32	8	32	16	2.1
Tulathromycin	0.5–4	1	2	16	0

* Clinical breakpoints were obtained from CLSI VET08 or CLSI M100 with the following clarifications: $ extrapolated from ampicillin. $$ Extrapolated from tetracycline. & Extrapolated from enrofloxacin. && Extrapolated from *Streptococcus suis*. § MIC is for trimethoprim in this table. §§ Extrapolated from *Staphylococus hyicus* and *Escherichia coli*.

Overall, 89.6% of the isolates (*n* = 43) were resistant to one or more antimicrobial agents, in such a way that 25.0% (*n* = 12) showed resistance to only one compound; 35.4% (*n* = 17) to two antimicrobial agents; 22.9% (*n* = 11) to three drugs and 6.2% (*n* = 3) to four antimicrobials simultaneously. The most common resistance pattern was observed for the two tetracyclines tested, with 12 isolates being resistant to both of them. On the other hand, only 10.4% (*n* = 5) of the isolates were susceptible to all 12 compounds evaluated (Table 2).

Table 2. Antimicrobial resistance profiles of 48 *Pasteurella multocida* strains in this study.

Number of Isolate	Number of Antimicrobial Agents	Resistance to
5	0	No antimicrobial resistance
2	1	Oxytetracycline
6	1	Sulphamethoxazole/trimethoprim
4	1	Tiamulin
12	2	Doxycycline + oxytetracycline
1	2	Marbofloxacin + oxytetracycline
3	2	Oxytetracycline + sulphamethoxazole/trimethoprim
1	2	Oxytetracycline + tiamulin
1	3	Amoxicillin + doxycycline + oxytetracycline
4	3	Doxcycline + oxytetracycline + sulphamethoxazole/trimethoprim
5	3	Doxcycline + oxytetracycline + tiamulin
1	3	Oxytetracycline + tiamulin + tilmicosin
1	4	Doxycycline + enrofloxacin + oxytetracycline + tiamulin
2	4	Doxycycline + oxytetracycline + sulphamethoxazole/trimethoprim + tiamulin

2.2. Description of Resistance Genes

Of the eight resistance genes examined, *tetB* was harbored by 39.6% of *P. multocida* isolates, while *tetA* was only borne by 12.5%. Globally, 22.9% of them showed one of the two tetracycline resistance genes, but none was positive to both simultaneously. With regard to β-lactam resistance genes, 27.1% of isolates were positive to bla_{ROB1}, while only 8.3% were to bla_{TEM}, in such a way that one third of isolates showed resistance to some of these two genes, and only one carried both bla_{ROB1} and bla_{TEM} genes. In addition, 41.7% of isolates showed the *ermC* gene, a figure that decreased until 22.9% to *msrE*; *ermA* was harboured by 16.7% and, finally, *mphE* was not found in any isolate. A total of 27.1% of isolates amplified one of the macrolide resistance genes; the same percentage amplified two of them, and 2.1% amplified three macrolide resistance genes at the same time.

2.3. *Analysis of the Association between the Presence of Resistance Genes and Antimicrobial Patterns*

Only in 19 cases (8.3% for the *tetA* gene, 29.2% for the *tetB* gene and 2.1% for the bla_{ROB1} gene) could a clear association be established between the resistance to a given antimicrobial agent and the detection of some of the genes being able to explain this lack of susceptibility (Table 3). Interestingly, this association was observed for tetracyclines in 18 of them (94.7%). On the contrary, the existence of 19 isolates carrying the *ermC* gene but being susceptible to the three macrolides evaluated, or the 15 isolates with the bla_{ROB1} gene but without resistance to amoxicillin must be highlighted (Table 3). Globally, the identification of resistance genes in 62 cases could not be associated with the susceptibility pattern observed for tetracyclines, β-lactams or macrolides (Table 3). Thus, no significant association between the presence of resistance genes and that of a resistant phenotype for one particular antimicrobial agent was observed (Table 4).

Table 3. Association between the presence of resistance genes and antimicrobial susceptibility patterns in 48 *Pasteurella multocida* isolates.

Resistance Gene	Number of Isolates	Resistance or Sensitivity	Resistance or Sensitivity to
tetA	3	Resistance	Tetracyclines *
tetA	1		Oxytetracycline
tetB	11		Tetracyclines *
tetB	3		Oxytetracycline
bla_{ROB1}	1		Amoxicillin
tetA	2	Sensitivity	Tetracyclines *
tetB	5		Tetracyclines *
bla_{ROB1}	15		Amoxicillin
ermA	8		Macrolides $
ermC	19		Macrolides $
msrE	12		Macrolides $
mphE	1		Macrolides $

* Tetracyclines are doxycycline and oxytetracycline. $ Macrolides are tildipirosin, tilmicosin and tulathromycin.

Table 4. *p*-values obtained after studying the association between resistance genes and a phenotype resistant for β -lactams, macrolides and tetracyclines in the 48 *Pasteurella multocida* isolates.

Antimicrobial Resistance Genes *		β-lactams	Macrolides $	Tetracyclines	
		Amoxicillin	Tilmicosin	Doxycycline	Oxitetracycline
β-lactam resistance genes	bla_{ROB1}	0.5536	-	-	-
	bla_{TEM}	0.8408	-	-	-
Macrolide resistance genes	*ermA*	-	0.7764	-	-
	ermC	-	0.6538	-	-
	msrE	-	0.7392	-	-
Tetracycline resistance genes	*tetA*	-	-	0.9131	0.9063
	tetB	-	-	0.5146	0.7255

* Only resistance genes to three antibiotic families were tested (β-lactams, macrolides and tetracyclines). $ Tilmicosin was the only macrolide tested because no resistant strains were obtained for tildipirosin and tulathromycin.

2.4. *Relationship between the Presence of Resistance Genes and Clusters based on Antimicrobial Susceptibility Pattern of 12 Antimicrobials*

P. multocida isolates were grouped into six clusters (Figure 1) and MIC values of these 48 isolates after a hierarchical clustering analysis for the 12 antimicrobial agents tested are shown in Table 5. Thus, cluster 1 shows low MIC values for most antimicrobials except for sulphamethoxazole (4 μg/mL) and oxytetracycline in six isolates. Cluster 2 shows low MIC values for all the antimicrobial families with the exception of pleuromutilins for most strains. Cluster 3 is similar to cluster 2 but MICs for amoxicillin and oxytetracycline were extremely high (8 µg/mL) and MICs for pleuromutilins were close to MIC_{50} for this isolate. Cluster 4 shows low MIC values for all antimicrobial families with the exception of quinolones for most strains. Cluster 5, which contains only one isolate, is similar to cluster 4, but the MIC values for tetracyclines and pleuromutilins were also high for this isolate. Finally, cluster 6 (one isolate) shows a peculiar susceptibility pattern with very high MICs for macrolides (64 µg/mL for tildipirosin, tilmicosin and tulathromycin), quinolones and tetracyclines (Figure 1 and Table 5). The presence of *tetA* and *ermA* genes was significantly associated with clusters 2 and 5 (p = 0.048) and clusters 2, 4 and 6 ($p < 0.0001$), respectively. For the remaining genes, no significant association with any of the clusters was seen.

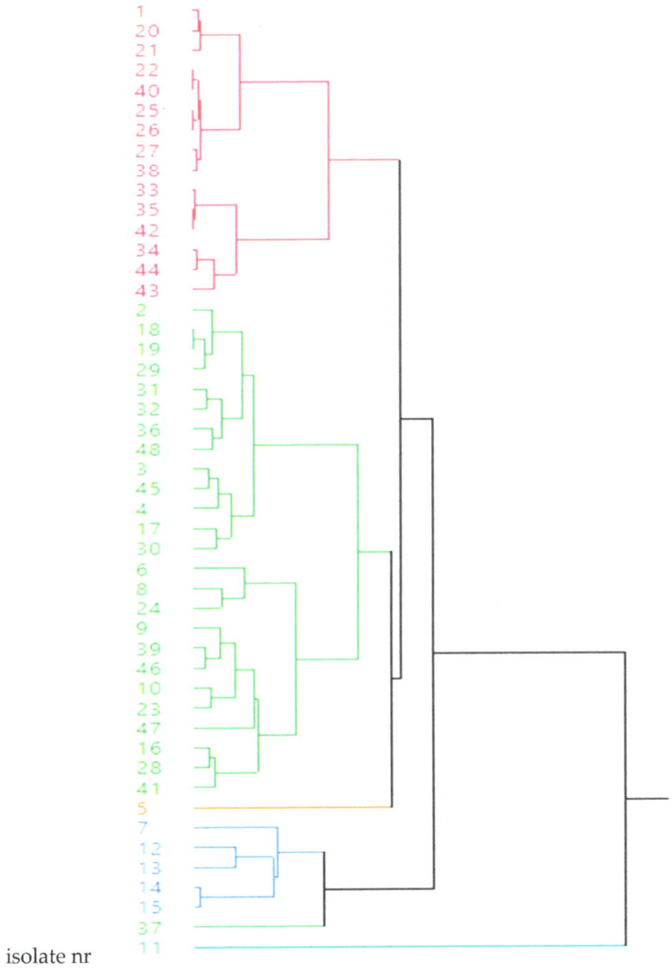

Figure 1. Dendrogram showing the results of 48 *Pasteurella multocida* isolates after a hierarchical clustering analysis of MIC values for the 12 antimicrobials tested.

Table 5. MIC values of the 48 *Pasteurella multocida* isolates grouped into six clusters after a hierarchical clustering analysis for the 12 antimicrobials tested.

Cluster	Isolate nr	MIC											
		Flor	Enrof	Amox	Marb	Ceft	Sulf	Tild	Dox	Oxitet	Tia	Tulat	Tilm
	38	0.5	0.03	0.25	0.03	0.06	4	0.5	0.25	0.5	16	1	2
	27	0.5	0.03	0.25	0.03	0.06	4	0.5	0.5	0.5	16	1	2
	22	0.5	0.03	0.25	0.03	0.06	4	0.5	0.5	0.5	16	1	4
	40	0.5	0.03	0.25	0.03	0.06	4	0.5	0.5	0.5	16	1	4
	25	0.5	0.03	0.25	0.03	0.06	4	0.5	0.5	1	16	1	4
	26	0.5	0.03	0.25	0.03	0.06	4	0.5	0.5	1	16	1	4
	34	0.5	0.03	0.25	0.03	0.06	4	0.5	1	8	16	1	2
1	44	0.5	0.03	0.25	0.03	0.06	4	0.5	1	8	16	1	4
	21	0.5	0.03	0.25	0.03	0.12	4	0.5	0.25	0.5	16	1	4
	20	0.5	0.03	0.25	0.03	0.12	4	0.5	0.5	0.5	16	1	2
	35	0.5	0.03	0.25	0.03	0.12	4	0.5	1	8	16	1	2
	42	0.5	0.03	0.25	0.03	0.12	4	0.5	1	8	16	1	2
	33	0.5	0.03	0.25	0.03	0.12	4	1	1	8	16	1	2
	43	0.5	0.03	0.5	0.03	0.06	4	0.5	2	8	16	1	4
	1	0.5	0.03	0.5	0.03	0.12	4	0.5	0.5	1	16	1	2
	17	0.5	0.03	0.25	0.03	0.06	0.06	0.5	1	2	2	1	2
	45	0.5	0.03	0.25	0.03	0.06	0.06	0.5	2	2	8	0.5	4
	3	0.5	0.03	0.25	0.03	0.06	0.06	1	2	4	8	1	8
	36	0.5	0.03	0.25	0.03	0.06	0.25	0.5	0.25	0.5	16	1	4
	29	0.5	0.03	0.25	0.03	0.06	0.06	1	2	2	16	1	8
	18	0.5	0.03	0.25	0.03	0.06	1	1	2	2	16	1	8
	19	0.5	0.03	0.25	0.03	0.06	1	1	2	2	16	1	8
	2	0.5	0.03	0.5	0.03	0.06	0.06	1	2	4	16	2	8
	31	0.5	0.03	0.25	0.03	0.06	0.25	2	1	2	16	2	16
	32	0.5	0.03	0.25	0.03	0.06	0.06	2	0.5	0.5	16	4	16
	46	0.5	0.03	0.25	0.03	0.06	1	1	0.25	0.5	32	1	8
	8	0.5	0.03	0.25	0.03	0.06	2	1	1	8	32	1	16
2	41	0.5	0.03	0.25	0.03	0.06	0.06	2	2	2	32	2	16
	24	0.5	0.03	0.25	0.03	0.06	0.06	2	2	8	32	2	16
	28	0.5	0.03	0.25	0.03	0.06	0.25	2	2	2	32	2	8
	16	0.5	0.03	0.25	0.03	0.06	1	2	2	4	32	2	8
	48	0.5	0.03	0.25	0.06	0.06	0.06	1	1	2	16	2	8
	4	0.5	0.03	0.5	0.03	0.06	0.06	2	2	2	8	2	16
	6	0.5	0.03	0.5	0.03	0.06	0.06	2	1	8	16	2	8
	39	0.5	0.03	0,5	0.03	0.06	0.12	2	0.5	0.5	32	2	8
	47	0.5	0.03	0,5	0.03	0.06	0.06	4	0.5	1	32	4	32
	30	0.5	0.06	0.12	0.12	0.06	0.06	1	1	2	8	1	4
	10	0.5	0.06	0.25	0.06	0.12	0.5	2	0.5	0.5	32	4	8
	9	0.5	0.06	0.25	0.12	0.06	1	2	0.25	0.5	32	4	16
	23	0.5	0.12	0.25	0.12	0.12	0.06	1	0.5	1	32	2	8
3	5	0.5	0.03	8	0.03	0.06	0.25	2	1	8	16	4	16
	7	0.5	0,03	0.5	0.03	0.25	0.12	0.5	0.5	1	16	2	4
	14	0.5	0.25	0.25	0.25	0.12	0.12	0.5	0.5	0.5	16	1	4
4	12	0.5	0.25	0.25	0.25	0.25	0.25	1	0.5	0.5	16	2	8
	15	0.5	0.25	0.5	0.25	0.12	0.12	0.5	0.5	1	16	2	4
	13	0.5	0.25	0.5	0.5	0.25	0.12	0.5	0.5	1	16	2	4
5	37	0.5	0.5	0.25	0.5	0.06	0.06	1	2	4	32	2	8
6	11	2	0.5	0.25	0.5	0.12	0.25	64	8	8	16	64	64

Flor: florfenicol; enrof: enrofloxacin; amox: amoxicillin; marb: marbofloxacin; ceft: ceftiofur; tild: tildipirosin; dox: doxycycline; oxitet: oxitetracycline; tia: tiamulin; tulat: tulathromycin; tilm: tilmicosin.

3. Discussion

Spain is one of the European countries with a higher antibiotic consumption in animals (2,964 tonnes of active substance in 2014) [15], and this fact must be taken into account in studies addressing the resistance percentages for antimicrobial agents in pathogenic bacteria. One of the critical points is the selection of antimicrobials to be tested in vitro for further use in swine production; in this study, the most frequently used antimicrobials for treating respiratory diseases in pigs were compared. Surprisingly, only one *P. multocida* isolate among the 48 tested was found to be resistant to amoxicillin in our investigation, opposite to the 13/32 resistant isolates (40.6%) reported also in Spain one year ago to ampicillin [16], a very similar β-lactam antibiotic. The resistance to this group of compounds has been linked mainly with the presence of the bla_{ROB1} resistance gene, not only in *P. multocida* [17] but alo in other genera and species of *Pasteurellaceae*, such as *Actinobacillus pleuropneumoniae* [18] or *Glässerella parasuis* [19]. In fact, the isolate resistant to amoxicillin harbored this resistance gene. On the other hand, eleven isolates showing the $bla_{ROB\text{-}1}$ gene, three bearing the bla_{TEM} gene and even another one sharing both genes were susceptible to amoxicillin; consequently, these genes were present but were not expressed in these isolates. Just as in our study, a lower appearance of bla_{TEM} compared to bla_{ROB1} has been previously observed [16,20]. A similar behavior has been reported in Spain for 30 years for ceftiofur, a broad-spectrum third-generation cephalosporin [16,21] which was approved for treatment of swine respiratory tract diseases approximately at that time. Its resistance has been linked to the bla_{TEM} gene [22]. Even though this gene has been detected in four *P. mutocida* isolates, all of them have shown susceptibility to ceftiofur.

The resistance rates for tetracyclines in this study were almost four times higher (for oxytetracycline) or almost three times higher (for doxycycline) than those reported only one year before also in Spain; however, detection of the *tetB* gene was similar in both investigations [19]. This one has been most frequently found the *tet* gene [19,23], not only in *P. multocida* but also in other *Pasteurellaceae*, such as *A. pleuropneumoniae* [9]. The presence of *tetB* gene suggests that the mechanism underlying the resistance to tetracyclines involves efflux pump proteins that move these compounds out of the bacteria, so causing the inactivity of tetracyclines against *P. multocida* [24]. The spread of this gene has been related with either its presence in transmissible plasmids and transposons, such as pB1001 and Tn*10*, respectively [11], or to clonal dissemination rather than horizontal transfer of plasmids [23].

As in a previous study [19], enrofloxacin and marbofloxacin behaved as two of the highest in vitro effective antibiotics against the isolates. Even so, one of the clinical strains (2.1%) was resistant to enrofloxacin, a percentage much smaller than the 22.5% found for this fluoroquinolone by Oh et al. in Brazil [23]. Florfenicol is a safe phenicol used exclusively for the treatment of pneumonias caused by *P. multocida*; in this way, it was completely active against these 48 isolates. Tiamulin is an antibiotic used in the treatment of several infections in swine. Although this compound was proposed as a proper antibiotic against animal *Pasteurella* spp. [20], the 25% level of resistance observed in this investigation, albeit lower than that reported two decades ago [21], does not advise its use against pneumonias caused by *P. multocida*.

Macrolides showed excellent effective results, with only one isolate (2.1%) being resistant to tilmicosin but not harboring any of the three macrolide resistance genes studied. Quite similar resistance rates were found in Spain for the last 30 years [21]; however, a substantially higher inefficacy (12.5%) was recently demonstrated for erythromycin [16].

Fourteen resistance *P. multocida* panels were obtained in this study (29.2% over 48 isolates), with a spread lower than that seen fifteen years ago (38.5%) [25], and especially lower than the 56.2% reported in the last five years [16]. Although the rate of isolates behaving as resistant to at least two of the antimicrobial agents here compared were almost 20 points below the rate reported in 2018 (84.4% vs. 64.5%) [16]; these results suggest the need for a restrictive use of antimicrobial agents in porcine husbandry, especially that of tetracyclines, sulphametoxozole/trimethoprim and tiamulin. Other investigators [26] showed 36.6% of *P. multocida* isolates being multirresistant in Brazil, a percentage considerably lower than that seen in this study. The multiresistance in *P. multocida* to tetracyclines and sulfonamides has been previously related, not with large plasmids as in most Gram-negative organisms, but with small plasmids of 4–6 kb in size [17].

On the basis of these results, the identification of the eight antimicrobial resistance genes does not enable us to foresee the behavior of the 48 *P. multocida* isolates to amoxicillin, doxycycline, oxytetracycline, tildiporison, tilmicosin and tulathromycin, as there is absence of a significant association between both parameters. To our knowledge, this is the first investigation in which such a noticeable mismatch between phenotypic and genetic characterization of resistances in *P. multocida* is reported. Similarly, after grouping isolates into six clusters according to their antimicrobial sensitivity behavior, only an association among these clusters and the presence or not of resistance genes could be established for the *tetA* and *ermA* genes. Nevertheless, this association was not linked to the antimicrobial susceptibility pattern described for each cluster. Thus, the presence of the *tetA* gene was significantly associated with clusters 2 and 5, and showed a very different pattern and it was not associated with resistance to tetracyclines in the case of cluster 2 for most isolates. Cluster 5 contained only one isolate and, therefore, this result must be assessed with caution. In the case of the *ermA* genes, its presence was significantly associated with clusters 2, 4 and 6 that had very different antimicrobial susceptibility patterns. Curiously, cluster 6 showed high MIC values for macrolides, and the *ermA* gene was present. In short, the presence of resistance genes cannot be associated with antimicrobial susceptibility for all the families tested. Therefore, these results clearly recommend carrying out phenotypic characterization in order to optimize the use of antimicrobials under field conditions. This point is critical taking into account a one-health approach in connection with the use of antimicrobials in livestock.

4. Material and Methods

4.1. Clinical Samples

Clinical samples were taken between 2017 and 2019 in farms in "Castilla y León" (north-western Spain) from diseased or recently deceased pigs with acute clinical signs of respiratory tract infections that had not been exposed to antimicrobial treatment for at least 15 days prior to sampling. Thus, the pigs included in the sampling procedure were three to 24 weeks old, with overt clinical signs such as loss of appetite, apathy, hyperthermia (>39.8 °C), and significantly increased mortality rates vs. baseline situation due mainly to respiratory disorders in intensive farms. In each case, at least two animals with these clinical signs were humanely sacrificed, and lung samples of these animals or from recently deceased pigs (<12 h) were drawn.

All experimental procedures were approved by the Ethics Committee for Animal Experimentation of the University of Lleida and performed in accordance with authorization 10343 issued by the Catalan Department of Agriculture, Livestock, Fisheries and Food (Section of biodiversity and hunting).

4.2. Bacterial Isolation and Identification

Clinical specimens were grown aseptically on Columbia blood agar base supplemented with 5% of defibrinated sheep blood (Oxoid), chocolate blood agar (GC II agar with IsoVitaleX, BD) and MacConkey agar (Biolife). All plates were incubated at 35–37 °C in aerobic conditions with 5–10% CO_2 for 24–48 h. Identification of isolates was carried out by matrix assisted laser desorption ionization-time of flight (MALDI-TOF) mass espectrometry (Biotyper System, Bruker Daltonics, Bremen, Germany) as previously described [24].

4.3. Antimicrobial Sensitivity Testing

Bacteria were cultured on Columbia blood agar and incubated at 35–37 °C in ambient air (or with 5–10% CO_2) for 18–24 h. MICs were determined using the broth microdilution method by means of customizing 96-well microtiter plates (Sensititre, Trek Diagnostic Systems Inc., East Grinstead, UK) containing 12/7 or 8 antimicrobials/concentrations, respectively, in accordance with the recommendations presented by the Clinical and Laboratory Standards Institut CLSI [16,17]. The antimicrobial agents tested were amoxicillin, ceftiofur, doxycycline, enrofloxacin, florfenicol, marbofloxacin, sulphamethoxazole/trimethoprim, oxytetracycline, tiamulin, tilmicosin, tildipirosin and tulathromycin. This panel was selected in order to represent the commonly used compounds for treatment of pig respiratory diseases in farms. Three to five colonies were picked and emulsified in demineralized water to obtain a turbidity of 0.5 McFarland standard (Sensititre™ nephelometer V3011). Suspensions were further diluted in cation-adjusted Mueller-Hinton broth to reach a final inoculum concentration of 5×10^5 CFU/mL. Then, the panel was reconstituted by adding 100 μL/well of the inoculum, and plates were incubated at 35 ± 2 °C for 18–24 h [27,28]. The antibiotic panels were read manually using Sensititre™ Vizion (V2021) and the MIC value was established as the lowest concentration inhibiting visible growth. A colony count and a purity check were performed for each clinical strain following CLSI and manufacturer recommendations. Moreover, control *P. multocida* strains were also included in all the susceptibility testing runs as quality control [27,28]. The MICs of the quality control strains had to be within acceptable CLSI ranges to authenticate the results obtained in the laboratory.

4.4. Determination of Antimicrobial Resistance Genes

Eight antibiotic resistance genes, corresponding to three antimicrobial families, were tested: tetracyclines (*tetA, tetB*), β-lactams (bla_{ROB1}, bla_{TEM}) and macrolides (*ermA, ermC, msrE, mphE*). The primers used are shown in Table 6. The PCRs were performed in an Eppendorf Mastercycler® thermocycler by using 0.2 mL tubes containing 47 μL of PCR master mix and 3 μL of DNA sample (primers used and annealing temperatures are shown in Table 6). A volume of 10 μL of each reaction mixture was analyzed by electrophoresis in an agarose gel. The PCR products were stained with RedSafe™ and visualized under UV light.

Table 6. Pimers used in the PCRs carried out for the detection of eight antimicrobial resistance genes in 48 *Pasteurella multocida* isolates.

Resistance Gene	Primer	Amplicon Size	Annealing Temperature	Reference
tetA	**F**: 5′-GTA ATT CTG AGC ACT GTC GC-3′ **R**: 5′-CTG CCT GGA CAA CAT TGT TT-3′	1057 pb	62 °C	[20]
tetB	**F**: 5′CCT TAT CAT GCC AGT CTT GC-3′ **R**: 5′ ACT GCC GTT TTT TTC GCC-3′	774 pb	50 °C	[20]
bla_{ROB1}	**F**: 5′ CAT TAA CGG CTT GTT CGC-3′ **R**: 5′-CTT GCT TTG CTG CAT CTT-3′	852 pb	55 °C	[20]
bla_{TEM}	**F**: 5′GAG TAT TCA ACA TTT TCG T-3′ **R**: 5′-ACC AAT GCT TAA TCA GTG A-3′	856 pb	55 °C	[20]

Table 6. *Cont.*

Resistance Gene	Primer	Amplicon Size	Annealing Temperature	Reference
ermA	**F**: 5′-ACG ATA TTC ACG GTT TAC CCA CTT-A-3′ **R**: 5-AAC CAG AAA AAC CCT AAA GAC ACG-3′	610 pb	53 °C	[20]
ermC	**F**: 5′-AAT-CGG CTC AGG AAA AGG-3′ **R**: 5′-ATC GTC ATT TCC TGC ATG-3′	562 pb	55 °C	[20]
msrE	**F**: 5′-TAT AGC GAC TTT AGC GCC AA-3′ **R**: 3′-GCC GTA GAA TAT GAG CTG AT-3′	271 pb	58 °C	[20]
mphE	**F**: 5′-ATG CCC AGC ATA TAA ATC GC-3′ **R**: 5′-ATA TGG ACA AAG ATAGCC CG-3′	295 pb	58 °C	[20]

4.5. Data Analysis

A strain was considered susceptible to one antimicrobial agent if its MIC value was below its clinical breakpoint. Clinical breakpoints from the CLSI were used when available [16,17] and they were extrapolated from clinical breakpoints of other organisms when data from the CLSI were not available (Table 1). Moreover, MIC distributions were used to define MIC_{50}, MIC_{90}, being determined respectively as the MICs inhibiting 50% and 90% of isolates.

4.6. Statistical Analysis

SPSS software version 2.1 was used to carry out the statistical analysis. In all the cases, *p*-values ≤0.05 were considered significant. A multivariate analysis was applied on the MIC of the 12 antimicrobials for all the strains. Thus, a dendrogram was generated using between-group linkage via Ward's hierarchical clustering that allows generating clusters of strains according to their antimicrobial susceptibility testing for all the antimicrobials together. A chi-square test was used to determine the association between the isolates harboring or not a resistance gene to a certain antimicrobial family and its association with the clusters determined based on hierarchical clustering analysis.

5. Conclusions

Ceftiofur, florfenicol, tildipirosin and tulathromycin were highly effective in vitro against the *P. multocida* isolates tested and, therefore, they remain suitable for the treatment of porcine respiratory infections due to this pathogen. However, the identification of β-lactam, tetracycline and macrolide resistance genes did not allow the prediction of antimicrobial resistances for these families. For this reason, knowledge of the antimicrobial susceptibility patterns (MICs) becomes essential to implement a prudent use of antimicrobials under field conditions.

Author Contributions: Conceptualization, C.-B.G.-M., L.F. and S.M.-M.; methodology, M.P.-R., E.P.-F. and A.V.; formal analysis, M.P.-R., L.F. and S.M.-M.; writing, C.-B.G.-M.; review and editing, L.F. and S.M.-M.; funding acquisition, C.-B.G.-M. and L.F. All authors have read and agreed to the final version of the manuscript.

Funding: Junta de Castilla y León (Consejería de Agricultura y Ganadería, Junta de Castilla y León, Spain) and Cost Action CA18217 (European Network for Optimization of Veterinary Antimicrobial Treatment).

Acknowledgments: This study was supported by the project "Caracterización fenotípica y genética de aislados de *Pasteurella multocida* en explotaciones porcinas de Castilla y León", financed by the "Consejería de Agricultura y Ganadería, Junta de Castilla y León", Spain, and by Cost Action CA18217: European Network for Optimization of Veterinary Antimicrobial Treatment.

Conflicts of Interest: The authors declare no conflict of interest.

References

1. Carr, J.; Chen, S.P.; Connor, J.F.; Kirkwood, R.; Segalés, S. Respiratory disorders. In *Pig Health*; Carr, J., Chen, S.P., Connor, J.F., Kirkwood, R., Segalés, S., Eds.; CRC Press Taylor & Francis: Boca Ratón, FL, USA, 2018; pp. 103–152.
2. Kachooel, A.; Ranjbar, M.M.; Kachooel, S. Evaluation of *Pasteurella multocida* serotype B:2 resistance to immune serum and complement system. *Vet. Res.* **2017**, *8*, 179–184.
3. De Alvis, M.C. Haemorrhagic septicaemia—A general review. *Br. Vet. J.* **1992**, *148*, 99–112. [CrossRef]
4. Tang, X.; Zhao, Z.; Hu, J.; Wu, B.; Cai, X.; He, Q.; Chen, H. Isolation, antimicrobial resistance, and virulence genes of *Pasteurella multocida* strains from swine in China. *J. Clin. Microbiol.* **2009**, *47*, 951–958. [CrossRef] [PubMed]
5. Fraile, L. *Antimicrobial Therapy in Swine*; Practical approach; Editorial Servet: Zaragoza, Spain, 2013.
6. Li, Y.; Cunha de Silva, G.; Li, Y.; Rossi, C.C.; Fernández-Crespo, R.; Williamson, S.M.; Langford, P.R.; Soares Bazzolli, D.M.; Bossé, J.T. Evidence of illegitimate recombination between two *Pasteurellaceae* plasmids resulting in a novel multi-resistance replicon, pM3362MDR in *Actinobacillus pleuropneumoniae*. *Front. Microbiol.* **2018**, *9*, 2489. [CrossRef]
7. Holmer, I.; Salomonsen, C.M.; Jorsal, S.E.; Astrup, L.B.; Jensen, V.F.; Høg, B.B.; Pedersen, K. Antibiotic resistance in porcine pathogenic bacteria and relation to antibiotic usage. *BMC Vet. Res.* **2019**, *15*, 449. [CrossRef]
8. Roberts, M.C. Tetracycline therapy: Update. *Clin. Infect. Dis.* **2003**, *36*, 462–467. [CrossRef]
9. Blanco, M.; Gutiérrez-Martín, C.B.; Rodríguez-Ferri, E.F.; Roberts, M.C.; Navas, J. Distribution of tetracycline resistance genes in *Actinobacillus pleuropneumoniae* isolates from Spain. *Antimicrob. Agents Chemother.* **2006**, *50*, 702–708. [CrossRef]
10. White, D.G.; Zhao, S.; Simjee, S.; Wagner, D.D.; McDermott, P.F. Antimicrobial resistance of foodborne pathogens. *Microbes Infect.* **2002**, *4*, 405–412. [CrossRef]
11. Michael, G.B.; Bossé, J.T.; Schwarz, S. Antimicrobial resistance in *Pasteurellaceae* of veterinary origin. *Microbiol. Spectr.* **2018**, *6*. [CrossRef]
12. Schwarz, S. Mechanisms of antimicrobial resistance in *Pasteurellaceae*. In *Pasteurellaceae. Biology, Genomics and Molecular Aspects*; Kuhnert, P., Christensen, H., Eds.; Caister Academic Press: Norfolk, UK, 2008; pp. 199–228.
13. Zeineldin, M.M.; Megahed, A.; Blair, B.; Burton, B.; Aldridge, B.; Lowe, J. Negligible impact of perinatal tulathromycin metaphylaxis on the development dynamics of fecal microbiota and their accompanying antimicrobial resistome in piglets. *Front. Microbiol.* **2019**, *10*, 726. [CrossRef]
14. González-Marín, C.; Spratt, D.A.; Millar, M.R.; Simmonds, M.; Kempley, S.T.; Allaker, R.P. Identification of bacteria and potential sources in neonates at risk of infection delivered by caesarean and vaginal birth. *J. Med. Microbiol.* **2012**, *61*, 31–41. [CrossRef] [PubMed]
15. ECDC/EFSA/EMA. *Second Joint Report on the Integrated Analysis of the Consumption of Antimicrobial Agents and Occurrence of Antimicrobial Resistance in Bacteria from Humans and Food-Producing Animals*; John Wiley and Sons Ltd.: Solna, Sweden, 2017; p. 134.

16. Petrocchi-Rilo, M.; Gutiérrez-Martín, C.B.; Méndez-Hernández, J.I.; Rodríguez-Ferri, E. Antimicrobial resistance of *Pasteurella multocida* isolates recovered from swine pneunomina in Spain throughout 2017 and 2018. *Vet. Anim. Sci.* **2019**, *7*, 100044. [CrossRef] [PubMed]
17. San Millán, A.; Escudero, J.A.; Gutiérrez, B.; Hidalgo, L.; García, N.; Llagostera, M.; Domínguez, L.; González-Zorn, B. Multiresistance in *Pasteurella multocida* is mediated by coexistence of small plasmids. *Antimicrob. Agents Chemother.* **2009**, *53*, 3399–3404. [CrossRef] [PubMed]
18. Matter, D.; Rossano, A.; Limat, S.; Vorlet-Fawer, L.; Brodard, I.; Perreten, V. Antimicrobial resistance profile of *Actinobacillus pleuropneumoniae* and *Actinobacillus porcitonsillarum*. *Vet. Microbiol.* **2007**, *122*, 146–156. [CrossRef]
19. San Millán, A.; Escudero, J.A.; Catalán, A.; Nieto, S.; Farelo, F.; Gibert, M.; Moreno, M.A.; Domínguez, L.; González-Zorn, L. β-lactam resistance in *Haemophilus parasuis* is mediated by plasmid pb1000 bearing bla_{ROB1}. *Antimicrob. Agents Chemother.* **2007**, *51*, 2260–2264. [CrossRef]
20. Dayao, D.A.E.; Gibson, J.S.; Blackall, P.J.; Turni, C. Antimicrobial resistance genes in *Actinobacillus pleuropneumoniae, Haemophilus parasuis* and *Pasteurella multocida* isolated from Australian pigs. *Austr. Vet. J.* **2016**, *94*, 227–231. [CrossRef]
21. Vera-Lizarazo, Y.A.; Rodríguez-Ferri, E.F.; Martín de la Fuente, A.J.; Gutiérrez-Martín, C.B. Evaluation of changes in antimicrobial susceptibility patterns of *Pasteurella multocida* subsp. *multocida* isolates from pigs in Spain in 1987–1988 and 2003–2004. *Am. J. Vet. Res.* **2006**, *67*, 663–668.
22. Chander, Y.; Oliveira, S.; Goyal, S.M. Characterization of ceftiofur resistance in swine bacterial pathogens. *Vet. J.* **2011**, *187*, 139–141. [CrossRef]
23. Oh, Y.H.; Moon, D.C.; Lee, Y.J.; Hyun, B.H.; Lim, S.K. Genetic and phenotypic characterization of tetracycline-resistant *Pasteurella multocida* isolated from pigs. *Vet. Microbiol.* **2019**, *233*, 159–163. [CrossRef]
24. Furian, T.Q.; Borges, K.A.; Laviniki, V.; da Silveira Rocha, S.L.; de Almeida, C.N.; do Nascimiento, V.P. Virulence genes and antimicrobial resistance of Pasteurella multocida isolated from poultry and swine. *Brazil. J. Microbiol.* **2016**, *47*, 210–216. [CrossRef]
25. Singhal, N.; Kumar, M.; Kanaujia, P.K.; Virdi, S.J. MALDI-TOF mass spectrometry: An emerging technology for microbial identification and diagnosis. *Front. Microbiol.* **2015**, *6*, 791. [CrossRef] [PubMed]
26. Jones, R.N.; Pfaller, M.A.; Rhomberg, P.R.; Walter, D.H. Tiamulin activity against fastidious and nonfastidious veterinary and human bacterial isolate: Initial development of in vitro susceptibility test methods. *J. Clin. Microbiol.* **2002**, *40*, 461–465. [CrossRef] [PubMed]
27. Clinical and Laboratory Standards Institute. *Performance Standards for Antimicrobial Disk and Dilution Susceptibility Tests for Bacteria Isolated from Animals, 2018*, 4th ed.; CLSI Supplement VET08; Wayne: Philadelphia, PA, USA.
28. Clinical and Laboratory Standards Institute. *Performance Standards for Antimicrobial Susceptibility Testing, 2018*, 28th ed.; CLSI Supplement M100; Wayne: Philadelphia, PA, USA.

antibiotics

MDPI

Article

Levers to Improve Antibiotic Treatment of Lambs via Drinking Water in Sheep Fattening Houses: The Example of the Sulfadimethoxine/Trimethoprim Combination

Aude A. Ferran, Marlène Z. Lacroix, Alain Bousquet-Mélou, Ivain Duhil and Béatrice B. Roques *

INTHERES, Université de Toulouse, INRAE, ENVT, 31300 Toulouse, France ; aude.ferran@envt.fr (A.A.F.); marlene.lacroix@envt.fr (M.Z.L.); alain.bousquet-melou@envt.fr (A.B.-M.); duhilivain@gmail.com (I.D.)

* Correspondence: beatrice.roques@envt.fr; Tel.: +33-5-61192320

Received: 17 July 2020; Accepted: 28 August 2020; Published: 31 August 2020

check for updates

Abstract: To limit the spread of bacterial diseases in sheep fattening houses, antibiotics are often administered collectively. Collective treatments can be delivered by drinking water but data on the drug's solubility in water or on plasma exposure of the animals are lacking. We first assessed the solubility of products containing sulfadimethoxine (SDM), associated or not with trimethoprim (TMP), in different waters. We then compared in lambs the SDM and TMP pharmacokinetic profiles after individual intravenous (IV) and oral administrations of SDM-TMP in experimental settings (n = 8) and after a collective treatment by drinking water with SDM-TMP or SDM alone in a sheep fattening house (n = 100 for each treatment). The individual water consumption during the collective treatments was also monitored to characterize the ingestion variability. We showed that TMP had a short terminal half-life and very low oral bioavailability, demonstrating that it would be unable to potentiate SDM by oral route. Conversely, SDM had a long terminal half-life of 18 h and excellent oral bioavailability. However, delivery by drinking water resulted in a very high interindividual variability of SDM plasma concentrations, meaning that although disease spread could be controlled at the group level, some individuals would inevitably be under- or over-exposed to the antibiotic.

Keywords: drinking water; antibiotic; lamb; trimethoprim; sulfonamides; pharmacokinetics; metaphylaxis

1. Introduction

The management of pulmonary diseases in sheep fattening houses often relies on the administration of antibiotics to sick animals but also to contaminated ones to prevent the spread of the infection. Indeed, it has been shown that early/metaphylactic antibiotic treatments are more efficacious than curative treatments administered only to clinically sick animals [1,2]. Due to the high density of animals in fattening houses, tens or hundreds of animals need to be treated during the epidemic stage of disease, which precludes individual administrations of the antibiotics by intramuscular or subcutaneous route.

In such cases, a collective oral treatment via the feed or drinking water is required even if, in the context of a prudent use of antimicrobials in veterinary medicine, mass medication is of major concern [3]. In the recent EMA (European Medicines Agency) categorization of antibiotics for prudent and responsible use in animals, oral group medications were classified as high risk for resistance selection, the risk being greater for medicated food than for drinking water [3]. Indeed, delivery of a drug in drinking water is more flexible than in feed. Medicated drinking water can be instantaneously prepared and the doses and volumes easily modulated every day [4]. However, most of the oral formulations available for sheep were developed for direct administration as a bolus in the animal's mouth and no or very few data are available on the drug's solubility and stability in water. Moreover, the drinking water in fattening houses can come from the municipal water supply or from underground water extracted from a well and can have very different chemical properties ranging from acidic to basic and different hardnesses which can impair drug's solubility. In a recent study by Vandael et al. [5], 33 out of 52 pig farmers reported some practical problems, such as solubility issues and precipitation, with drinking water medication.

In addition to solubility and stability issues in the pipelines, group medication exhibits additional variability associated with individual drinking behaviors, which can lead to overexposure or underexposure of animals to the antibiotic. In pigs, Soraci et al. [6] showed that the plasma exposure of animals to fosfomycin varied considerably between pigs after administration in the feed or drinking water and that this interindividual variability, lower for drinking water, could be partly explained by the social rank of the animal. However, apart from ensuring adequate access of the animals to the water, interindividual variability is probably very difficult to manage in the field. Therefore, any factor that might contribute to poor plasma exposure to antibiotics, such as product solubility or dosage regimen, needs to be carefully optimized to limit treatment failures and the selection of antibiotic resistance.

A combination of sulfonamides and diaminopyrimidines has long been used in veterinary medicine to manage bacterial and protozoal infections and is frequently employed to control respiratory infections in cattle and sheep [7]. These antibiotics have been classified as low risk by EMA [3] and are considered suitable for first-line treatments in veterinary medicine. Sulfonamides and diaminopyrimidines are considered as primarily bacteriostatic but become synergistic and bactericidal when used in combination by inhibiting different steps of tetrahydrofolate biosynthesis [8]. Many sulfonamides (sulfadiazine, sulfadimethoxine, sulfamethoxypyridazine, sulfamethoxazole, sulfadoxine or sulfadimidine) are available in combination with trimethoprim (TMP) in veterinary medicine while only sulfamethoxazole is registered in combination with TMP in human medicine. The terminal half-life of TMP is less than one hour in sheep [9,10] whereas very different half-lives have been reported for the various sulfonamides. Sulfadiazine or sulfathiazole with half-lives in sheep of 4 h [10] and 1.1 h [11] respectively are considered as short-acting sulfonamides while sulfadimethoxine (SDM) with a half-life of 12.5 h in cattle [12] is a long-acting one. Whatever the pharmacokinetic properties of drugs, most of the formulations registered in animals contain a 5:1 ratio for sulfonamides and TMP, which was originally extrapolated from human medicine even though data on the relevance of this ratio in veterinary species are very sparse. The main advantage of a long half-life is that fluctuations in the concentrations during the dosing interval are low, requiring less frequent administrations, while the drawback can be the delay for plasma concentrations to reach steady-state [13]. The bioavailability after administration by oral route can also differ, with bioavailabilities ranging from 12 to 68% in dwarf goats for some sulfonamides [14] and from 44 to 84% in goats for others [15]. In sheep, the oral bioavailabilities reported for sulfadiazine and sulfamethazine are around 69% [10] and 58% [16], respectively. No value for the bioavailability of TMP after oral route in ruminants were found but Shoaf et al. [17] reported very low concentrations after oral treatment in 12-week old calves.

In this study, we investigated the exposure of sheep to SDM and TMP after administration of the SDM-TMP combination or SDM alone at the recommended doses in the drinking water. We first compared the oral and intravenous pharmacokinetic profiles of the drugs in experimental settings and then assessed, in field conditions, the drug concentrations in the drinking water and in lamb plasma after delivery of the drug via the drinking water. In vitro solubility assays were performed to identify and investigate the factors limiting adequate drug exposure, by comparing the oral pharmacokinetic profiles in pre-ruminating and ruminating lambs, assessing the drug concentrations in the troughs, and by monitoring individual drinking behaviors.

2. Results

2.1. Solubility in Water of Formulations Containing the SDM-TMP Combination or SDM Alone

One of the two tested SDM-TMP formulations, Trisulmix® Powder, was not soluble in water after 2 h at RT or at +30 °C. Dissolution of this formulation was facilitated by adding the organic diluent (Trisulmix® Powder:Super Diluant Virbac®, 3:1), but as soon as water was added, the product precipitated whatever the pH or hardness of the water.

The same SDM-TMP combination in liquid form, Trisulmix® Liquid, was more soluble than the powder form as, without the organic diluent, only a very slight deposit was observed at RT and at +4 °C for almost all the pH and hardness conditions. However, a heavy precipitate was observed for hard water (50 °f) at pH 5.5. Addition of the organic diluent (Trisulmix® Liquid:Super Diluant Virbac® 2:1) led to excellent solubility after 2 h at RT or +4 °C whatever the pH and hardness conditions.

The SDM formulation tested, Emericid® Sulfadimethoxine, was soluble in water at RT and +4 °C even if the solution appeared cloudier as pH and—especially—water hardness were increased.

Thus, the Trisulmix® Liquid formulation mixed with the organic diluent was used both to determine the pharmacokinetic parameters of SDM and TMP in experimental settings and in the first field experiment. The second field experiment in the sheep fattening house was carried out with Emericid® Sulfadimethoxine.

2.2. Pharmacokinetic Parameters of SDM and TMP in Experimental Settings

Pharmacokinetic profiles of SDM and TMP were obtained for 8 lambs after successive administrations of SDM-TMP by oral, intravenous, and again by oral routes. The SDM plasma concentration profiles are shown in Figure 1. The SDM concentrations remained above the LOQ of the assay (0.25 μg/mL) until 72 h after SDM-TMP administration, both by oral and intravenous routes. The pharmacokinetic parameters of SDM obtained after non-compartmental analysis are presented in Table 1. For the 8 sheep tested, the peak SDM plasma concentration (C_{max}) ranged from 6.91 to 35.62 μg/mL for the oral routes. The terminal half-lives ($t_{1/2}$) ranged from 14.00 to 31.65 h and from 13.19 to 19.34 h for the oral routes and the intravenous route, respectively. Only the terminal half-life differed significantly between the first and second oral routes ($p < 0.05$) while the $AUC_{0\text{-}inf}$ (Area Under Curve from time 0 extrapolated to infinite time), the apparent clearance (Cl/F), the C_{max}, the time at which this concentration was reached (T_{max}), the apparent volume of distribution at steady-state (Vss/F) and the bioavailability of SDM were not significantly different ($p > 0.05$) suggesting that the effect of lamb age and ruminal status on SDM pharmacokinetic parameters was negligible.

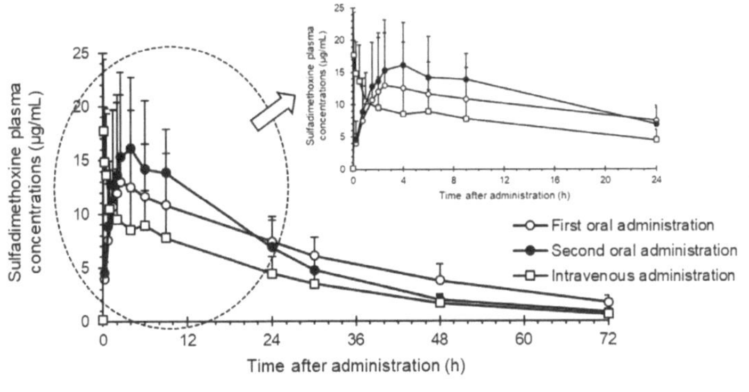

Figure 1. Sulfadimethoxine (SDM) plasma concentrations (mean ± SD) after single administrations of a SDM-trimethoprim (TMP) combination orally (Trisulmix® Liquid, 24.7 mg/kg SDM + 5.3 mg/kg TMP, open circles = first oral administration, closed circles = second oral administration) or intravenously (Trisulmix® Injectable, 24.7 mg/kg SDM + 5.3 mg/kg TMP, open squares) to eight lambs.

Table 1. Pharmacokinetic parameters of SDM (mean ± SD) after single administrations of a SDM-TMP combination orally (Trisulmix® Liquid, 24.7 mg/kg SDM + 5.3 mg/kg TMP) or intravenously (Trisulmix® Injectable, 24.7 mg/kg SDM + 5.3 mg/kg TMP) to eight lambs.

Pharmacokinetic Parameters	Oral Administration 1 «Pre-ruminant» Status	Intravenous Administration	Oral Administration 2 «Ruminant» Status
C_{max_obs} (µg/mL)	16.00 ± 9.86	-	17.81 ± 6.20
T_{max} (h)	5.14 ± 2.31	-	4.69 ± 2.83
$AUC_{0\text{-}inf}$ (µg.h/mL)	489.8 ± 169.7	282.9 ± 99.8	417.1 ± 116.2
Cl or Cl/F (mL/min/kg)	0.75 ± 0.28	1.12 ± 0.35	0.88 ± 0.23
$t_{1/2}$ (h)	24.24 ± 4.36	17.26 ± 2.25	17.77 ± 5.36 *
Vss or Vss/F (L/kg)	1.57 ± 0.62	1.72 ± 0.61	1.33 ± 0.49
F	1.09 ± 0.23	-	1.25 ± 0.21

C_{max_obs} = observed peak plasma SDM concentration, T_{max} = time at which the C_{max} is reached, $AUC_{0\text{-}inf}$ = Area Under Curve from time 0 extrapolated to infinite time, Cl = clearance and Cl/F = apparent clearance, $t_{1/2}$ = terminal half-life, Vss = volume of distribution at steady-state and Vss/F = apparent volume of distribution at steady-state, F = bioavailability. Significantly different between the two oral administrations: * $p < 0.05$.

The TMP plasma concentrations profiles are shown in Figure 2. After the intravenous administration, the TMP plasma concentrations remained above the LOQ of 0.01 µg/mL only up to 2 h. The pharmacokinetic parameters of TMP obtained after non-compartmental analysis of the intravenous profiles are presented in Table 2. The terminal half-life ranged from 0.32 to 1.03 h. After the oral administrations, because the TMP plasma concentrations were below the LOQ in 76 samples out of 144 during the first 24 h, the pharmacokinetic parameters could not be precisely estimated. For two animals out of eight, the concentrations were below the LOQ for all sampling times after the first oral administration. The highest concentration obtained in one sheep after oral administration was 0.084 µg/mL.

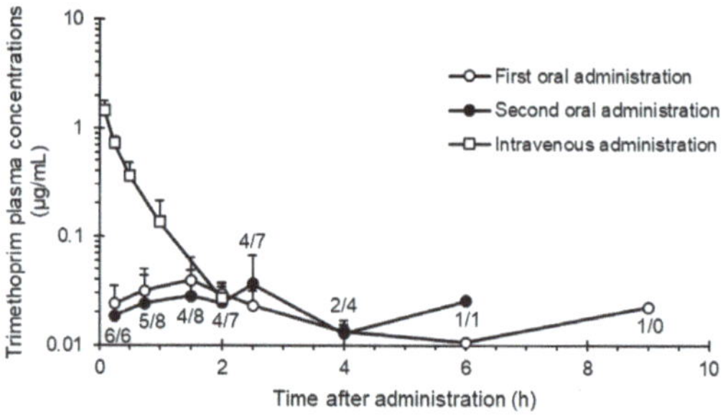

Figure 2. TMP plasma concentrations (mean ± SD) after single administrations of a SDM-TMP combination orally (Trisulmix® Liquid, 24.7 mg/kg SDM + 5.3 mg/kg TMP, open circles = first oral administration, closed circles = second oral administration) or intravenously (Trisulmix® Injectable, 24.7 mg/kg SDM + 5.3 mg/kg TMP, open squares) to eight lambs. For the intravenous administrations, concentrations were above the LOQ (Limit of Quantification) of 0.01 µg/mL from 0.08 to 2 h for all lambs and below the LOQ for all the other sampling times. For the oral administrations, the number of samples with concentrations above the LOQ are indicated on the graph (x/x = numbers of samples > LOQ for the first oral route/numbers of samples > LOQ for the second oral route).

Table 2. Pharmacokinetic parameters of TMP (mean ± SD) after a single administration of a SDM-TMP combination intravenously (Trisulmix® Injectable, 24.7 mg/kg SDM + 5.3 mg/kg TMP) to eight lambs.

Pharmacokinetic Parameters	Intravenous Administration
$AUC_{0\text{-}inf}$ (ng.h/mL)	644.0 ± 157.2
Cl (mL/min/kg)	178.7 ± 36.05
$t_{1/2}$ (h)	0.47 ± 0.23
Vss (L/kg)	5.58 ± 2.34

$AUC_{0\text{-}inf}$ = Area Under Curve from time 0 extrapolated to infinite time, Cl = clearance and Cl/F = apparent clearance, $t_{1/2}$ = terminal half-life, Vss = volume of distribution at steady-state. The pharmacokinetic parameters of TMP after a single oral administration of an SDM-TMP combination (Trisulmix® Liquid) could not be estimated.

2.3. Individual Water Consumption in Fattening Houses

For the first field experiment, the individual daily water consumption over the 10 days of recordings for animals weighing around 24 kg on average (min: 15.2 kg, max: 35.7 kg) ranged from 0 to 9.8 L and from 0 to 7.1 L for pen 1 (without blood samplings) and pen 2 (with blood samplings), respectively (Figure 3). The average volumes consumed over the period were 2.0 ± 1.3 and 2.1 ± 1.1 L/d for pen 1 and pen 2, respectively, which was slightly lower than the expected volume of 2.5 L/d. Individual daily water consumption varied considerably from one lamb to another for the same day of treatment and from one day to another for the same lamb. The average daily water consumption did not decrease following addition of the SDM-TMP combination to the drinking water, suggesting that palatability of the treatment was not a problem. In the same way as for individual daily water consumption, the circadian cycle was different for each lamb (Figure 4). However, a trend was detected for all lambs with a higher water intake between 10 a.m. and 8 p.m. and a lower one overnight. Two consumption peaks could be observed at around 12 p.m. and 4 p.m.

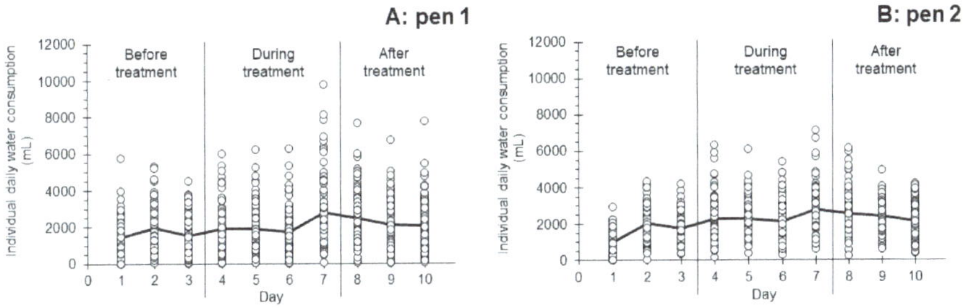

Figure 3. Individual daily water consumption of 96 lambs in pen 1 (4 lambs were not detected at the drinking troughs) and 98 lambs in pen 2 (1 lamb was not detected and 1 lamb died during the experiment), 3 days before, 4 days during and 3 days after the administration of a SDM-TMP combination (Trisulmix® Liquid, 37.4 mg/kg/24 h SDM + 8.0 mg/kg/24 h TMP) in the drinking water. Each circle corresponds to the daily water consumption of one lamb. The solid line links the average daily water consumption.

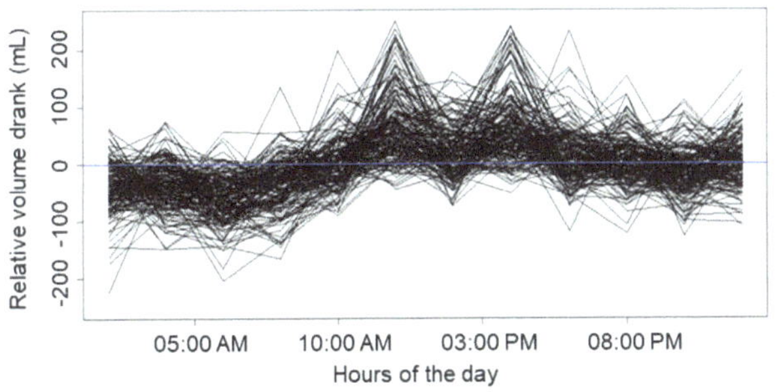

Figure 4. Individual circadian rhythms for water consumption of all lambs in pens 1 and 2 for the first field experiment.

2.4. Drug Concentrations in Drinking Troughs

2.4.1. First Field Experiment with the SDM-TMP Combination

On the first treatment day, the solution in the metering pump was apparently homogeneous and no deposit was observed in the drinking troughs. However, a deposit gradually accumulated over the next three days of treatment. The deposit found in the metering pump and drinking troughs on the 4th and last day of treatment is shown in Scheme 1. The SDM and TMP concentrations in the metering pump were calculated so that the lambs received 37.4 mg/kg BW/24 h of SDM and 8.0 mg/kg BW/24 h of TMP, according to a theoretical water intake of 2.5 L per animal and per day, with the metering pump set at 4%. According to these settings, the theoretical concentrations of SDM and TMP in the troughs should be equal to 374 and 80 µg/mL, respectively. The SDM concentrations in the drinking troughs increased from the 1st to 3rd day of treatment, becoming more stable and close to 100% of the theoretical concentration on the 3rd and 4th day of treatment (Table 3). After the end of treatment, SDM quickly disappeared from the watering system. The TMP concentrations recorded in the drinking troughs were well below the desired concentration with a maximum of 25.7 ± 15.9% of the theoretical concentration on the 4th day of treatment. Besides, 3 days after the end of treatment, the TMP concentrations in the troughs remained similar to the concentrations obtained during the treatment.

Table 3. Percentage of the theoretical concentrations of SDM and TMP (mean ± SD and [range]) found in the drinking troughs before, during and after the SDM-TMP treatment of 200 lambs for 4 days via the drinking water (Trisulmix® Liquid, 37.4 mg/kg/24 h SDM + 8.0 mg/kg/24 h TMP). Before and during the SDM-TMP treatment, water was collected from all the drinking troughs (n = 4, two in two different pens). Just before treatment end and after the SDM-TMP treatment, water was collected from one drinking trough/pen (n = 2) and the two obtained values are reported separately.

During Treatment	Sampling Time	Mean (± SD)% [Min–Max] of the Theoretical Concentrations SDM Theoretical Concentration = 374 µg/mL TMP Theoretical Concentration = 80 µg/mL	
		SDM	TMP
1st day of treatment	Before treatment T_1	-	-
	T_1 + 1 h	2.0 ± 2.2% [0.8–5.4]	2.2 ± 1.4% [1.0–4.1]
	T_1 + 4 h	15.7 ± 13.6% [0.5–33.4]	5.7 ± 5.2% [0.7–12.1]
	T_1 + 8 h	50.5 ± 21.3% [23.2–74.5]	16.8 ± 8.3% [11.2–29.1]
	T_1 + 12 h	**92.1 ± 7.5%** [81.1–97.8]	5.7 ± 2.1% [3.6–8.5]
2nd day of treatment	Before treatment T_2	27.2 ± 20.6% [9.7–56.7]	10.5 ± 3.8% [5.4–14.4]
	T_2 + 1 h	55.2 ± 24.6% [29.5–83.8]	15.2 ± 9.1% [6.7–25.5]
	T_2 + 4 h	84.2 ± 3.7% [78.8–87.2]	8.8 ± 2.8% [6.0–12.3]
	T_2 + 8 h	**100.9 ± 2.5%** [98.6–103.7]	6.6 ± 0.6% [5.8–7.3]
	T_2 + 12 h	76.4 ± 16.5% [59.4–97.5]	9.4 ± 2.7% [5.4–11.1]
3rd day of treatment	Before treatment T_3	24.2 ± 16.4% [11.7–46.3]	13.2 ± 4.0% [8.3–17.6]
	T_3 + 1 h	**124.7 ± 42.4%** [65.3–158.0]	4.5 ± 3.1% [1.7–8.9]
	T_3 + 4 h	**106.7 ± 31.5%** [70.9–145.7]	5.0 ± 2.9% [2.6–9.2]
	T_3 + 8 h	**118.9 ± 33.6%** [76.2–158.0]	4.2 ± 1.6% [2.9–6.3]
4th day of treatment	Before treatment T_4	**125.6 ± 12.4%** [110.5–137.8]	3.3 ± 1.0% [2.0–4.3]
	T_4 + 1 h	79.0 ± 19.7% [61.6–96.3]	9.2 ± 6.1% [4.7–17.7]
	T_4 + 8 h	**94.7 ± 1.2%** [93.5–95.7]	5.3 ± 0.9% [4.6–6.6]
	T_4 + 12 h	67.2 ± 18.8% [44.0–82.5]	25.7 ± 15.9% [5.6–43.7]
Before treatment end	T_4 + 24 h	66.3/66.6%	10.3/29.6%
After treatment	**Sampling time**	**Mean (±SD)% of theoretical concentrations remaining in the drinking troughs after treatment/theoretical concentrations in the drinking troughs before treatment end ***	
1 day after	-	1.2/2.2%	10.8/31.9%
2 days after	-	7.5/8.4%	69.7/182.7%
3 days after	-	6.0/6.9%	51.7/180.7%

The theoretical concentrations in the drinking troughs were estimated for a metering pump set at 4% and a theoretical concentration in the metering pump of 9.35 g/L for SDM and 2 g/L for TMP. The theoretical concentration in the metering pump was calculated with the following equation:

$$\text{Concentration in the metering pump (mg/L)} = \frac{\text{Dose (mg/kg/day)} \times \text{Average lamb weight (kg)}}{\text{Average water consumption per lamb}\left(\frac{\text{L}}{\text{day}}\right) \times \text{pump percentage}}$$

with an average lamb weight of 25 kg, an average water consumption per lamb of 2.5 L/day and a pump dilution percentage of 0.04. The mean observed values above 90% are highlighted in bold. * After treatment, a percentage of the theoretical concentrations in the drinking troughs relative to the concentration in the metering pump could not be determined as the theoretical concentration in the metering pump was zero. Thus, the percentage expressed here represents the percentage of SDM or TMP remaining in the drinking troughs relative to the concentrations in the drinking troughs before the end of the treatment.

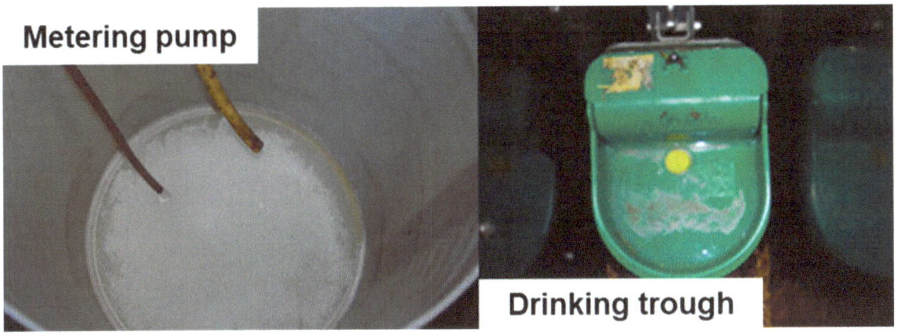

Scheme 1. Deposit found in the metering pump and in the drinking troughs on the 4th and last day of treatment of lambs via the drinking water with an SDM-TMP combination (Trisulmix® Liquid, 37.4 mg/kg/24 h SDM + 8.0 mg/kg/24 h TMP). The metering pump was set at 4%. The theoretical concentrations in the metering pump and in the drinking troughs during treatment were 9.35 g/L for SDM + 2 g/L for TMP and 374 mg/L for SDM + 80 mg/L for TMP, respectively.

2.4.2. Second Field Experiment with SDM Alone

For all treatment days, the solution in the metering pump appeared homogeneous and no deposit was observed in the drinking troughs (Scheme 2). The SDM concentrations in the metering pump were calculated so that the lambs received 55.68 mg/kg BW of SDM on the 1st day and 27.84 mg/kg BW/24 h of SDM for the 4 next days, according to a theoretical water intake of 2.5 L per animal and per day, with the metering pump set at 10%. By using these settings and considering the effective daily concentrations in the metering pump, the theoretical concentrations of SDM in the troughs should be equal to 483, 299, 289, 268 and 238 μg/mL for the 1st to 5th days of treatment, respectively. The SDM concentrations in the drinking troughs were stable and close to 100% of the theoretical concentration from the 1st day of treatment (Table 4). No SDM was found in the drinking troughs when the treatment was stopped and the pipes were flushed.

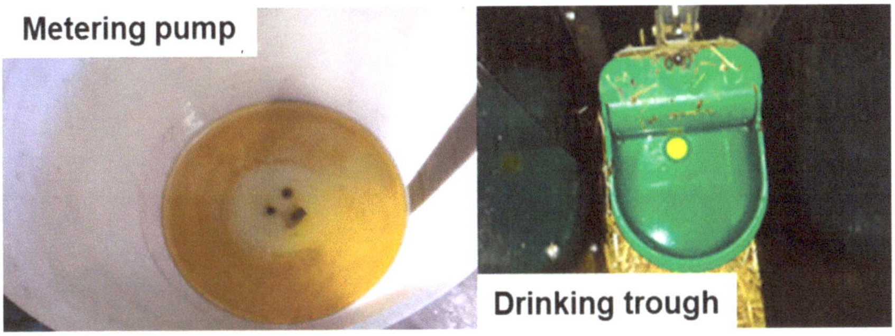

Scheme 2. Deposit found in the metering pump and in the drinking troughs on the 5th and last day of treatment of lambs via the drinking water with SDM (Emericid® Sulfadimethoxine, 55.68 mg/kg for the first day and 27.84 mg/kg/24 h from the 2nd to the 5th day). The metering pump was set at 10%. The average SDM observed concentrations in the metering pump during the five treatment days were 4.83 g/L for the first day of treatment and 2.73 g/L for the other 4 days. The average SDM theoretical concentrations in the drinking troughs during the five treatment days were 483 μg/mL for the first day of treatment and 273 μg/mL for the other 4 days.

Table 4. Percentage of the theoretical concentrations of SDM found in drinking troughs during the SDM treatment of 200 lambs for 5 days via the drinking water (Emericid® Sulfadimethoxine, 55.68 mg/kg SDM the 1st day and 27.84 mg/kg/24 h SDM from the 2nd to the 5th day). Depending on the sampling time, percentages were given as mean ± SD and [range] when water was collected from all the drinking troughs (n = 4, two in two different pens) and as two separate values when water was collected in only one drinking trough/pen (n = 2). No SDM was found in the drinking troughs as soon as the treatment was stopped and the pipes were flushed (not shown in the table).

During Treatment	Sampling Time	Number of Drinking Troughs Tested	Mean (±SD)% [Min–Max] of the Theoretical Concentrations
1st day of treatment	T_1 + 1 h	n = 2, one per/pen	81.8/92.5%
	T_1 + 3 h	n = 4, two per pen	**91.1 ± 10.9%** [74.9–98.3]
	T_1 + 5 h	n = 2	86.7/93.2%
	T_1 + 7 h	n = 4	**92.1 ± 1.5%** [90.2–93.8]
	T_1 + 9 h	n = 2	89.9/95.6%
	T_1 + 12 h	n = 4	**90.9 ± 3.0%** [87.3–94.7]
2nd day of treatment	Before treatment T_2	n = 4	**98.4 ± 5.4%** [93.8–106.0]
	T_2 + 1 h	n = 2	104.4 /115.3%
	T_2 + 3 h	n = 4	88.8 ± 22.2% [55.7–103.5]
	T_2 + 5 h	n = 2	98.7/102.3%
	T_2 + 7 h	n = 4	**92.9 ± 6.5%** [86.4–101.3]
	T_2 + 9 h	n = 2	99.3/100.6%
	T_2 + 12 h	n = 4	**92.6 ± 6.6%** [83.1–97.2]
3rd day of treatment	Before treatment T_3	n = 4	**97.3 ± 0.8%** [96.4–98.4]
	T_3 + 1 h	n = 2	103.5/106.2%
	T_3 + 3 h	n = 4	**103.5 ± 0.9%** [102.5–104.6]
	T_3 + 5 h	n = 2	104.9/106.5%
	T_3 + 7 h	n = 4	**92.3 ± 27.3%** [52.6–114.9]
	T_3 + 9 h	n = 2	79.6/115.5%
4th day of treatment	Before treatment T_4	n = 4	**110.0 ± 17.0%** [94.7–131.1]
	T_4 + 1 h	n = 2	91.7/96.9%
	T_4 + 3 h	n = 4	**95.7 ± 0.5%** [94.9–96.0]
	T_4 + 5 h	n = 2	91.4/95.6%
	T_4 + 7 h	n = 4	**92.3 ± 0.3%** [91.9–92.7]
	T_4 + 9 h	n = 2	94.1/94.7%
	T_4 + 12 h	n = 4	**92.2 ± 2.7%** [89.1–94.7]
5th day of treatment	Before treatment T_5	n = 4	65.0 ± 37.2% [32.5–102.0]
	T_5 + 1 h	n = 2	97.5/99.1%
	T_5 + 3 h	n = 4	**92.1 ± 8.5%** [80.0–98.1]
	T_5 + 5 h	n = 2	89.8/99.4%
	T_5 + 7 h	n = 4	**98.0 ± 1.4%** [96.5–99.5]
	T_5 + 9 h	n = 2	101.5/105.3%
	T_5 + 12 h	n = 4	**98.0 ± 2.9%** [94.7–100.8]

The theoretical concentrations in the drinking troughs were estimated for a metering pump set at 10% and the observed concentrations in the metering pump for each treatment day. Then, the theoretical concentrations in the drinking troughs after each treatment renewal were estimated from the daily observed concentrations in the metering pump and were 483, 299, 289, 268 and 238 µg/mL from the 1st to 5th days of treatment, respectively. The mean observed values above 90% are highlighted in bold.

2.5. Individual Pharmacokinetics of SDM and TMP Administered in Combination via the Drinking Water

The TMP plasma concentrations were below the LOQ of 1 µg/mL for all 100 lambs regardless of the day of collection. The SDM plasma concentrations are presented in Figure 5. They were between 2.61 and 68.90 µg/mL (35.8 ± 14.2 µg/mL) on the 2nd day of treatment, between 19.35 and 124.45 µg/mL (73.9 ± 21.9 µg/mL) on the 3rd day of treatment and between 21.94 and 156.15 µg/mL (95.0 ± 22.6 µg/mL) on the 4th day of treatment, demonstrating that the average SDM concentrations were nearly 3 fold higher on the 4th day than on the 2nd day of treatment.

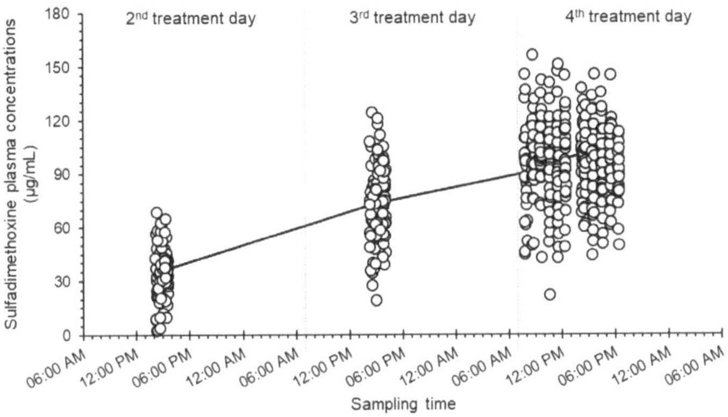

Figure 5. Individual SDM plasma concentrations for the 100 lambs in pen 2 that received an SDM-TMP combination (Trisulmix® Liquid, 37.4 mg/kg/24 h SDM + 8.0 mg/kg/24 h TMP) for 4 days in the drinking water. The stock solution in the metering pump was renewed every morning around 07:00 am. Each circle corresponds to the plasma concentration for one lamb. The solid line links the average plasma concentrations.

2.6. Individual Pharmacokinetics of SDM Administered Alone via the Drinking Water

To limit the time required for SDM plasma concentrations to reach steady-state, in the second field experiment we planned to start with a loading dose of 55.68 mg/kg BW SDM on the 1st day followed by a dose of 27.84 mg/kg BW/24 h SDM from the 2nd to the 5th day. Since TMP actually hardly reached the troughs and seemed to precipitate, a formulation that only contained SDM (Emericid® Sulfadimethoxine, Virbac, Carros, France) was selected for this experiment.

The individual SDM plasma concentrations obtained in the lambs are presented in Figure 6. They were similar for the 5 days of treatment and ranged from 1.28 to 73.24 µg/mL on the 1st day of treatment (38.1 ± 13.8 µg/mL), from 12.97 to 81.94 µg/mL (50.2 ± 13.6 µg/mL) on the 2nd day of treatment, from 9.35 to 89.22 µg/mL (49.8 ± 13.2 µg/mL) on the 3rd day of treatment, from 17.05 to 98.49 µg/mL (60.2 ± 13.8 µg/mL) on the 4th day of treatment, and from 14.84 to 75.51 µg/mL (49.0 ± 12.0 µg/mL) for the 5th day of treatment.

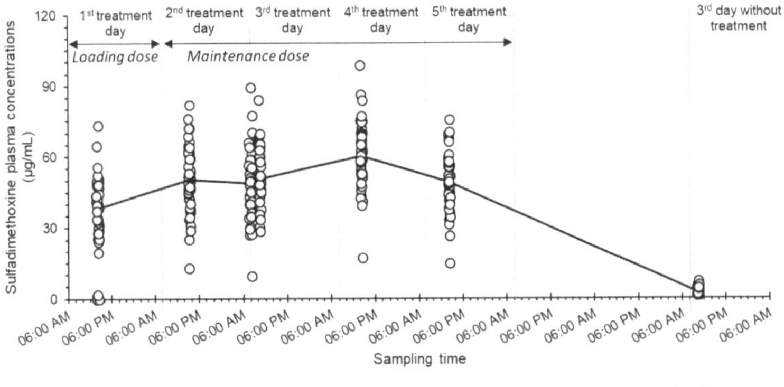

Figure 6. Individual SDM plasma concentrations for lambs (n = 100) that received a SDM treatment (Emericid® Sulfadimethoxine, 55.68 mg/kg for the first day and 27.84 mg/kg/24 h from the 2nd to the 5th day) for 5 days in the drinking water. Each circle corresponds to the plasma concentration for one lamb. On the third day after the last treatment day, the SDM plasma concentrations were above the LOQ (Limit of Quantification) of 1 µg/mL for 36 out of 50 lambs. The solid line links the average plasma concentrations.

3. Discussion

Although several products containing a combination of sulfonamide and TMP have been registered for oral route in sheep, little if any information is available on their pharmacokinetic properties, especially when administered via the drinking water, which implies that the blood exposure of animals to the drugs after such treatments is uncertain. To promote a rational use of antibiotics and avoid useless antibiotic consumption, a better knowledge is required of the animal's blood exposure to drugs after treatments via the drinking water.

The first issue with using drinking water to deliver a drug is the drug's solubility which needs to be very high, considering the very concentrated stock solution required upstream of the metering pump. For many drugs/formulations, no information is available about solubility at the time of registration, even though precipitation can occur in water especially at low temperature, extreme (mainly alkaline) pH, or in hard water. In this study, the low in vitro solubility of one of the drugs, even after addition of a diluent, excluded it from further experiments. A recent review on water medication reported that this problem of solubility in the stock solution could also occur for other antimicrobial drugs [18]. In our study, one product was soluble at high concentrations for 2 h at +4 °C in the laboratory and the solution seemed homogeneous in the metering pump with no deposit on the first treatment day but eventually a deposit appeared both in the pump and the drinking troughs as the days went by. These observations demonstrate that an apparent solubility at the time of stock solution preparation may not be sufficient to ensure solubility in the pipelines throughout the treatment period. Stability of the drug in the stock solutions is another issue because these solutions are usually prepared once or at most twice a day in farms. Here, SDM seemed to remain stable since the expected concentration was found in the troughs at all sampling times during the treatment with SDM alone.

The need to obtain drug solubility and stability data before administering a new treatment in drinking water is therefore paramount. However, to comply with EMA recommendations, relatively old drugs (sulfonamides, tetracyclines, penicillins, etc.), for which solubility and pharmacokinetics data are usually poor, are preferentially selected for oral medication.

To determine the exposure of animals to SDM-TMP, we first examined the plasma concentration profiles obtained after individual administration of the SDM-TMP combination (Trisulmix® Liquid for oral administration and Trisulmix® Injectable for intravenous administration) in experimental settings. The dose ratio of SDM:TMP in these formulations is 5:1, which is the most common. This ratio was first established in human medicine to ensure the greatest synergistic effect on bacteria and the ratio of peak plasma concentrations of sulfamethoxazole:TMP in human patients was thus 20:1 [19–21]. To be able to use this same dose ratio in veterinary medicine, the pharmacokinetic profiles of the drugs would need to be similar in animals and humans to preserve the synergistic effect. However, several studies have shown that TMP pharmacokinetics are highly dependent on the species examined. For example, the half-life of TMP is 10–14 h in humans [22], whereas it is about 35–44 min in sheep [9,10]. We also found a similar half-life of 0.47 ± 0.23 h after IV administration. Indeed, TMP is supposed to be extensively metabolized by the liver in cattle and goats [23]. Being a weak base, TMP can also be trapped in tissues and in the rumen where it can then be degraded by the local microflora. The same mechanisms could also explain the very low bioavailability already observed after oral route in ruminants [17,23] and confirmed here in experimental settings. Thus, the very short half-life of TMP suggests that the contribution of TMP as a potentiator of SDM would be very poor in sheep, whatever the route of administration, and the very low oral bioavailability reinforces this drawback when the drug is given orally. In addition, our results indicate that the presence of TMP in the SDM-TMP formulation could decrease the solubility of the product. Indeed, deposits were observed in the pipelines, the expected concentrations of TMP were never attained in the troughs and, more importantly, residual TMP concentrations were observed for several days after the end of treatment in the troughs. This sustained presence of TMP in the ducts could exert selective pressure on the bacterial biofilms formed in the pipelines and favor the selection of antimicrobial resistance in the farm environment. Although SDM exhibited a far better behavior as it rapidly attained the expected concentrations in the troughs and rapidly disappeared from the pipes at the end of the treatment, these concentrations were much more variable when SDM was combined with TMP than when administered alone.

Different pharmacokinetic profiles after oral administration have been reported for sulfonamides in ruminants. Some sulfonamides such as sulfadimidine (=sulfamethazine), sulfanilamide or sulfamerazine have low bioavailabilities by oral route whereas others such as sulfamethoxazole, sulfatroxazole, or sulfadiazine have oral bioavailabilities exceeding 70% in adult goats or calves [14,15,17]. Previous studies have also shown that age and diet can affect the disposition of sulfonamides with, for example, a slight decrease in bioavailability observed in animals fed with grain as compared to animals receiving milk [17]. In this study, the bioavailability of SDM by oral route was complete for both pre-ruminant and ruminant lambs, implying that the oral route would be suitable for lambs of any age. SDM is reported to have a long half-life in many species, with a half-life of 12.5 h in cattle [12]. In our study, a similar terminal half-life was found in lambs with averages of 21.0 and 17.3 h after administration by oral and intravenous routes, respectively. This long terminal half-life can decrease the intra-individual variability of SDM concentrations but can also increase the time required to attain the steady-state concentrations [13]. Considering a half-life of 17 h, an administration once a day and equation 5 [13], the plasma concentrations of SDM at steady state should have been 1.6-fold higher than the concentrations observed on the 1st day of treatment. Under our conditions, we found a greater difference between the 2nd and 4th days of treatment, the average plasma concentrations in lambs being 2.7-fold higher on the 4th day than on the 2nd day. One explanation could be that the SDM concentrations in drinking troughs were lower than expected on the first days of treatment with the SDM-TMP combination. Another explanation could be that the lambs delayed water consumption and thus antibiotic intake on the 1st day of treatment. Low exposure to SDM during the first days of treatment is not desirable, because efficacy against the pathogens might be delayed and allow the spread of the disease over a longer period. Moreover, underexposure to antibiotics, while being useless to control the pathogens, can promote the selection of resistance. To address this issue of low concentrations at the beginning of treatment, we first tried to improve the supply of SDM to the drinking troughs. As TMP concentrations in drinking troughs were very low, we suspected that TMP precipitates and could at the same time lower the SDM solubility. We thus decided to administer SDM alone, expecting the subsequent solubility and concentrations in the drinking troughs to be closer to those required from the very beginning of the treatment. As the terminal half-life of SDM was quite long, we therefore planned a loading dose (twice the maintenance dose) for the 1st day of treatment. This new dosing regimen led to very similar average plasma concentrations of 38.1 (1st day), 50.2 (2nd day), 49.8 (3rd day), 60.2 (4th day) and 49.0 (5th day) μg/mL, with a 1.3-fold difference between the 1st and 5th day at the population level.

The individual plasma concentrations of SDM in lambs ranged from 1.28 to 98.49 μg/mL (49.8 ± 14.6 μg/mL) during the 5-day treatment. Such high intra- and inter-individual variabilities can result in ineffective treatments or toxicity in some animals with extremely low or high exposures. The measurements of water consumption did not reveal any decrease in consumption in the pens at the start of treatment suggesting that the taste of the drug was accepted by the animals. Individual water consumption by pigs is reported to be influenced by numerous factors including stress, boredom, environmental temperature, disease, feed type and constituents and water flow rates [18], but in our study, despite the same age, weight, environment, food and health status, the individual consumption varied considerably between the lambs. Soraci et al. [6] showed that consumption in healthy animals was also dependent on social rank, even if the effect was lower for water than for feed consumption. Here, the estimated individual daily drinking volumes ranged from 0 to 9.8 L implying that the individual daily doses, for a SDM concentration in the drinking troughs of 374 μg/mL, ranged from 0 to 147 mg/kg BW while the targeted one was 37.4 mg/kg BW. These different doses probably explain most of the observed inter-individual variability in plasma concentrations but the time-development of drinking behavior of each lamb, with either frequent or infrequent visits to the troughs, could also accentuate this variability. In pigs, one or two peaks of water consumption were observed over each

24-h period [18]. We also observed a similar trend with two peaks, mainly during daytime, in the lamb population. However, at the individual level, some lambs behaved very differently, drinking frequently throughout the day for no obvious reason. Under epidemic conditions, the variability between animals can be even higher due to a potential influence of the disease on drinking behavior and additional studies should be carried out to check if sick animals are at least as exposed to drugs as healthy animals. Success of the treatment at the population level will then rely on attaining a defined target value for the relevant pharmacokinetic/pharmacodynamic index, which is dependent both on exposure to the drug and on the MIC of pathogens, in a sufficiently high proportion of the animals within the group. Here, we showed that the synergy of SDM and TMP was lost in sheep, due to the absence of TMP in sheep plasma, and that the efficacy of SDM alone to control pathogenic bacteria should therefore be considered. Unfortunately, most of the published susceptibility data on respiratory pathogens such as *Mannheimia haemolytica* and *Pasteurella multocida* are provided for the sulfamethoxazole/TMP combination [24] and very few data are available for sulfonamides alone. In any case, even if adequate exposure to the drug at the population level would control disease spread within the herd, a second-line treatment would be required for a few animals due to unavoidable individual underexposure to the drug.

4. Materials and Methods

4.1. Solubility in Water of Formulations Containing the SDM-TMP Combination or SDM Alone

Solubility in drinking water of two different formulations of SDM-TMP (Trisulmix® Powder and Trisulmix® Liquid, Coophavet, Ancenis, France) and one formulation of SDM alone (Emericid® Sulfadimethoxine, Virbac, Carros, France) was assessed in water with different combinations of pH (5.5, 6.5, 7.5 or 8.5) and hardness (10 °f, 30 °f and 50 °f), representative of those found in sheep fattening houses. A carbonate buffer was first prepared, the pH was then adjusted with HCl 2 M or NaOH 10 M and the hardness with $CaCO_3$ to create the different testing conditions.

Based on the labelled doses of 30 mg/kg BW SDM and 6.5 mg/kg BW TMP for Trisulmix® Powder and Trisulmix® Liquid, the predicted water consumption per animal (1 L/10 kg BW/day) and the pump dilution rate of 10%, the maximum concentration calculated for the different formulation in the metering pump were 17 g of Trisulmix® Powder and 17 mL of Trisulmix® Liquid per liter of water. Based on the labelled dose of 55.68 mg/kg BW for Emericid® Sulfadimethoxine, the predicted water consumption per animal (1 L/10 kg BW/day) and the pump dilution rate of 6%, the maximum concentration calculated for the formulation in the metering pump was 43.2 mL of Emericid® per liter of water.

The solubility of the different formulations was first tested after 2 h at room temperature (RT), then at +4 °C if the product was soluble at RT or at +30 °C if the product was not soluble at RT. For formulations containing the SDM-TMP combination, the experiments were carried out in the presence or not of an organic diluent (Super Diluant Virbac®, Virbac, Carros, France) which is sometimes recommended to increase drug solubility in the dosing pump in sheep fattening houses. For all the tests, the level of product solubility was determined visually. The most soluble formulations were used to determine the pharmacokinetic parameters of SDM and TMP in experimental settings and for the treatment of animals in fattening houses.

4.2. Animals

All the lambs were Lacaune or Lacaune crossbreds supplied by the agricultural cooperative Arterris (Castelnaudary, France). The experimental protocols were authorized by the French Ministry of Research under the number #4637_2016032217062253 on 11 May 2017 for the laboratory experiment done at the INTHERES animal facility and the number #11919_2017102415533573 on 26 June 2018 for the two experiments conducted in a sheep fattening house managed by the agricultural cooperative Arterris.

4.3. Pharmacokinetic Parameters of SDM and TMP in Experimental Settings

Eight, 1-month-old lambs (4 males and 4 females) were weaned on the day of their arrival in the animal facility as they would have been on entering the fattening house. They were fed ad libitum with a starter feed for 10 days and then with a maintenance feed, these feeds being the same as those used in the fattening house and free of antibiotics. The lambs also had free access to water and straw. They received one dose of diclazuril on arrival and another one 10 days later (Vecoxan® 2.5 mg/mL, 1 mg/kg BW, Elanco, Sèvres, France) to reduce the risks of coccidiosis. Six days after their arrival and weaning, the 8 lambs (13.5 ± 1.8 kg BW) received an oral bolus of SDM-TMP (Trisulmix® Liquid, 24.7 mg/kg BW SDM + 5.3 mg kg BW TMP). Blood samples were collected just before drug administration and 0.25, 0.75, 1.5, 2, 2.5, 4, 6, 9, 24, 30, 48 and 72 h after administration. Seven days later, the lambs (15.1 ± 2.1 kg BW) received an intravenous bolus of SDM-TMP (Trisulmix® Injectable, 24.7 mg/kg BW SDM + 5.3 mg/kg BW TMP, Coophavet, Ancenis, France). Blood samples were collected just before administration and 0.08, 0.25, 0.5, 1, 2, 4, 6, 9, 24, 30, 48 and 72 h after administration, to determine the oral bioavailability of SDM and TMP. Finally, again seven days later (that is 14 days after the first oral administration and 20 days after weaning), the oral administration was repeated on the same lambs (17.6 ± 2.8 kg BW) to determine whether the pharmacokinetics of SDM and TMP could be influenced by the lamb's ruminal status. Each 2 mL blood sample was taken from one jugular vein (for the intravenous administration, jugular opposed to the one used for the administration) and collected in heparinized tubes. The samples were then centrifuged at 3000× *g* for 10 min at +4 °C, and the collected plasma stored at −20 °C before assay.

4.4. Individual Pharmacokinetics of SDM and TMP in Combination and Individual Water Consumption in Fattening Houses

Two hundred lambs, around 40 days old, were dosed with Trisulmix® Liquid (37.4 mg/kg BW/24 h SDM + 8.0 mg/kg BW/24 h TMP) for 4 days via drinking water. A sufficient volume of stock solution was prepared once a day in the metering pump to supply the drug in the pipelines over 24 h. The metering pump was set at 4%. Dissolution of the SDM-TMP was facilitated by adding Super Diluant Virbac® to the metering pump (Trisulmix® Liquid:Super Diluant Virbac®, 1:1). The treated lambs were allocated to two pens of 100 lambs (50 males and 50 females), each pen being equipped with two constant-level drinking troughs. The lambs in pen 1 were neither sampled nor handled, in order to assess water consumption before, during and after treatment with limited human influence, while the lambs in pen 2 were sampled several times to quantify the plasma SDM and TMP concentrations. The individual water consumption was determined in real time for all the lambs in pens 1 and 2 from three days before treatment to three days after the end of treatment using water meters connected to the drinking troughs which detected the RFID chip in the lamb ear tags. Lamb access to the drinking troughs was adapted to allow only one lamb at a time. Water samples were taken throughout the duration of treatment from the two drinking troughs in each of the two pens (n = 4) before, and 1 h, 4 h (except on the 4th day), 8 h and 12 h (except on the 3rd day) after the renewal of the treatment in the metering pump each morning, and from one drinking trough in each of the two pens once per day for 4 days after the treatment. The water samples were collected in vials stored at +4 °C until the assays. The lambs in pen 2 were divided into 4 batches of 25 lambs. One blood sample per lamb was taken on the 2nd and 3rd days of treatment and four blood samples per lamb, taken between 07:30 and 18:30 at 12 sampling times with 25 sampled lambs at each time, were obtained on the 4th day of treatment. The blood samples were collected in heparinized tubes, centrifuged at 3000× *g* for 10 min at +4 °C, and the collected plasma stored at −20 °C.

4.5. Individual Pharmacokinetics of SDM Alone in Fattening Houses

The number and characteristics of the treated animals were identical to those in the first experiment. This time, the 200 lambs were dosed with Emericid® Sulfadimethoxine (55.68 mg/kg BW SDM on the 1st day and 27.84 mg/kg BW/24 h SDM from the 2nd to 5th day) for 5 days via the drinking water.

A sufficient volume of stock solution was prepared once a day in the metering pump to supply the drug in the pipelines over 24 h. The pump was set at 10%. Water samples were taken throughout the duration of treatment: from the metering pump before and 3 h after renewal of the treatment, from the drinking troughs several times during the treatment, twice on the day the treatment was stopped and once every two days for 5 days after the treatment. One blood sample was obtained from the lambs of batch 1 (n = 50) in pen 2 on the 1st, 3rd and 4th days of treatment and the 3rd day (Day 8) after the end of treatment. One blood sample was obtained from the lambs of batch 2 (n = 50) in pen 2 on the 2nd, 3rd and 5th days of treatment and the 5th day (Day 10) after the end of treatment. The plasma and water samples were processed as previously described.

4.6. *SDM and TMP Assays*

4.6.1. SDM and TMP Assays in Plasma in the Laboratory Experiment

SDM and TMP plasma concentrations were determined by LC/MS with an Acquity ultra performance liquid chromatography (UPLC®) coupled to a Xevo® triple quadrupole mass spectrometer (Waters, Milford, MA, USA). Plasma samples (50 µL) were spiked with 150 µL of IS (Internal Standard) sulfapyridine at 0.1 µg/mL in trichloracetic acid (TCA 5%) and centrifuged for 10 min, at 20,000× *g* and +4 °C. The analytes were separated on a C18 column (Cortecs UPLC C18+, 2.1 × 50 mm, 1.6 µm, Waters) with an H2O, 0.1% HCOOH/AcN gradient elution (t(0 min): 10% AcN, t(0–2 min): 60% AcN ; t(2–2.10 min): 10% AcN ; t(2.10–3 min): 10% AcN). Samples were detected by multiple reactions monitoring (MRM) with a positive electrospray ionization. The MRM transitions monitored were m/z: 250 > 156, m/z: 291 > 230 and m/z: 311 > 108 for sulfapyridine, TMP and SDM, respectively, with collision energies of 16, 24 and 32 eV. The retention times were 1.38, 0.79 and 0.76 for SDM, TMP and IS, respectively. The performance of the method was checked in terms of linearity, inter- and intra-day precision and accuracy, and sensitivity. Six calibration points containing SDM and TMP at concentrations ranging from 0.01 to 5 µg/mL for TMP and from 0.25 to 50 µg/mL for SDM were extracted and assayed over three days. Both linear ($Y = aX + b$) and quadratic ($Y = aX^2 + bX + c$) models were tested with 1, $1/X$ and $1/X^2$ (X = nominal concentration) weightings with these resulting calibration curves. Three approaches were evaluated to select the best model of calibration: (1) the inspection of the residual distribution plotting against nominal concentrations, (2) the lack-of-fit test to check the goodness-of-fit of the model, and (3) the calculation of the relative concentration residuals (RCR%) between the nominal concentration and the concentration obtained with the model, which should be lower than ± 15%. The best calibration fit was obtained with a quadratic model weighted by $1/X^2$ (X = concentration) for both molecules with RCR% were lower than 15% for all concentrations. The LOQ (limit of quantification) was evaluated with five replicates of plasma samples spiked at 0.25 µg/mL for SDM and 0.01 µg/mL for TMP. They were set as the lowest concentration level of the calibration curve that can be quantified with an acceptable repeatability and accuracy (CV% lower than 20% and accuracy range 80–120%). The accuracies and the intra- and inter-day precisions of the method were evaluated with five replicates of three quality control (QC) samples at three concentration levels (0.025, 0.25 and 2.5 µg/mL for TMP and 0.25, 2.5 and 25 µg/mL for SDM) over three days. Intra and inter-day precision were expressed with coefficient of variation percent (CV%) and calculated with an ANOVA. The intra-day CV% precision was below 11% and 8% and the inter-day CV% precisions were below 19% and 18% for TMP and SDM, respectively. The accuracies ranged from 104% to 121% for TMP, and from 81% to 93% for SDM.

4.6.2. SDM and TMP Assays in Plasma and Drinking Water in the Field Experiments

As a very low level of TMP was detected in the plasma with the previous method and during the previous experiment, and SDM response in the field experiment saturated the MS signal with the previous method, a LC/UV method was developed solely for SDM in plasma. This method using higher concentration levels was also adapted to quantify TMP and SDM in water.

Briefly, SDM and TMP were determined by LC/UV with an Acquity ultra performance liquid chromatography (UPLC®) coupled to a diode array detector (Waters, Milford, MA, USA). The analytes were detected at 270 nm and were eluted under the same conditions as described for the laboratory experiment. SDM was extracted from plasma (100 µL) with 300 µL of IS sulfapyridine at 10 µg/mL diluted in TCA 5% and centrifuged for 10 min, at 20,000× *g* and +4 °C. The performance of the method was evaluated with a calibration ranging from 1 to 500 µg/mL using a linear model weighted by 1/X and three QC samples (3, 30 and 300 µg/mL). The accuracy ranged from 83% to 104% and intra-day CV% precision was below 13% and inter-day CV% precision was below 14%. The LOQ was set at 1 µg/mL with an intra-day CV precision of 6% and an accuracy of 106%. In water, 100 µL of samples were directly diluted with 300 µL of TCA 5%. As the run took only 3 min, all samples were processed on the same day. The calibration curve ranged from 5 to 1000 µg/mL and from 0.5 to 100 µg/mL for SDM and TMP, respectively.

4.7. Pharmacokinetic and Statistical Analyses

For the laboratory experiment, the non-compartmental analysis was conducted with Phoenix® software (Phoenix, WinNonlin 64, NLME 1.6, Certara L. P., Pharsight, St-Louis, MO, USA). As (i) the clearance after the intravenous administration was higher than the apparent clearance after the oral administrations and (ii) we cannot exclude a carryover effect between the different administrations, the bioavailabilities by oral route were corrected by addition of the terminal half-life term for each route of administration in the calculation [25]. The bioavailabilities by oral route were thus determined with Equation (1):

$$F = \frac{AUC_{oral}}{AUC_{iv}} \times \frac{t_{1/2,iv}}{t_{1/2,oral}} \times \frac{Dose_{iv}}{Dose_{oral}} \qquad (1)$$

where AUC_{oral} and AUC_{iv} are the Area Under Curve from time 0 extrapolated to infinite time after oral and intravenous administrations, $t_{1/2,\,iv}$ and $t_{1/2,\,oral}$ are the terminal half-life after intravenous and oral administrations, and $Dose_{iv}$ and $Dose_{oral}$ are the actual dose administered by intravenous and oral route.

The influence of ruminal status on the SDM pharmacokinetic parameters after an oral administration was analyzed by a non-parametric test (Wilcoxon test) with R® software (R 3.4.3, R Development Core Team, Vienna, Austria).

5. Conclusions

In conclusion, we showed that, beyond this example of sulfonamides and TMP, medication via the drinking water will require investigation of a drug's solubility and pharmacokinetics as well as animal behavior to avoid inadequate exposure at the population level and to remain compliant with a rational use of antibiotics in veterinary medicine.

Author Contributions: Conceptualization, M.Z.L., A.B.-M., A.A.F. and B.B.R.; methodology, M.Z.L., A.B.-M., I.D., A.A.F. and B.B.R.; formal analysis, M.Z.L., I.D., and B.B.R.; writing—original draft preparation, M.Z.L., A.A.F. and B.B.R.; writing—review and editing, M.Z.L., A.B.-M., I.D., A.A.F. and B.B.R.; supervision, A.B.-M.; project administration, M.Z.L., A.B.-M. and B.B.R.; funding acquisition, A.B.-M. All authors have read and agreed to the published version of the manuscript.

Funding: This work was funded by the Occitanie Pyrénées-Méditerranée Region and BPI France.

Acknowledgments: The authors thank the agricultural cooperatives ARTERRIS and UNICOR, partners of the OVIBOOST project and strongly involved in the experiments in sheep fattening houses. One part of this research is supported by COST Action CA18217–European Network for Optimization of Veterinary Antimicrobial Treatment

Conflicts of Interest: The authors declare no conflict of interest. The funders had no role in the design of the study; in the collection, analyses, or interpretation of data; in the writing of the manuscript, or in the decision to publish the results.

References

1. Lhermie, G.; Ferran, A.A.; Assié, S.; Cassard, H.; El Garch, F.; Schneider, M.; Woerhlé, F.; Pacalin, D.; Delverdier, M.; Bousquet-Mélou, A.; et al. Impact of timing and dosage of a fluoroquinolone treatment on the microbiological, pathological, and clinical outcomes of calves challenged with mannheimia haemolytica. *Front. Microbiol.* **2016**, *7*, 237. [CrossRef]
2. Vasseur, M.V.; Lacroix, M.Z.; Toutain, P.-L.; Bousquet-Melou, A.; Ferran, A.A. Infection-stage adjusted dose of beta-lactams for parsimonious and efficient antibiotic treatments: A Pasteurella multocida experimental pneumonia in mice. *PLoS ONE* **2017**, *12*, e0182863. [CrossRef]
3. EMA: Categorisation of Antibiotics in the European Union. EMA/CVMP/CHMP/682198/2017. 2019. Available online: https://www.ema.europa.eu/en/documents/report/categorisation-antibiotics-european-union-answer-request-european-commission-updating-scientific_en.pdf (accessed on 31 August 2019).
4. Ferran, A.A.; Roques, B.B. Can oral group medication be improved to reduce antimicrobial use? *Vet. Rec.* **2019**, *185*, 402–404. [CrossRef]
5. Vandael, F.; Filippitzi, M.-E.; Dewulf, J.; Daeseleire, E.; Eeckhout, M.; Devreese, M.; Croubels, S. Oral group medication in pig production: Characterising medicated feed and drinking water systems. *Vet. Rec.* **2019**, *185*, 405. [CrossRef]
6. Soraci, A.L.; Amanto, F.; Tapia, M.O.; de la Torre, E.; Toutain, P.-L. Exposure variability of fosfomycin administered to pigs in food or water: Impact of social rank. *Res. Vet. Sci.* **2014**, *96*, 153–159. [CrossRef] [PubMed]
7. Giguère, S.; Prescott, J.F.; Dowling, P.M. (Eds.) *Antimicrobial Therapy in Veterinary Medicine: Giguère/Antimicrobial Therapy in Veterinary Medicine*; John Wiley & Sons, Inc.: Hoboken, NJ, USA, 2013; ISBN 978-1-118-67501-4.
8. Minato, Y.; Dawadi, S.; Kordus, S.L.; Sivanandam, A.; Aldrich, C.C.; Baughn, A.D. Mutual potentiation drives synergy between trimethoprim and sulfamethoxazole. *Nat. Commun.* **2018**, *9*, 1003. [CrossRef] [PubMed]
9. Atef, M.; Al-Khayyat, A.A.; Fahd, K. Pharmacokinetics and tissue distribution of trimethoprim in sheep. *Zbl. Vet. Med. A* **1978**, *25*, 579–584. [CrossRef] [PubMed]
10. Batzias, G.C.; Delis, G.A.; Koutsoviti-Papadopoulou, M. Bioavailability and pharmacokinetics of sulphadiazine, N4-acetylsulphadiazine and trimethoprim following intravenous and intramuscular administration of a sulphadiazine/trimethoprim combination in sheep. *Vet. Res. Commun.* **2005**, *29*, 699–712. [CrossRef] [PubMed]
11. Bevill, R.F.; Koritz, G.D.; Dittert, L.W.; Bourne, D.W. Disposition of sulfonamides in food-producing animals V: Disposition of sulfathiazole in tissue, urine, and plasma of sheep following intravenous administration. *J. Pharm. Sci.* **1977**, *66*, 1297–1300. [CrossRef]
12. Boxenbaum, H.G.; Fellig, J.; Hanson, L.J.; Snyder, W.E.; Kaplan, S.A. Pharmacokinetics of sulphadimethoxine in cattle. *Res. Vet. Sci.* **1977**, *23*, 24–28. [CrossRef]
13. Toutain, P.L.; Bousquet-Melou, A. Plasma terminal half-life. *J. Vet. Pharmacol. Ther.* **2004**, *27*, 427–439. [CrossRef] [PubMed]
14. Rátz, V.; Maas, R.; Semjén, G.; van Miert, A.S.; Witkamp, R.F. Oral bioavailability of sulphonamides in ruminants: A comparison between sulphamethoxazole, sulphatroxazole, and sulphamerazine, using the dwarf goat as animal model. *Vet. Quart.* **1995**, *17*, 82–87. [CrossRef] [PubMed]
15. Elbadawy, M.; Ishihara, Y.; Aboubakr, M.; Sasaki, K.; Shimoda, M. Oral absorption profiles of sulfonamides in Shiba goats: A comparison among sulfadimidine, sulfadiazine and sulfanilamide. *J. Vet. Med. Sci.* **2016**, *78*, 1025–1029. [CrossRef] [PubMed]
16. Bulgin, M.S.; Lane, V.M.; Archer, T.E.; Baggot, J.D.; Craigmill, A.L. Pharmacokinetics, safety and tissue residues of sustained-release sulfamethazine in sheep. *J. Vet. Pharmacol. Ther.* **1991**, *14*, 36–45. [CrossRef] [PubMed]
17. Shoaf, S.E.; Schwark, W.S.; Guard, C.L. The effect of age and diet on sulfadiazine/trimethoprim disposition following oral and subcutaneous administration to calves. *J. Vet. Pharmacol. Ther.* **1987**, *10*, 331–345. [CrossRef]
18. Little, S.B.; Crabb, H.K.; Woodward, A.P.; Browning, G.F.; Billman-Jacobe, H. Review: Water medication of growing pigs: Sources of between-animal variability in systemic exposure to antimicrobials. *Animal* **2019**, *13*, 3031–3040. [CrossRef]

19. Bushby, S.R.M. Trimethoprim-sulfamethoxazole: In vitro microbiological aspects. *J. Infect. Dis.* **1973**, *128*, S442–S462. [CrossRef]
20. Masters, P.A.; O'Bryan, T.A.; Zurlo, J.; Miller, D.Q.; Joshi, N. Trimethoprim-sulfamethoxazole revisited. *Arch. Intern. Med.* **2003**, *163*, 402. [CrossRef]
21. Root, R.K. (Ed.) *Clinical Infectious Diseases: A Practical Approach*; Oxford University Press: Oxford, UK, 2000; ISBN 978-0-19-514349-2.
22. Gleckman, R.; Blagg, N.; Joubert, D.W. Trimethoprim: Mechanisms of action, antimicrobial activity, bacterial resistance, pharmacokinetics, adverse reactions, and therapeutic indications. *Pharmacotherapy* **1981**, *1*, 14–20. [CrossRef]
23. Nielsen, P.; Romvary, A.; Rasmussen, F. Sulphadoxine and trimethoprim in goats and cows: Absorption fraction, half-lives and the degrading effect of the ruminal flora. *J. Vet. Pharmacol. Ther.* **1978**, *1*, 37–46. [CrossRef]
24. El Garch, F.; de Jong, A.; Simjee, S.; Moyaert, H.; Klein, U.; Ludwig, C.; Marion, H.; Haag-Diergarten, S.; Richard-Mazet, A.; Thomas, V.; et al. Monitoring of antimicrobial susceptibility of respiratory tract pathogens isolated from diseased cattle and pigs across Europe, 2009–2012: VetPath results. *Vet. Microbiol.* **2016**, *194*, 11–22. [CrossRef] [PubMed]
25. Toutain, P.L.; Bousquet-Melou, A. Bioavailability and its assessment. *J. Vet. Pharmacol. Ther.* **2004**, *27*, 455–466. [CrossRef] [PubMed]

antibiotics

MDPI

Article

Extended-Spectrum β-Lactamase-Producing *Enterobacterales* Shedding by Dogs and Cats Hospitalized in an Emergency and Critical Care Department of a Veterinary Teaching Hospital

Anat Shnaiderman-Torban [1], Shiri Navon-Venezia [2,3,†], Efrat Kelmer [1], Adar Cohen [1], Yossi Paitan [4,5], Haya Arielly [5] and Amir Steinman [1,*,†]

1 Koret School of Veterinary Medicine (KSVM), The Robert H. Smith Faculty of Agriculture, Food and Environment, The Hebrew University of Jerusalem, Rehovot 7610001, Israel; ashnaiderman@gmail.com (A.S.-T.); kelmere1@gmail.com (E.K.); adarkohen@gmail.com (A.C.)

2 Department of Molecular Biology, Faculty of Natural Science, Ariel University, Ariel 40700, Israel; shirinv@ariel.ac.il

3 The Miriam and Sheldon Adelson School of Medicine, Ariel University, Ariel 40700, Israel

4 Department of Clinical Microbiology and Immunology, Sackler Faculty of Medicine, Tel Aviv University, Tel Aviv 6997801, Israel; yossi.paitan@clalit.org.il

5 Clinical Microbiology Lab, Meir Medical Center, Kfar Saba 4428164, Israel; Ariellyhaya@clalit.org.il

* Correspondence: amirst@savion.huji.ac.il; Tel.: +972-3-9688544

† Equal contribution.

Received: 28 July 2020; Accepted: 26 August 2020; Published: 27 August 2020

Abstract: Extended-spectrum β-lactamase-producing *Enterobacterales* (ESBL-PE) gut shedding in human medicine is considered as a major reservoir for ESBL-associated infections in high risk patients. In veterinary medicine, data regarding ESBL-PE gut shedding on admission to emergency and critical care department is scarce. We aimed to determine ESBL-PE shedding rates by dogs and cats in this setting and to determine the risk factors for shedding, at two separate periods, three-years apart. Rectal swabs were collected from animals, on admission and 72 h post admission, enriched and plated on Chromagar ESBL plates, followed by bacterial identification. ESBL phenotype was confirmed and antibiotic susceptibility profiles were determined (Vitek 2). Medical records were reviewed for risk factor analysis (SPSS). Overall, 248 animals were sampled, including 108 animals on period I (2015–2016) and 140 animals on period II (2019). In both periods combined, 21.4% of animals shed ESBL-PE on admission, and shedding rates increased significantly during hospitalization (53.7%, *p*-value < 0.001). The main ESBL-PE species were *Escherichia coli* and *Klebsiella pneumoniae*, accounting for more than 85% of the isolates. In a multivariable analysis, previous hospitalization was a risk factor for ESBL-PE gut shedding (*p*-value = 0.01, Odds ratio = 3.05, 95% Confidence interval 1.28–7.27). Our findings demonstrate significant ESBL-PE gut shedding among small animals in the emergency and critical care department, posing the necessity to design and implement control measures to prevent transmission and optimize antibiotic therapy in this setting.

Keywords: ESBL-PE; antibiotic resistance; companion animals; emergency and critical care

1. Introduction

Extended-spectrum β-lactamases (ESBL) enzymes enable bacteria to hydrolyze penicillins, cephalosporins and monobactams, thus conferring resistance which is limiting the therapeutic options [1]. ESBL producing *Enterobacterales* (ESBL-PE) colonize various body sites, such as the intestinal and urinary tract, and may cause infections in these body systems, as well as pneumonia and bloodstream infections [2]. In human medicine, ESBL-PE gut shedding by patients is considered as a major reservoir for ESBL-associated infections both in the community and in hospitals [3]. Furthermore, according to several studies in human hospitals, ESBL-PE gut colonization increases the risk of a subsequent ESBL-PE infection in high-risk patients [4,5]. This was recently demonstrated in a study from Switzerland, where ESBL-PE colonization on admission to the intensive care unit in the University Hospital Basel was associated with subsequent ESBL-PE infection [6]. The suggested pathomechanism is transition of colonizing bacteria from the impaired intestinal tract to the bloodstream [2], which highlights the importance of ESBL-PE colonized patients not only as reservoirs but also as high-risk patients for developing infections. Therefore, on hospital admission, sampling is essential for both identification of patients at risk for developing ESBL-PE infection and for the prevention of ESBL-PE spread among other high-risk patients [7].

In the recent years, several studies described ESBL-PE colonization and infection in dogs and cats [8,9]. Infections caused by ESBL-PE in dogs and cats include abscesses and wounds, otitis, upper respiratory tracts diseases, gastro-intestinal infections and cystitis [8,10]. Colonization was also described worldwide, with rates ranging from 6% to 24% in different geographical regions and different cohorts [11–14]. Recent studies described co-carriage of ESBL producing *Escherichia coli (E. coli)* and *Klebsiella pneumoniae (K. pneumoniae)* strains in humans and dogs of the same household [15,16]. These findings highlight the importance of investigating shedding rates and risk factors for shedding by dogs and cats in both veterinary and 'one health' perspectives.

Several studies investigated ESBL-PE gut shedding and infection rates in healthy and in hospitalized dogs and cats [17], but data regarding shedding rates and risk factors of ESBL-PE on admission to the emergency and critical care department is scarce. This data is crucial to understand the epidemiology of ESBL-PE shedding in emergency veterinary medicine, in specific in an emergency and critical care department setup, in which patients are in life-threatening situations that require intensive medical treatments. Understanding ESBL-PE gut shedding in this cohort is essential to design control measures and prevent the environmental spread of ESBL-PE, and for the identification of animals at high risk for ESBL-PE infection.

In this study, we aimed to determine the ESBL-PE gut shedding rates in dogs and cats admitted to the emergency and critical care department, at two different periods, three-years apart. The analyses included identification of the ESBL-PE bacterial species, their antibiotic susceptibility patterns, and the risk factors for shedding on admission and during hospitalization in this department.

2. Results

2.1. Population Characteristics

Shedding of ESBL-PE in dogs and cats admitted to the small animal emergency and critical care department was studied during two periods. During period I, 108 patients were sampled on admission and 20 patients were re-sampled 72 h post admission (Figure 1). Of those animals that were sampled on admission, 87 were dogs, which belonged to 33 different breeds, and 21 were cats, all belonged to one breed. The most common cause of admission was having a gastrointestinal disease (31.7%), 28.9% of the animals were treated with antibiotics within the previous year and 13% were hospitalized in the previous year, with a median hospitalization length of two days (Supplementary Table S1).

During Period II, 140 patients were sampled and 21 patients were re-sampled 72 h post admission (Figure 1). Of those animals that were sampled on admission, 102 were dogs, which belonged to 34 different breeds, and 38 were cats, which belonged to eight different breeds. The most common cause of admission was having a gastrointestinal disease (24.1%), similarly to period I. Antibiotic treatment within the previous year was documented in 28.4% of animals, and 20.9% of animals were hospitalized in the previous year. The median hospitalization length was three days (Supplemental Table S1).

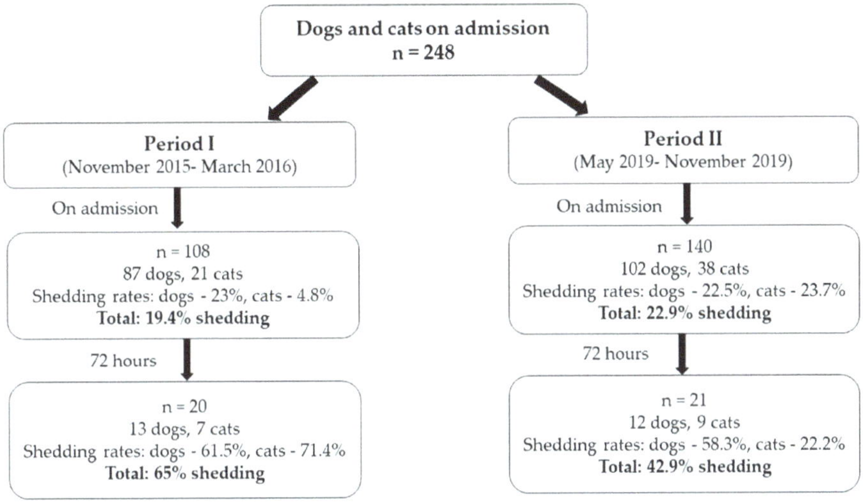

Figure 1. Gut shedding of ESBL-PE in dogs and cats admitted to the small animal emergency and critical care department during two periods-study design.

Overall, 28.6% of all the sampled animals were treated with antibiotics within a year prior to admission to the department (Supplementary Table S1). The most prevalent antibiotic therapy was β-lactams, excluding carbapenems that were not used at all (Table 1). The population characteristics in both periods (I and II) was almost similar. The only significant difference was that previous admission to a veterinary clinic was higher ($p = 0.008$) during period II (Supplementary Table S1).

Table 1. Previous antibiotic treatments in dogs and cats prior to admission to the small animal emergency and critical care department.

Period	Animal	Antibiotic Therapy Within A Year Prior To Admission (% Valid Percentage) [1]					
		Penicillins [2]	Amoxicillin-Clavulanate	Cephalosporins [3]	Quinolones	Doxycycline	Metronidazole
I	Dogs ($n = 87$)	13.5	4.1	4.1	4.1	1.4	4.2
	Cats ($n = 21$)	13.3	13.3	0	13.3	0	13.3
	Total ($n = 108$)	13.5	5.7	3.4	5.7	1.1	5.7
II	Dogs ($n = 102$)	4.9	8.5	3.7	3.7	6.1	3.7
	Cats ($n = 38$)	0	9.7	6.5	0	3.2	0
	Total ($n = 140$)	3.5	8.8	4.5	2.7	5.3	2.7
I & II	Dogs ($n = 189$)	9	6.9	3.9	3.9	3.9	3.9
	Cats ($n = 59$)	4.3	11.9	4.3	4.3	2.2	4.3
	Total ($n = 248$)	8	7.6	4.1	4	3.5	4.1

[1] Valid percent-missing data was removed from the denominator. [2] Including: amoxicillin, ampicillin and penicillin.
[3] Including: cefazolin and cefalexin.

2.2. ESBL-PE Gut Shedding Rates

Data on the ESBL-PE gut shedding rates in animals during the two study periods is presented in Table 2. Overall, for both periods combined, the ESBL-PE gut shedding rates increased during hospitalization (72 h post admission), from 21.4% to 53.7% ($p < 0.001$).

Table 2. ESBL-PE gut shedding rates on admission to small animal emergency and critical care department and following 72 h of hospitalization.

Period	Animal	ESBL Gut Shedding Rate		
		on Admission % (Frequency, 95% CI)	**At 72 h % (Frequency, 95% CI)**	**p-Value [1]**
I	Dogs (n = 87)	23 (20/87, 14.6–33.3)	61.5 (8/13, 31.6–86.1)	0.007 *
	Cats (n = 21)	4.8 (1/21, 0.1–23.8)	71.4 (5/7, 29–96.3)	0.001 *
	Total (n = 108)	19.4 (21/108, 12.5–28.2)	65 (13/20, 40.8–84.6)	<0.001 *
II	Dogs (n = 102)	22.5(23/102, 14.9–31.9)	58.3 (7/12, 27.7–84.8)	0.014 *
	Cats (n = 38)	23.7 (9/38, 11.4–40.2)	22.2 (2/9, 2.8–60)	1
	Total (n = 140)	22.9 (32/140, 16.2–30.7)	42.9 (9/21, 21.8–69.0)	0.062
I & II	Dogs (n = 189)	22.8 (43/189, 17–29.4)	60 (15/25, 39.7–78.9)	<0.001 *
	Cats (n = 59)	16.9 (10/59, 8.4, 29)	43.8 (7/16, 19.8–70.1)	0.04 *
	Total (n = 248)	21.4 (n = 53/248, 16.4–27.0)	53.7 [1] (n = 22/41, 37.4–69.3)	<0.001 *

[1] A comparison between ESBL-PE gut shedding rate on admission and at 72 h post admission, in the same raw. All other comparisons, between the same animal species in different periods or between cats and dogs on the same period- were not significantly different. * $p < 0.05$.

In order to determine the acquisition and the persistence of ESBL-PE during hospitalization in the emergency and critical care department, we re-sampled all animals that were still hospitalized 72 h after admission (41 animals in both periods). Of these that were non-ESBL-PE carriers on admission (n = 27), 59.3% remained negative and 40.7% acquired ESBL-PE (*de novo* shedders) during hospitalization; of the ESBL-PE on admission shedders (n = 14), 71.4% remained positive and 28.6% turned negative during hospitalization. The total acquisition rate of ESBL-PE during hospitalization was 26.8% (11/41, nine animals in period I and two animals in period II).

2.3. *Distribution of the ESBL-PE Bacterial Species*

2.3.1. On Admission

On admission, during period I, 26 ESBL-PE isolates were recovered belonging to three bacterial species with *E. coli* being the major species–69.2%, following with *K. pneumoniae*–23.1% and *Citrobacter freundii*–7.7%. During Period II, 39 bacteria were isolated, including five bacterial species: 64.1% *E. coli,* 23.1% *K. pneumonia,* 7.7% *Enterobacter cloacae,* 2.55% *Cronobacter sakazakii* and 2.6% *Citrobacter freundii.* The relative prevalence of the ESBL-PE species on admission was similar between periods I and II, therefore we present the overall prevalence combining period I and II. The most prevalent species on admission were *E. coli* (66.2%, 43/65, 95% CI 53.4–77.4) and *K. pneumoniae* (23.1%, 15/65, 95% CI 13.5–35.2) (Figure 2A).

2.3.2. During Hospitalization

During hospitalization (72 h post admission), during period I, 19 bacterial isolates were isolated, including five bacterial species: 52.6% *E. coli,* 26.3% *K. pneumoniae,* 10.5% *Enterobacter cloacae,* 5.3% *Citrobacter freundii* and 5.3% *Proteus mirabilis.* During Period II, 13 bacterial isolates were isolated, including three bacterial species: 61.5% *K. pneumoniae,* 30.8% *E. coli* and 7.7% *Enterobacter cloacae.* There were no statistical differences in the prevalence of the bacterial species between period I and II. Overall, combining periods I and II, the most prevalent bacterial species during hospitalization were *E. coli* and *K. pneumoniae,* accounting for 84.6% of all the isolates. We noticed a significant decrease in *E. coli* prevalence during hospitalization (p = 0.048), compared to on admission, and no significant change in the prevalence of the other bacterial species. The increase in *K. pneumoniae* prevalence (1.8-fold) was insignificant (p = 0.096).

Data describing the ESBL-PE species recovered from hospitalized animals, some of which acquired more than one species, and their susceptibility patterns are summarized (Supplementary Table S2). Of 41 animals that were re-sampled at 72 h, 24.4% (n = 10/41) acquired *K. pneumoniae*, 24.4% (n = 10/41) acquired *E. coli*, two animals (a cat and a dog) acquired *Enterobacter cloacae*, and single animals acquired *Proteus mirabilis* and *Citrobacter freundii*. *Escherichia coli* was persistent in three dogs (7.3%, 3/41, 95% CI 15.4–19.2) and *K. pneumoniae* was persistent in one dog (2.4%, 1/41, 95% CI 0.6–15.4) (Figure 2B).

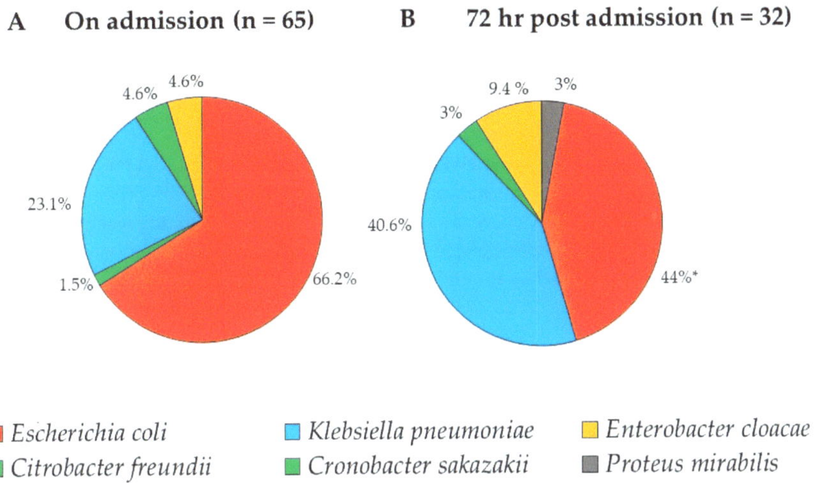

Figure 2. Bacterial species isolated from dogs and cats on admission (I, n = 65) and 72 h post admission (II, n = 33) to the small animal emergency and critical care department. * A significant decrease in *E. coli* prevalence (p = 0.048).

2.4. Susceptibility Patterns of the ESBL-PE Isolates

During period I, there was a significant decrease in resistance rates to amoxicillin-clavulanate and a significant increase in resistance rates to ofloxacin ($p < 0.05$, Table 3). During period II, there was a significant increase in resistance rates to ofloxacin and nitrofurantoin ($p < 0.05$).

Table 3. Antibiotic resistance rates of ESBL-PE isolates originated from dogs and cats hospitalized in an emergency and critical care department in two periods.

Period	Sampling (Number of Isolates)	AMC (95% CI)	OFL (95% CI)	AMK (95% CI)	GEN (95% CI)	TMS (95% CI)	NIT (95% CI)	MDR (95% CI)
Period I	Admission (n = 26)	100 (86.7–100)	44 (24.4–65.1)	3.8 (0.1–19.6)	15.4 (4.4–34.9)	65.4 (44.3–82.8)	7.7 (0.9–25.13)	69.2 (48.2–85.7)
	72 h post admission (n = 19)	69.2 [1] (38.6–90.9)	87.5 [3] (61.7–98.5)	0 (0–17.7)	41.2 (18.4–67.1)	88.2 (63.6–98.5)	5.9 (0.2–28.7)	94.4 (72.7–99.9)
Period II	Admission (n = 39)	28.2 [2] (15–44.9)	53.9 (37.2–69.9)	0 (0–9)	38.5 (23.4–55.4)	71.8 (55.1–85)	17.95 (7.5–33.5)	61.5 (44.6–77.6)
	72 h post admission (n = 13)	46.2 (19.2–74.9)	100 [4] (73.5–100)	0 (0–24.7)	38.5 (13.9–68.4)	84.6 (54.5–98.1)	53.85 [5,6] (25.2–80.8)	92.3 [7] (64–99.8)

[1] A significant decrease in resistance rate to AMC (amoxicillin-clavulanate) during period I (admission versus 72 h post admission), $p < 0.001$. [2] A significant decrease in resistance rate to AMC between period I and II, on admission, $p < 0.001$. [3] A significant increase in resistance rate to OFL (ofloxacin) during period I, $p = 0.008$. [4] A significant increase in resistance rate to OFL during period II, $p = 0.004$. [5] A significant increase in resistance rate to NIT (nitrofurantoin) during period II, $p = 0.026$. [6] A significant increase in resistance rate to NIT between period I and II, 72 h post admission, $p = 0.009$. [7] A significant increase in multidrug resistance rate 72 h post admission, on period II, $p = 0.044$.

Comparing resistance rates to different antibiotics between period I and II on hospital admission, there was a significant decrease in resistant rates to amoxicillin-clavulanate and a significant increase in resistance rates to nitrofurantoin ($p < 0.05$, Table 3). Other resistance rates between the periods were not significantly different, on both admission and 72 h post admission (Table 3).

There was a significant increase in multi-drug resistance rates between admission and hospitalization on period II (Table 3). All bacterial isolates were susceptible to imipenem.

2.5. *Risk Factor Analysis for ESBL-PE Gut Shedding*

2.5.1. Period I

In a univariable analysis of dogs, the following categorical variables were associated with ESBL-PE gut shedding on admission: hepatic disease and respiratory disease ($p < 0.05$, Table 4). These variables, as well as cardiovascular disease were analyzed in a logistic regression model and were found to be non-significant ($p > 0.05$, Table 5). In a univariable analysis of cats, no variables were significantly associated with gut shedding. In a univariable analysis of dogs and cats together, hepatic disease, respiratory disease and the animal species were included in a logistic regression model ($p < 0.2$, Table 4). Respiratory disease was identified as the only risk factor for ESBL-PE gut shedding on admission (Table 5).

2.5.2. Period II

In a univariable analysis of dogs, the following variables were associated with ESBL-PE gut shedding on admission: hematologic disease, respiratory disease and weight ($p < 0.05$, Table 4). These variables, as well as amoxicillin-clavulanate treatment, were analyzed in a logistic regression model. The variable "weight" was identified as a risk factor for ESBL-PE gut shedding (Table 5). In a univariable analysis of cats, admission to a veterinary clinic in the previous year, hospital admission in the previous year and weight were associated with ESBL-PE gut shedding on admission ($p < 0.05$, Table 4. These variables were non-significant in a logistic regression model ($p > 0.05$, Table 5).

In a univariable analysis of dogs and cats together, ESBL-PE gut shedding on admission was associated with shedding 72 h post admission, previous hospital admission, respiratory disease and weight ($p < 0.05$, Table 4). These variables (excluding shedding 72 h post admission), as well as admission to a veterinary clinic in the previous year, injury, and a hematological disease were analyzed in a logistic regression model. Weight was identified as a risk factor for shedding on admission (Table 5).

2.5.3. Periods I and II

In a univariable analysis of dogs, weight was significantly associated with ESBL-PE gut shedding on admission ($p < 0.05$, Table 4). In a univariable analysis of cats, hospital admission in the previous year was significantly associated with ESBL-PE gut shedding on admission (Table 4). In a logistic regression model, including also weight, admission to a veterinary clinic in the previous year and injury, none of these variables were identified as risk factors for ESBL-PE gut shedding (Table 5).

In a univariable analysis of dogs and cats together, ESBL-PE gut shedding on admission was significantly associated with animal weight and with hospital admission in the previous year ($p < 0.05$, Table 3). These variables, as well as injury, were analyzed in a logistic regression model. Hospital admission in the previous year was identified as a risk factor for ESBL-PE gut shedding on admission (Table 5).

Table 4. Univariable analyses for ESBL-PE gut shedding on hospital admission to the small animal emergency and critical care department.

Period		Period I			Period II			Period I & II		
Variables (*p*-Value)		Dogs	Cats	Dogs & Cats	Dogs	Cats	Dogs & Cats	Dogs	Cats	Dogs & Cats
Demographics	Species [1]			0.07 [6]			0.89			0.38
	Gender [2]	0.52	0.41	0.42	0.29	0.41	0.7	0.87	0.23	0.98
	Breed	0.82	1	0.62	0.63	0.64	0.62	0.75	0.78	0.77
	Age	0.87	NI [5]	0.94	0.36	0.27	0.74	0.44	0.23	0.81
	Weight	0.8	0.57	0.45	0.01 *,6	0.08	0.03 *,6	0.04 *,6	0.19 [6]	0.048 *,6
Medical background	Previous admission to a veterinary clinic [3]	0.26	1	0.22	1	0.03 *,6	0.16 [6]	0.52	0.17 [6]	0.89
	Previous hospitalization [3]	1	1	1	0.24	0.03 *,6	0.02 *,6	0.313	0.02 *,6	0.035 *,6
	Length of illness before admission	0.4	NI	0.35	0.88	0.77	0.93	0.66	0.77	0.49
Previous antibiotic treatments [3]	Antibiotic treatment (yes/no)	0.73	0.4	0.54	0.92	1	0.74	0.85	1	0.92
	Penicillins [4]	0.66	0.13	0.37	1	NI	1	1	0.28	0.51
	Amoxicillin-clavulanate	0.42	0.13	0.16	0.19 [6]	1	0.12 [6]	0.69	1	0.74
	Cephalosporines	1	NI	1	1	1	0.59	0.6	1	0.36
	Quinolones	0.42	0.13	0.16	0.55	NI	0.53	0.35	0.28	0.18
	Doxycycline	1	NI	1	0.33	1	0.61	0.35	1	0.62
	Metronidazole	0.43	1	1	0.55	NI	0.53	0.35	1	0.652
Clinical syndrome on admission	Neurological disease	0.73	1	1	0.56	0.63	0.4	0.4	1	0.45
	Injury	1	1	1	0.45	0.31	0.12 [6]	0.57	0.19 [6]	0.11 [6]
	Cardiovascular disease	0.07 [6]	1	0.21	1	0.66	0.76	0.22	0.67	0.58
	Hematologic disease	0.68	0.053	1	0.028 *,6	1	0.14 [6]	0.25	0.51	0.27
	Gastro-intestinal disease	0.54	1	0.59	0.49	1	0.46	0.37	1	0.4
	Endocrinopathy	NI	NI	NI	1	1	0.57	1	1	0.58
	Hepatic disease	0.046 *,6	1	0.09 [6]	0.57	1	0.68	0.62	1	0.72

Table 4. *Cont.*

	Period	Period I			Period II			Period I & II		
	Variables (p-Value)	**Dogs**	**Cats**	**Dogs & Cats**	**Dogs**	**Cats**	**Dogs & Cats**	**Dogs**	**Cats**	**Dogs & Cats**
Clinical syndrome on admission	Reproduction related disease	1	NI	1	0.59	NI	0.59	0.2	NI	0.21
	Respiratory	0.02 *[,6]	1	0.055 [6]	0.04 *[,6]	1	0.04 *[,6]	0.82	0.67	0.8
	Orthopedic	0.68	1	1	1	0.56	0.3	0.53	0.58	0.26
	Intoxication	1	NI	1	0.41	1	0.54	0.66	1	0.68
	Ophthalmological	1	1	1	0.57	0.22	1	0.6	0.3	1
	Tumor	0.29	NI	0.46	0.59	0.56	0.95	0.62	1	0.55
	Urinary-tract disease	1	1	0.73	1	0.37	0.56	0.8	0.42	0.94
Outcomes	Hospital discharge (yes/no)	0.73	0.08	0.75	0.76	0.37	0.8	0.55	1	0.78
	ESBL-PE gut shedding 72 h post admission	1	1	1	0.24	0.17	0.03 *	0.23	0.6	1
	Length of stay	0.48	0.56	0.45	0.14 [7]	0.9	0.23	0.44	1	0.55
	Length of stay excluding dead	0.52	[8]	0.27	0.28	0.57	0.57			0.96

[1] Only for dogs and cat analyses. [2] Four categories: intact male, intact female, castrated male and spayed female. [3] During the previous year. [4] Including amoxicillin and amoxicillin-clavulanate. [5] NI—not identified, there is not enough data for analysis. [6] Included in a multivariable analysis due to $p \leq 0.2$. [7] "Length of stay" was not included in a multivariable analysis, since this is an outcome and not a risk factor. [8] The distribution of this variable is the same across categories of ESBL-PE gut shedding at admission, therefore this test cannot be computed. * $p \leq 0.05$.

Table 5. Logistic regression analyses for ESBL-PE gut shedding on hospital admission to the small animal emergency and critical care department.

Period	**Period I**		**Period II**			**Periods I & II**	
Variable (*p*-Value, OR, 95% CI)	**Dogs**	**Dogs & Cats**	**Dogs**	**Cats**	**Dogs & Cats**	**Cats**	**Dogs & Cats**
Species [1]	NI [3]	0.09 OR = 0.16 0.02–1.35	NI	NI	NI	NI	NI
Previous admission to a veterinary clinic [2]	NI	NI	NI	0.999	0.14 OR = 0.19 95% CI 0.03–1.47	0.774 OR = 0.7 95% CI 0.6–7.6	NI
Previous hospital admission [2]	NI	NI	NI	0.92 OR = 0.76 0.002–232	0.095 OR = 5.82 1.28–7.27	0.56 OR = 0.7 95% CI 0.6–7.6	**0.01 *** **OR = 3.05** **1.28–7.27**
Amoxicillin-clavulanate before admission [2]	NI	NI	>0.99	NI	0.999	NI	NI
Injury on admission	NI	NI	NI	NI	0.999	0.999	0.4 OR = 0.51 0.11–2.4
Cardiovascular disease on admission	0.42 OR = 2.05 0.36–11.74	NI	NI	NI	NI	NI	NI
Hematologic disease on admission	NI	NI	0.12 OR = 4.35 0.68–27.84	NI	0.35 OR = 2.54 0.36–17.86	NI	NI
Hepatic disease on admission	1	0.069	NI	NI	NI	NI	NI
Respiratory disease on admission	0.08 OR = 3.43 0.87–13.49	**0.029 *** **OR = 3.63** **1.15–11.5**	>0.99	0.99	0.998	NI	NI
Weight (Kg)	NI	NI	**0.014 *** **OR = 1.07** **1.01–1.13**	0.07 OR = 3.69 0.89–15.26	**0.011 *** **OR = 1.1** **1.02–1.19**	0.3 OR = 1.33 0.78–2.25	0.07 OR = 1.02 0.99–1.05

[1] Only for dogs & cats analyses. [2] During the previous year. [3] NI—Not Included due to $p > 0.2$ in the univariable analysis (Table 4). * $p < 0.05$.

3. Discussion

This study investigated the prevalence and risk factors for ESBL-PE gut shedding by dogs and cats on admission to an emergency and critical care department in a veterinary teaching hospital, during two periods. To our knowledge, this study is unique as it focusses specifically on shedding of antibiotic resistant ESBL-PE and defines risk factors for gut shedding in this population. Understanding the burden of ESBL-PE shedding in complicated animal patients in the hospital vicinity is highly valuable for designing control measures. Minimizing resistance spread and the identification of patients at risk for developing ESBL-PE infection is still understudied in veterinary medicine.

Overall, during the two periods, we screened 248 dogs and cats on admission. The veterinary referral center studied here is the largest emergency center in the country and treats animals from all over the country. Data regarding dogs and cats was collected and analyses were performed in several perspectives—(i) the two time periods, (ii) dogs versus cats and (iii) combined analyses—taking into consideration both animal species and the two-time periods. Although we investigated two different animal species, we chose to examine the combined data of dogs and cats in addition to a separate species analyses, due to similar housing conditions in the community, similar animal-human contact and similar hospitalization conditions.

The overall ESBL-PE shedding rate on admission was 21.4% and was insignificantly different between the periods. Shedding rate on admission does not necessarily represent the healthy companion animal community, since these animals were referred to a tertiary referral center, 63.2% of them were previously treated in a veterinary clinic and 17.7% were hospitalized in the previous year. This shedding rate is similar to what was found among horses in the same veterinary hospital, where ESBL-PE shedding upon hospital admission was 19.6% [18]. Data from human medicine reported in Israel more than a decade ago, indicated lower ESBL-PE shedding rates upon hospital admission of 13.7% [19] and 10.7% in another study [20]. The comparison to human population is important in the perspective of 'one health', since companion animals live in close contact to humans, but these studies were performed in different periods and in dissimilar set-ups, and therefore, further studies are warranted for a reliable comparison.

Analyzing the data during the two periods revealed similarities between the two periods with respect to the population characteristics and the ESBL-PE shedding rates, both on admission and 72 h post admission (Supplementary Table S1). Although the two periods are three-years apart, we did not find an increase in the prevalence of ESBL-PE gut shedding (Supplementary Table S1), nor in the antibiotic usage (Table 1). In a recent European study, investigating the antimicrobial usage and resistance in companion animals, 19% of animals received at least one antimicrobial treatment six months preceding sampling, with the most frequently used antimicrobial was amoxicillin-clavulanate [21]. In our study, 28.6% of animals were treated one-year preceding sampling, and β-lactams, excluding carbapenems were the most frequently used group. The comparable result may imply similar antibiotic stewardships in companion animals' medicine in the recent years.

During hospitalization, the ESBL-PE gut shedding rate increased significantly to 53.7%, overall ESBL-PE acquisition rate was 26.8%, *E. coli* acquisition rate was 24.4% and persistent in 7.3% of the animals. These findings could be the result of acquisition of resistant bacteria or mobile genetic elements from the hospital environment. Alternatively, these could be the result of an increase in resistant bacteria that were undetected in the gastrointestinal flora as was previously suggested [18,22]. In a similar study in a veterinary teaching hospital in the United States, multidrug resistant (MDR) *E. coli* was acquired in 6.8% of the animals and was persistent in 3% [22]. However, data on ESBL-producing *E. coli* was not examined in this later study. These different trends are interesting findings that could have been driven by a number of factors, including different population characteristics, antibiotic stewardships and variation in the study design. Despite the arising numbers of different studies regarding ESBL-PE shedding and infections in a variety of companion animals' cohorts, there is a lack of evidence regarding the association between ESBL-PE shedding and infections. In human medicine,

ESBL-PE gut shedding has been identified as a risk factor for infection [4,6] and this should be further studied in animals as well.

The main ESBL-PE species were *E. coli* and *K. pneumoniae*, as previously reported in companion animals [13,23,24]. There was no significant change in species prevalence between on-admission and during hospitalization, in both periods and between periods. The only significant difference was the decrease in *E. coli* prevalence post admission, when combining both periods, alongside with insignificant increase in *K. pneumoniae* prevalence. In similar studies conducted in the large animal department in the same veterinary teaching hospital and during similar time periods, the main ESBL-PE species found were *E. coli* and *K. pneumoniae*, but there were significant changes in bacterial species distribution, including new species that were acquired during hospitalization [18,25]. This may be due to differences in pathologies and antibiotic stewardships between the small and large animals as well as differences in hospitalization facilities, and therefore calls for further investigation.

We found differences in bacterial antibiotic resistance patterns between periods I and II (Table 3). In ESBL-PE isolates obtained 72 h post admission during period II we found a significant increase MDR and specifically in resistance rates to ofloxacin and nitrofurantoin. Nitrofurantoin is not widely used in veterinary medicine owing to its pharmacokinetics and adverse clinical effects [26]. However, nitrofurantoin is commonly used for treatment of uncomplicated urinary tract infection in otherwise healthy young women [27]. Co-selection of resistance to aminoglycosides, quinolones and tetracycline is prevalent among ESBL-producers as was previously described in human ESBL isolates and in environmental samples [28–30]. Fluoroquinolones are frequently used in veterinary medicine [31], and therefore further research is needed to ascertain the gravity of quinolones resistance and the overall MDR among nosocomial veterinary pathogens.

In human medicine, several studies were conducted on carriage of ESBL-PE on admission to emergency and intensive care units. Shedding rates varied dramatically between reports in different countries from 4 to 62.5% [6,32,33] and risk factors for ESBL-PE shedding included elderly age, cirrhosis, broad-spectrum antibiotic treatment, urinary or intra-abdominal infections and residence in overcrowded households districts [34,35]. Hospitalization in the previous year was identified as a risk factor for ESBL-PE shedding in dogs and cats in both periods (p =0.01, OR = 3.05, 95% CI 1.28–7.27, Table 5), as reported before in human medicine [20,36]. This is an important finding and should be considered in decision making for implementing active surveillance in veterinary clinics. The duration of ESBL-PE carriage was beyond the scope of this study. In human medicine, ESBL-PE shedding duration varies significantly between different populations, from 59 days to over one year [37–39]. A longitudinal study on ESBL-PE carriage in healthy dogs presented duration of at least six months [40], but data regarding duration following hospital discharge is lacking. Additional studies are required in order to predict suspected ESBL-PE shedding animals on admission.

The limitations of this study include a small sample size collected in each period, small number of cats and a retrospective medical data collection. Even though the statistical analysis revealed significant risk factors, a larger sample size may have resulted in the identification of additional risk factors that could differentiate between ESBL-PE gut shedding among dogs and cats. Unfortunately, data regarding ESBL-PE infection in these animals was not available, therefore conclusions regarding the association between ESBL-PE colonization and infection could not be drown. Another limitation is that we only selected one colony from each of the colors/morphology for our analysis, which may result in missing information about other clones. This study emphasizes the importance of applying an active surveillance policy for ESBL-PE shedding in small animals admitted to emergency and critical care department in veterinary hospitals. Future studies should include a larger cohort and further investigate the association between ESBL-PE shedding and infections caused by these antibiotic resistant pathogens.

4. Materials and Methods

4.1. Study Design

We conducted a case-control study in the small animal emergency and critical care department in the Koret School of Veterinary Medicine-Veterinary Teaching Hospital (KSVM-VTH), during two time periods, three years apart: period I (November 2015–March 2016) and period II (May 2019–November 2019). During period I, 108 patients (87 dogs and 21 cats) were sampled on admission and 20 patients (13 dogs and 7 cats) were re-sampled 72 h post admission. During period II, 140 patients (102 dogs and 38 cats) were sampled on admission and 21 patients (12 dogs and 9 cats) were re-sampled 72 h post admission. All animals that survived and were not discharged were re-sampled 72 h post-admission. The study was approved by the Internal Research Committee of the KSVM, Israel (Protocol KSVM-VTH/15_2015). Sampling of all animals required owners' approval and was performed on admission prior to any medical treatment or procedure in the hospital.

4.2. Isolation of ESBL-PE Gut Shedding and Species Identification

Rectal specimens were collected using bacteriological swabs (Meus s.r.l., Piove di Sacco, Italy) and were inoculated directly into a Luria Bertani infusion enrichment broth (Hy-Labs, Rehovot, Israel) to increase the sensitivity of ESBL-PE detection [17]. After incubation at 37 °C (18–24 h), enriched samples were plated onto Chromagar ESBL plates (Hy-Labs, Rehovot, Israel), at 37 °C for 24 h. Colonies that appeared after overnight incubation at 37 °C were recorded, and one colony of each distinct color and/or morphology was re-streaked onto a fresh Chromagar ESBL plate to obtain a pure culture. Pure isolates were stored at −80 °C for further analysis.

Isolates were subjected to Vitek-MS (BioMérieux, Inc., Marcy-l'Etoile, France) for species identification or to Vitek-2 (BioMérieux, Inc., Marcy-l'Etoile, France) for species identification and/or antibiotic susceptibility testing (AST-N270 Vitek-2 card). Species identification by Vitek-MS was performed according to the manufacturer instructions. Briefly, isolated colony was sampled onto the MS slid followed by addition of 1μL VITEK MS CHCA, the slide was inserted, after drying, into the Vitek-MS for identification. Positive identification after spectrum analysis with Confidence Level above 95 was considered as good identification. Species identification and/or antibiotic susceptibility testing by Vitek-2 using the VITEK 2 GN card for identification and the AST-N270 card for susceptibility testing according to the manufacturer instructions. In addition, susceptibility of ofloxacin and imipenem were analyzed using disc diffusion assay (Oxoid, Basingstoke, UK) according to the Clinical and Laboratory Standards Institute (CLSI) guidelines [41,42]. ESBL production was tested and confirmed with the CLSI confirmatory test using both CTX (30 mg) and CAZ (30 mg) (Oxoid, Basingstoke, UK) disks alone and in combination with CA (10 mg) (Sensi-Discs BD, Breda, The Netherlands). The test was considered positive when an increase in the growth-inhibitory zone around either the CTX or the CAZ disk with CA was 5 mm or greater of the diameter around the disk containing CTX or CAZ alone. Results were interpreted according to the CLSI guidelines [41,42]. Isolates were defined MDR based on an in vitro resistance to three or more classes of antimicrobial agents [43]. A nosocomial ESBL-PE acquisition was defined when an animal became an ESBL-PE shedder during hospitalization, or when a new ESBL-PE species was isolated at 72 h post admission compared to admission. A persistent ESBL-PE species was defined when the same animal shed this species on admission and at 72 h post admission.

4.3. Demographic and Medical Data

Medical records were reviewed for the following information: signalment (species, age, sex and breed); weight; admission to any veterinary clinic within the previous year (yes/no); admission to the hospital within the previous year (yes/no); clinical signs on admission; duration of illness before admission; antibiotic therapy within a year prior to hospitalization (yes/no and also divided by antibiotic classes); hospitalization length of stay and short-term outcome.

4.4. Statistical and Risk Factor Analyses

Statistical analyses were performed using the IBM STATISTICS SPSS software (SPSS Version 24; SPSS Inc, Chicago, IL, USA). Data distribution was examined by testing whether the Skewness and kurtosis equal zero and by performing the Shapiro-Wilk's test. Continuous variables were analyzed using t-tests or Mann-Whitney U-tests, according to the distribution of the variable. Categorical variables were analyzed using the Fisher's exact test or the Pearson chi-square test, as appropriate. In all statistical analyses, $p \leq 0.05$ indicated significance. A multiple logistic regression model, using the ENTER method, was applied for ESBL-PE shedding using variables with $p \leq 0.2$ [44]. Due to the retrospective design, prevalence and rate were calculated as valid percentage, whereas missing data was removed from mechanism. Rates and confidence intervals were calculates using the WinPepi software (version 11.62) [45].

5. Conclusions

This study substantiates the significance of ESBL-PE shedding by dogs and cats on admission to an emergency and critical care department, and during hospitalization. Further studies and active surveillance should focus on community-onset, nosocomial ESBL-PE shedding and association with ESBL-PE infection.

Supplementary Materials: The following are available online at http://www.mdpi.com/2079-6382/9/9/545/s1, Table S1: Characterization of dogs and cats admitted to the emergency and critical care department. Table S2: ESBL-PE species recovered from hospitalized animals sampled on admission and 72 h post admission to the small animal emergency and critical care department.

Author Contributions: Conceptualization: A.S., S.N.-V. and A.S.-T.; methodology: Y.P., H.A. and A.S.-T.; software: A.S.-T.; validation: A.S., S.N.-V. and A.S.-T.; formal Analysis: A.S., S.N.-V. and A.S.-T.; investigation: A.S.-T., A.C. and E.K.; resources: A.S., S.N.-V. and Y.P.; data Curation: A.S.-T.; writing—original draft preparation: A.S.-T., A.S. and S.N.-V.; writing—review and editing: all authors; visualization: A.S., S.N.-V. and A.S.-T.; supervision, project administration and funding acquisition: A.S. and S.N.-V. All authors have read and agreed to the published version of the manuscript.

Funding: This research received no external funding.

Acknowledgments: The authors would like to thank the clinicians and technicians of the Koret School of Veterinary Medicine—Veterinary Teaching Hospital, emergency and critical care department for their assistance in sample collection. Part of this research was supported by Cost Action CA18217: European Network for Optimization of Veterinary Antimicrobial Treatment.

Conflicts of Interest: The authors declare no conflict of interest.

References

1. Pitout, J.D.; Laupland, K.B. Extended-spectrum β-lactamase-producing *Enterobacteriaceae*: An emerging public-health concern. *Lancet Infect. Dis.* **2008**, *8*, 159–166. [CrossRef]
2. Biehl, L.M.; Schmidt-Hieber, M.; Liss, B.; Cornely, O.A.; Vehreschild, M.J.G.T. Colonization and infection with extended spectrum beta-lactamase producing *Enterobacteriaceae* in high-risk patients—Review of the literature from a clinical perspective. *Crit. Rev. Microbiol.* **2016**, *42*, 1–16. [CrossRef]
3. Dickstein, Y.; Temkin, E.; Ish Shalom, M.; Schwartz, D.; Carmeli, Y.; Schwaber, M.J. Trends in antimicrobial resistance in Israel, 2014–2017. *Antimicrob. Resist. Infect. Control* **2019**, *8*, 96. [CrossRef]
4. Bert, F.; Larroque, B.; Paugam-Burtz, C.; Dondero, F.; Durand, F.; Marcon, E.; Belghiti, J.; Moreau, R.; Nicolas-Chanoine, M.-H. Pretransplant fecal carriage of extended-spectrum β-lactamase-producing *Enterobacteriaceae* and infection after liver transplant, France. *Emerg. Infect. Dis.* **2012**, *18*, 908–916. [CrossRef]
5. Liss, B.J.; Vehreschild, J.J.; Cornely, O.A.; Hallek, M.; Fätkenheuer, G.; Wisplinghoff, H.; Seifert, H.; Vehreschild, M.J.G.T. Intestinal colonisation and blood stream infections due to vancomycin-resistant enterococci (VRE) and extended-spectrum beta-lactamase-producing *Enterobacteriaceae* (ESBLE) in patients with haematological and oncological malignancies. *Infection* **2012**, *40*, 613–619. [CrossRef]

6. Martinez, A.E.; Widmer, A.; Frei, R.; Pargger, H.; Tuchscherer, D.; Marsch, S.; Egli, A.; Tschudin-Sutter, S. ESBL-colonization at ICU admission: Impact on subsequent infection, carbapenem-consumption, and outcome. *Infect. Control Hosp. Epidemiol.* **2019**, *40*, 408–413. [CrossRef]
7. Tacconelli, E.; Cataldo, M.A.; Dancer, S.J.; De Angelis, G.; Falcone, M.; Frank, U.; Kahlmeter, G.; Pan, A.; Petrosillo, N.; Rodríguez-Baño, J.; et al. ESCMID guidelines for the management of the infection control measures to reduce transmission of multidrug-resistant Gram-negative bacteria in hospitalized patients. *Clin. Microbiol. Infect.* **2014**, *20*, 1–55. [CrossRef]
8. Bortolami, A.; Zendri, F.; Maciuca, E.I.; Wattret, A.; Ellis, C.; Schmidt, V.; Pinchbeck, G.; Timofte, D. Diversity, Virulence, and Clinical Significance of Extended-Spectrum β-Lactamase- and pAmpC-Producing Escherichia coli From Companion Animals. *Front. Microbiol.* **2019**, *10*, 1260. [CrossRef]
9. Zogg, A.L.; Simmen, S.; Zurfluh, K.; Stephan, R.; Schmitt, S.N.; Nüesch-Inderbinen, M. High Prevalence of Extended-Spectrum β-Lactamase Producing *Enterobacteriaceae* Among Clinical Isolates From Cats and Dogs Admitted to a Veterinary Hospital in Switzerland. *Front. Vet. Sci.* **2018**, *5*, 62. [CrossRef]
10. Piccolo, F.L.; Belas, A.; Foti, M.; Fisichella, V.; Marques, C.; Pomba, C. Detection of multidrug resistance and extended-spectrum/plasmid-mediated AmpC beta-lactamase genes in *Enterobacteriaceae* isolates from diseased cats in Italy. *J. Feline Med. Surg.* **2020**, *22*, 613–622. [CrossRef]
11. Karkaba, A.; Hill, K.; Benschop, J.; Pleydell, E.; Grinberg, A. Carriage and population genetics of extended spectrum β-lactamase-producing Escherichia coli in cats and dogs in New Zealand. *Vet. Microbiol.* **2019**, *233*, 61–67. [CrossRef]
12. Umeda, K.; Hase, A.; Matsuo, M.; Horimoto, T.; Ogasawara, J. Prevalence and genetic characterization of cephalosporin-resistant *Enterobacteriaceae* among dogs and cats in an animal shelter. *J. Med. Microbiol.* **2019**, *68*, 339–345. [CrossRef]
13. Melo, L.C.; Oresco, C.; Leigue, L.; Netto, H.M.; Melville, P.A.; Benites, N.R.; Saras, E.; Haenni, M.; Lincopan, N.; Madec, J.-Y. Prevalence and molecular features of ESBL/pAmpC-producing *Enterobacteriaceae* in healthy and diseased companion animals in Brazil. *Vet. Microbiol.* **2018**, *221*, 59–66. [CrossRef]
14. Zhang, P.L.C.; Shen, X.; Chalmers, G.; Reid-Smith, R.J.; Slavic, D.; Dick, H.; Boerlin, P. Prevalence and mechanisms of extended-spectrum cephalosporin resistance in clinical and fecal *Enterobacteriaceae* isolates from dogs in Ontario, Canada. *Vet. Microbiol.* **2018**, *213*, 82–88. [CrossRef]
15. Marques, C.; Belas, A.; Aboim, C.; Cavaco-Silva, P.; Trigueiro, G.; Gama, L.T.; Pomba, C. Evidence of Sharing of *Klebsiella pneumoniae* Strains between Healthy Companion Animals and Cohabiting Humans. *J. Clin. Microbiol.* **2019**, *57*, e01537-18. [CrossRef]
16. Van den Bunt, G.; Fluit, A.C.; Spaninks, M.P.; Timmerman, A.J.; Geurts, Y.; Kant, A.; Scharringa, J.; Mevius, D.; Wagenaar, J.A.; Bonten, M.J.M.; et al. Faecal carriage, risk factors, acquisition and persistence of ESBL-producing *Enterobacteriaceae* in dogs and cats and co-carriage with humans belonging to the same household. *J. Antimicrob. Chemother.* **2020**, *75*, 342–350. [CrossRef]
17. Murk, J.-L.A.N.; Heddema, E.R.; Hess, D.L.J.; Bogaards, J.A.; Vandenbroucke-Grauls, C.M.J.E.; Debets-Ossenkopp, Y.J. Enrichment broth improved detection of extended-spectrum-beta-lactamase-producing bacteria in throat and rectal surveillance cultures of samples from patients in intensive care units. *J. Clin. Microbiol.* **2009**, *47*, 1885–1887. [CrossRef]
18. Shnaiderman-Torban, A.; Navon-Venezia, S.; Dor, Z.; Paitan, Y.; Arielly, H.; Ahmad, W.A.; Kelmer, G.; Fulde, M.; Steinman, A. Extended-Spectrum β-lactamase-Producing *Enterobacteriaceae* Shedding in Farm Horses Versus Hospitalized Horses: Prevalence and Risk Factors. *Animals* **2020**, *10*, 282. [CrossRef]
19. Ben-Ami, R.; Schwaber, M.J.; Navon-Venezia, S.; Schwartz, D.; Giladi, M.; Chmelnitsky, I.; Leavitt, A.; Carmeli, Y. Influx of Extended-Spectrum β-Lactamase—Producing *Enterobacteriaceae* into the Hospital. *Clin. Infect. Dis.* **2006**, *42*, 925–934. [CrossRef]
20. Shitrit, P.; Reisfeld, S.; Paitan, Y.; Gottesman, B.-S.; Katzir, M.; Paul, M.; Chowers, M. Extended-spectrum beta-lactamase-producing *Enterobacteriaceae* carriage upon hospital admission: Prevalence and risk factors. *J. Hosp. Infect.* **2013**, *85*, 230–232. [CrossRef]
21. Joosten, P.; Ceccarelli, D.; Odent, E.; Sarrazin, S.; Graveland, H.; Van Gompel, L.; Battisti, A.; Caprioli, A.; Franco, A.; Wagenaar, J.A.; et al. Antimicrobial Usage and Resistance in Companion Animals: A Cross-Sectional Study in Three European Countries. *Antibiotics* **2020**, *9*, 87. [CrossRef]

22. Hamilton, E.; Kruger, J.M.; Schall, W.; Beal, M.; Manning, S.D.; Kaneene, J.B. Acquisition and persistence of antimicrobial-resistant bacteria isolated from dogs and cats admitted to a veterinary teaching hospital. *J. Am. Vet. Med. Assoc.* **2013**, *243*, 990–1000. [CrossRef]
23. Hong, J.S.; Song, W.; Park, H.-M.; Oh, J.-Y.; Chae, J.-C.; Shin, S.; Jeong, S.H. Clonal Spread of Extended-Spectrum Cephalosporin-Resistant *Enterobacteriaceae* Between Companion Animals and Humans in South Korea. *Front. Microbiol.* **2019**, *10*. [CrossRef]
24. Gandolfi-Decristophoris, P.; Petrini, O.; Ruggeri-Bernardi, N.; Schelling, E. Extended-spectrum β-lactamase-producing *Enterobacteriaceae* in healthy companion animals living in nursing homes and in the community. *Am. J. Infect. Control* **2013**, *41*, 831–835. [CrossRef]
25. Shnaiderman-Torban, A.; Paitan, Y.; Arielly, H.; Kondratyeva, K.; Tirosh-Levy, S.; Abells-Sutton, G.; Navon-Venezia, S.; Steinman, A. Extended-Spectrum β-Lactamase-Producing *Enterobacteriaceae* in Hospitalized Neonatal Foals: Prevalence, Risk Factors for Shedding and Association with Infection. *Animals* **2019**, *9*, 600. [CrossRef]
26. Hartmann, F.A.; Fox, L.; Fox, B.; Viviano, K. Diagnostic and therapeutic challenges for dogs with urinary tract infections caused by extended-spectrum β-lactamase-producing Escherichia coli. *J. Am. Vet. Med Assoc.* **2018**, *253*, 850–856. [CrossRef]
27. Gardiner, B.J.; Stewardson, A.J.; Abbott, I.J.; Peleg, A.Y. Nitrofurantoin and fosfomycin for resistant urinary tract infections: Old drugs for emerging problems. *Aust. Prescr.* **2019**, *42*, 14–19. [CrossRef]
28. FarajzadehSheikh, A.; Veisi, H.; Shahin, M.; Getso, M.; Farahani, A. Frequency of quinolone resistance genes among extended-spectrum β-lactamase (ESBL)-producing Escherichia coli strains isolated from urinary tract infections. *Trop. Med. Health* **2019**, *47*, 19. [CrossRef]
29. Wiener, E.S.; Heil, E.L.; Hynicka, L.M.; Johnson, J.K. Are Fluoroquinolones Appropriate for the Treatment of Extended-Spectrum β-Lactamase-Producing Gram-Negative Bacilli? *J. Pharm. Technol.* **2016**, *32*, 16–21. [CrossRef]
30. Tacão, M.; Moura, A.; Correia, A.; Henriques, I. Co-resistance to different classes of antibiotics among ESBL-producers from aquatic systems. *Water Res.* **2014**, *48*, 100–107. [CrossRef]
31. Ekakoro, J.E.; Okafor, C.C. Antimicrobial use practices of veterinary clinicians at a veterinary teaching hospital in the United States. *Vet. Anim. Sci.* **2019**, *7*, 100038. [CrossRef]
32. Kiddee, A.; Assawatheptawee, K.; Na-udom, A.; Boonsawang, P.; Treebupachatsakul, P.; Walsh, T.R.; Niumsup, P.R. Risk Factors for Extended-Spectrum β-Lactamase-Producing *Enterobacteriaceae* Carriage in Patients Admitted to Intensive Care Unit in a Tertiary Care Hospital in Thailand. *Microb. Drug Resist.* **2019**, *25*, 1182–1190. [CrossRef]
33. Massart, N.; Camus, C.; Benezit, F.; Moriconi, M.; Fillatre, P.; Le Tulzo, Y. Incidence and risk factors for acquired colonization and infection due to extended-spectrum beta-lactamase-producing Gram-negative bacilli: A retrospective analysis in three ICUs with low multidrug resistance rate. *Eur. J. Clin. Microbiol. Infect. Dis.* **2020**, *39*, 889–895. [CrossRef]
34. Razazi, K.; Rosman, J.; Phan, A.-D.; Carteaux, G.; Decousser, J.-W.; Woerther, P.L.; de Prost, N.; Brun-Buisson, C.; Dessap, A.M. Quantifying risk of disease due to extended-spectrum β-lactamase producing *Enterobacteriaceae* in patients who are colonized at ICU admission. *J. Infect.* **2020**, *80*, 504–510. [CrossRef]
35. Otter, J.A.; Natale, A.; Batra, R.; Auguet, O.T.; Dyakova, E.; Goldenberg, S.D.; Edgeworth, J.D. Individual- and community-level risk factors for ESBL *Enterobacteriaceae* colonization identified by universal admission screening in London. *Clin. Microbiol. Infect.* **2019**, *25*, 1259–1265. [CrossRef]
36. Detsis, M.; Karanika, S.; Mylonakis, E. ICU Acquisition Rate, Risk Factors, and Clinical Significance of Digestive Tract Colonization With Extended-Spectrum Beta-Lactamase-Producing *Enterobacteriaceae*: A Systematic Review and Meta-Analysis. *Crit. Care Med.* **2017**, *45*, 705–714. [CrossRef]
37. Birgand, G.; Armand-Lefevre, L.; Lolom, I.; Ruppe, E.; Andremont, A.; Lucet, J.-C. Duration of colonization by extended-spectrum β-lactamase-producing *Enterobacteriaceae* after hospital discharge. *Am. J. Infect. Control* **2013**, *41*, 443–447. [CrossRef]
38. Li, B.; Zhong, Y.; Fu, X.; Qiu, Y.; Wang, S.; Yang, A.J.; Huang, X. Duration of Stool Colonization in Healthy Medical Students with Extended-Spectrum-β-Lactamase-Producing *Escherichia coli*. *Antimicrob. Agents Chemother.* **2012**, *56*, 4558–4559. [CrossRef]

39. Nordberg, V.; Jonsson, K.; Giske, C.G.; Iversen, A.; Aspevall, O.; Jonsson, B.; Camporeale, A.; Norman, M.; Navér, L. Neonatal intestinal colonization with extended-spectrum β-lactamase–producing *Enterobacteriaceae*—A 5-year follow-up study. *Clin. Microbiol. Infect.* **2018**, *24*, 1004–1009. [CrossRef]
40. Baede, V.O.; Wagenaar, J.A.; Broens, E.M.; Duim, B.; Dohmen, W.; Nijsse, R.; Timmerman, A.J.; Hordijk, J. Longitudinal Study of Extended-Spectrum-β-Lactamase- and AmpC-Producing *Enterobacteriaceae* in Household Dogs. *Antimicrob. Agents Chemother.* **2015**, *59*, 3117–3124. [CrossRef]
41. Clinical and Laboratory Standards Institute (CLSI). *Performance Standards for Antimicrobial Susceptibility Testing*, 26th ed.; Clinical and Laboratory Standards Institute: Wayne, PA, USA, 2016.
42. Clinical and Laboratory Standards Institute (CLSI). *Performance Standards for Antimicrobial Susceptibility Testing*, 29th ed.; Clinical and Laboratory Standards Institute: Wayne, PA, USA, 2019.
43. Falagas, M.E.; Karageorgopoulos, D.E. Pandrug resistance (PDR), extensive drug resistance (XDR), and multidrug resistance (MDR) among Gram-negative bacilli: Need for international harmonization in terminology. *Clin. Infect. Dis.* **2008**, *46*, 1121–1122. [CrossRef]
44. Gilliver, S.; Valveny, N. How to interpret and report the results from multivariable analyses. *MEW* **2016**, *25*, 37–42.
45. Abramson, J.H. WINPEPI updated: Computer programs for epidemiologists, and their teaching potential. *Epidemiol. Perspect. Innov.* **2011**, *8*, 1. [CrossRef]

antibiotics

MDPI

Article

Antimicrobial Susceptibility Pattern of Porcine Respiratory Bacteria in Spain

Anna Vilaró [1], Elena Novell [1], Vicens Enrique-Tarancón [1], Jordi Balielles [1], Carles Vilalta [2], Sonia Martinez [3] and Lorenzo José Fraile Sauce [4,*]

[1] Grup de Sanejament Porcí, 25192 Lleida, Spain; micro@gsplleida.net (A.V.); elena@gsplleida.net (E.N.); Vicens@gsplleida.net (V.E.-T); Jordi@gsplleida.net (J.B.)
[2] Freelance researcher, Arbeca, 25192 Lleida, Spain; cvilalta@umn.edu
[3] Departamento de Sanidad Animal, Universidad de León, 24006 León, Spain; smarm@unileon.es
[4] Departament de Ciència Animal, Escola Tècnica Superior d'Enginyeria Agrària, University of Lleida-Agrotecnio, 25198 Lleida, Spain
* Correspondence: lorenzo.fraile@ca.udl.cat; Tel.: +34-973702814

Received: 19 June 2020; Accepted: 9 July 2020; Published: 11 July 2020

Abstract: The monitoring of antimicrobial susceptibility of pig pathogens is critical to optimize antimicrobial treatments and prevent development of resistance with a one-health approach. The aim of this study was to investigate the antimicrobial susceptibility patterns of swine respiratory pathogens in Spain from 2017 to 2019. Bacterial isolation and identification were carried out following standardized methods from samples coming from sacrificed or recently deceased pigs with acute clinical signs compatible with respiratory tract infections. Minimum inhibitory concentration (MIC) values were determined using the broth microdilution method containing a total of 10 and 7–8 antimicrobials/concentrations respectively, in accordance with the recommendations presented by the Clinical and Laboratory Standards Institute (CLSI). The obtained antimicrobial susceptibility varies between pig respiratory pathogens. *Actinobacillus pleuropneumoniae* (APP) and *Pasteurella multocida* (PM) were highly susceptible (≥90%) to ceftiofur, florfenicol and macrolides (tilmicosin, tildipirosin and tulathromycin). However, the antimicrobial susceptibility was intermediate (>60% but <90%) for amoxicillin and enrofloxacin in the case of APP and sulfamethoxazole/trimethropim and tiamulin in the case of PM. Both bacteria showed low (<60%) antimicrobial susceptibility to doxycycline. Finally, *Bordetella bronchiseptica* was highly susceptible only to tildipirosin and tulathromycin (100%) and its susceptibility for florfenicol was close to 50% and <30% for the rest of the antimicrobial families tested. These results emphasize the need of determining antimicrobial susceptibility in pig respiratory cases in order to optimize the antimicrobial treatment in a case-by-case scenario.

Keywords: antimicrobial susceptibility; swine; respiratory pathogens

1. Introduction

The Porcine Respiratory Disease Complex (PRDC) is a syndrome that results from a combination of infectious and non-infectious factors [1]. *Actinobacillus pleuropneumoniae* (APP), *Pasteurella multocida* (PM), *Mycoplasma hyopneumoniae* (MH), *Bordetella bronchiseptica* (BB) and *Glaesserella (Haemophilus) parasuis* (GP) are the most common bacterial agents involved. Porcine reproductive and respiratory syndrome virus (PRRSV), swine influenza virus (SIV) and porcine circovirus type 2 virus (PCV2) are the most prevalent viral agents [1–6]. On the other hand, many non-infectious predisposing factors are also involved in PRDC, such as poor environmental conditions, density, stressors, season of the year, genetic background and production flow (all-in-all out versus continuous flow) [7–9]. As a general approach, preventive medicine programs should be based on applying measures to control PRDC in a cost-effective way, such as improving environmental conditions, decreasing density and stressors, combined with vaccination against the major viral and bacterial infectious etiologic factors [10]. However, if such measures are not in place or fail, the use of antimicrobials may be needed.

The use of antimicrobials could be necessary to control bacteria involved in PRDC with a therapeutic or metaphylactic (group medication) goal. In particular, the objective of antimicrobial therapy is to provide an effective drug to obtain a fast, clinical recovery from the infection in affected animals but reducing the probability of generating antimicrobial resistance [11]. However, its use is one of the factors involved in the emergence and spread of bacterial antimicrobial resistance (AR) from pig origin worldwide [12,13]. Resistant bacteria in humans, food, environment and animals are interconnected, and exchange may continuously take place between these ecological niches. For this reason, AR needs to be addressed with a one-health perspective and action plans have been adopted to address this problem [14]. These plans are based on the development of programs to monitor the usage of antimicrobial agents in pig medicine and the occurrence of antimicrobial resistance in pigs at the European level [15,16]. In veterinary medicine, Antimicrobial Susceptibility Testing (AST) data could predict the clinical outcome of antimicrobial treatment, allowing a rational choice of these drugs to treat bacterial infections [11,17]. Antimicrobial susceptibility is usually measured using minimum inhibitory concentration (MIC) that is the lowest antimicrobial concentration that inhibits the growth of the target bacteria in vitro. Moreover, it is necessary to have valid clinical breakpoints (CB) to correctly interpret the MIC value obtained for each clinical case. Thus, all the clinical cases with MIC values below CB could be correctly treated with one antimicrobial at the common registered dose [11].

The Spanish national program to control antimicrobial resistance has been adopted to reduce the risk of developing antimicrobial resistance since 2014 [16]. One of the points of the program is focused on reducing the antimicrobial consumption in livestock in order to reduce the prevalence of resistant bacteria. This antimicrobial consumption has been steadily decreasing in the last years according to the available European data [15]. Unfortunately, there is little knowledge of antimicrobial susceptibility patterns for animal pathogenic bacteria in Spain. In this study, we present antimicrobial susceptibility patterns for some of the most important pig respiratory pathogenic bacteria, collected during the period 2017–2019 in Spain.

2. Results

Four-hundred samples were received from sow, wean-to-finish and fattening farms across Spain suffering clinical respiratory cases. In the case of sow farms, the samples were obtained from their nursery facilities. Bacterial isolation (APP, PM and BB) was only possible in 80.3% (321/400) of the cases, and in 22% (88/400) of them, it was possible to isolate more than one bacteria. The isolation of APP and PM and PM and BB was possible in 17.5% (70/400) and 4.5% (18/400) of the cases, respectively.

MIC_{50}, MIC_{90} and antimicrobial susceptibility for 162, 130 and 29 strains of APP, PM and BB are described in Tables 1–3, respectively. The number of GP isolates was low (35 strains) and it was not possible to determine the MIC value because we were unable to grow GP strains with the microdilution technique in our laboratory. The MIC distribution observed for each microorganism and drug are shown in Figures 1–5.

Table 1. *Bordetella bronchiseptica* (BB), MIC_{50}, MIC_{90}, current recommended clinical breakpoints (CB) and antimicrobial susceptibility. The MIC_{50} and MIC_{90} were determined from the MIC distribution from 29 BB strains isolated from respiratory clinical cases. The antimicrobial susceptibility was calculated as the percentage of bacterial isolates below CB.

Antimicrobial	MIC_{50} (μg/mL)	MIC_{90} (μg/mL)	Clinical Breakpoint (CB) [1] (μg/mL)	Antimicrobial Susceptibility Based On CB
Amoxicillin	16	16	0.5	0
Ceftiofur	4	4	2	0
Doxycycline	1	2	0.5	27.7
Enrofloxacin	0.5	0.5	0.25	20.7
Florfenicol	2	4	2	51.7
Sulfamethoxazole/ trimethropim [&]	4	8	0.5	3.4
Tiamulin	64	64	16	0
Tildipirosin	4	8	8	100
Tilmicosin	32	64	16	27.6
Tulathromycin	8	8	16	100

[1] Florfenicol, tildipirosin and tulathromycin CB were obtained from CLSI M100 2018 and CLSI VETO8 4th ed., 2018. The rest of the CB were extrapolated from *Pasteurella multocida* (Table 3). [&] MIC represented in the table is for trimethropin. Sulfamethoxazole/trimethropim ratio tested is 19:1.

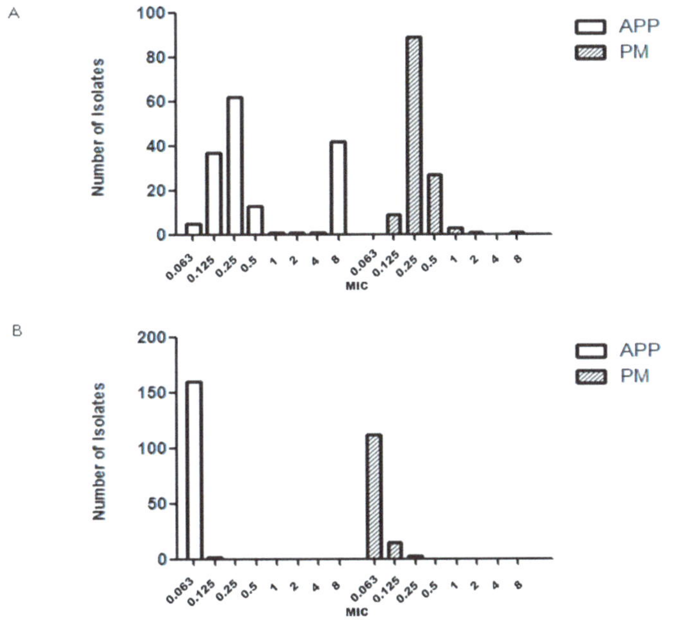

Figure 1. Minimum inhibitory concentration (MIC, μg/mL) distribution of amoxicillin (**A**) and ceftiofur (**B**) for *Actinobacillus pleuropneumoniae* (APP) and *Pasteurella multocida* (PM) isolated from lungs of pigs with respiratory symptoms.

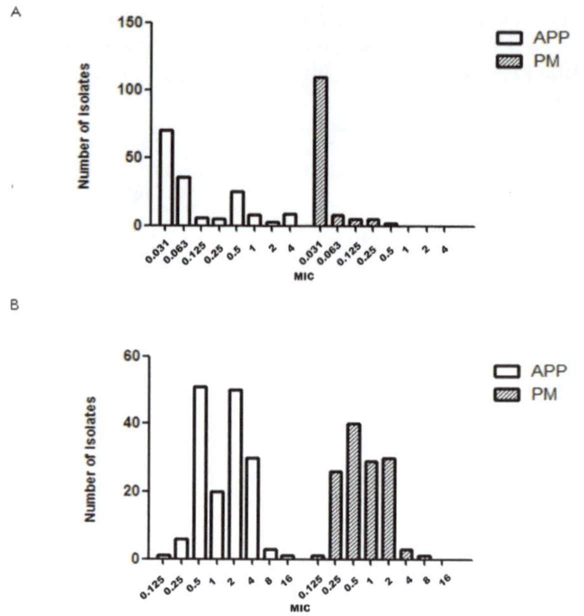

Figure 2. Minimum inhibitory concentration (MIC, µg/mL) distribution of enrofloxacin (**A**) and doxycycline (**B**) for *Actinobacillus pleuropneumoniae* (APP) and *Pasteurella multocida* (PM) isolated from lungs of pigs with respiratory symptoms.

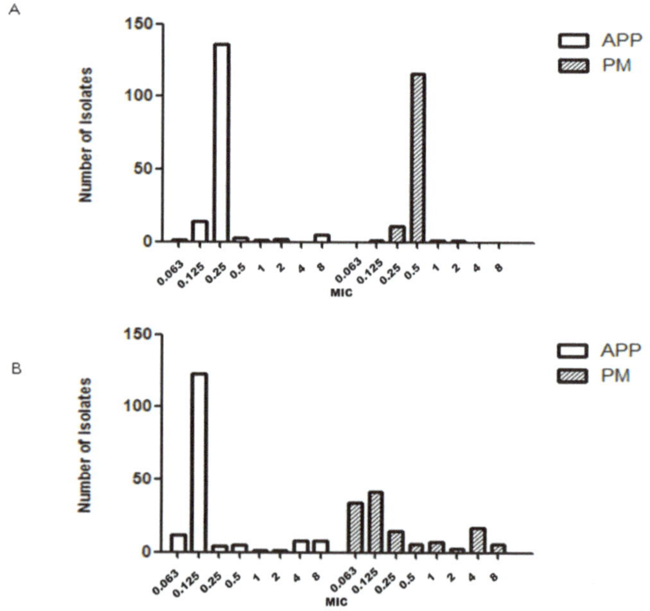

Figure 3. Minimum inhibitory concentration (MIC, µg/mL) distribution of florfenicol (**A**) and sulfamethoxazole/trimethoprim (**B**) for *Actinobacillus pleuropneumoniae* (APP) and *Pasteurella multocida* (PM) isolated from lungs of pigs with respiratory symptoms. In the case of sulfametoxazole/trimethoprim, the MIC value for trimethoprim is represented.

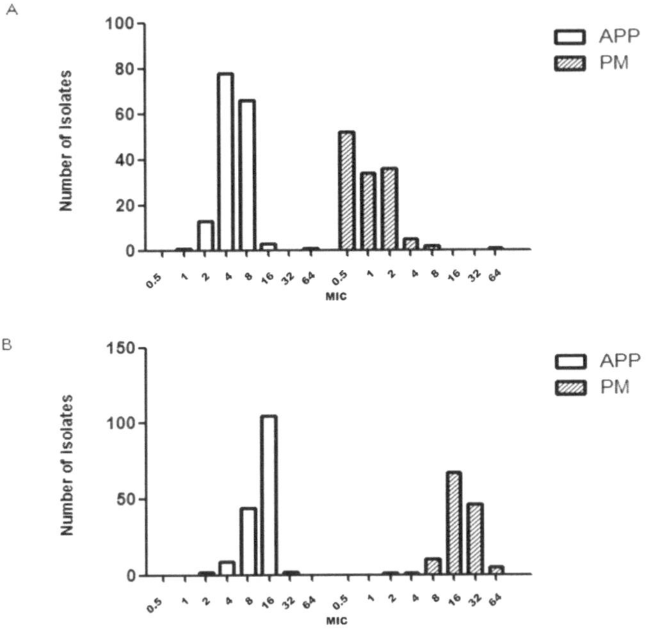

Figure 4. Minimum inhibitory concentration (MIC, μg/mL) distribution of tildipirosin (**A**) and tiamulin (**B**) for *Actinobacillus pleuropneumoniae* (APP) and *Pasteurella multocida* (PM) isolated from lungs of pigs with respiratory symptoms.

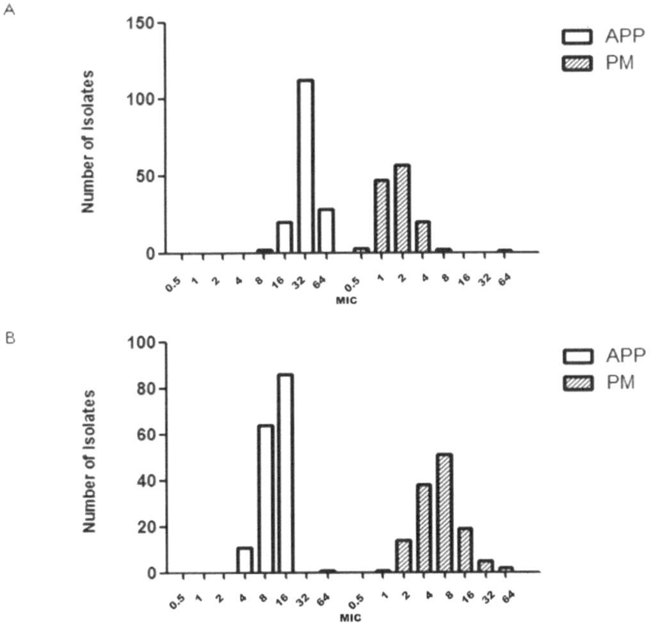

Figure 5. Minimum inhibitory concentration (MIC, μg/mL) distribution of tulathromycin (**A**) and tilmicosin (**B**) for *Actinobacillus pleuropneumoniae* (APP) and *Pasteurella multocida* (PM) isolated from lungs of pigs with respiratory symptoms.

APP and PM MIC distributions were very similar for ceftiofur (Figure 1B) and florfenicol (Figure 3A). On the other hand, the APP and PM MIC distributions were different for the following antimicrobials: amoxicillin (Figure 1A), enrofloxacin (Figure 2A), sulfamethoxazole/trimethoprim (Figure 3B), doxycycline (Figure 2B), tildipirosin and tiamulin (Figure 4A,B) and tulathromycin and tilmicosin (Figure 5A,B).

The isolates of APP were highly susceptible (≥90%) to macrolides (tildipirosin, tulathromycin and tilmicosin), tiamulin, florfenicol, sulfamethoxazole/trimethropim and ceftiofur. However, the antimicrobial susceptibility was intermediate (around 72%) for amoxicillin and enrofloxacin and low (35.7%) for doxycycline. *Pasteurella multocida* showed high susceptibility (≥90%) to macrolides (tildipirosin, tulathromycin and tilmicosin), florfenicol, enrofloxacin, amoxicillin and ceftiofur. However, PM antimicrobial susceptibility was intermediate (74.7%) for sulfamethoxazole/trimethropim and tiamulin (60.8%) and low (51.5%) for doxycycline. Thus, in general terms, APP and PM were susceptible to many families of antimicrobials, whereas BB was highly susceptible (100%) only to tildipirosin and tulathromycin. On the other hand, BB susceptibility for florfenicol was close to 50% and <30% for the rest of the antimicrobial families tested (Tables 1–3).

3. Discussion

There is a scarcity of updated information about antimicrobial susceptibility among porcine pathogens in Spain because there is no official program for their surveillance. The current study aims to address this gap by determining antimicrobial susceptibility, through determining MICs, of ten antimicrobials to three major respiratory tract pathogens recovered, prior to antibiotic treatment, from diseased pigs across Spain. In this case, we have focused on the antimicrobials most frequently used to treat respiratory disease in pigs.

The measurement of antimicrobial susceptibility is carried out by MIC determination that is more reproducible and comparable between laboratories [11] than disk diffusion techniques due to concerns about disk quality, performance issues [18,19] and variability intrinsically associated to some antimicrobials for the disk diffusion technique [20]. The MIC is the lowest antimicrobial concentration that inhibits in vitro the growth of the target bacteria in specific conditions of in vitro incubation. In this study, the antimicrobial susceptibility has been determined using international guidelines on antimicrobial susceptibility determination [21,22] that cannot be directly compared with other studies only based on disk diffusion techniques [20]. This methodology does not emulate the natural biophase in which bacteria grow in vivo, such as blood, interstitial or intracellular fluid. In any case, antimicrobial sensitivity testing in vitro is used to provide information concerning the efficacy of antimicrobial agents in vivo and thus determine whether an antibiotic is suitable or not to treat a specific condition [23], but MIC determination, as any technique, has weaknesses that should be outweighed [24]. Thus, there is an interesting scientific discussion about the usefulness of MIC to foresee the clinical outcome. Some authors recently have proposed to consider both pathogen- (MIC) and patient-specific drug exposure information to predict treatment success in humans. If both pieces of information are taken into account, it will change how antimicrobials are selected and it will allow optimizing the treatment through precision medicine [25]. Unfortunately, this approach is far away from the "everyday" veterinary medicine, where posology regimens of antimicrobials are fixed for each animal species and bacteria to be treated (registered dose for a veterinary medicinal product). Furthermore, the selection of the antimicrobial is even stricter due to the existence of withdrawal periods in livestock to assure food safety that exclude off-label use of antimicrobials to apply precision medicine [25].

Comparison of antimicrobial susceptibility from other laboratories must be carried out with caution due to inconsistencies in methodology (MIC versus disk diffusion technique), selection of antimicrobial substances in the test panel and variations in interpretation criteria for clinical breakpoints. In our study, the isolates of APP were highly susceptible for macrolides (tildipirosin, tilmicosin and tulathromycin), tiamulin, florfenicol, sulfamethoxazole/trimethropim and ceftiofur.

However, the antimicrobial susceptibility was intermediate for amoxicillin and enrofloxacin, and low for doxycycline. This antimicrobial susceptibility pattern described for APP in this study agrees with results obtained by Spanish researchers with strains collected from 1997 [26]. These results could be surprising due to the historic consumption of antimicrobials in Spain and the authors recommend not directly linking the use of antimicrobials with the presence of antimicrobial resistance for any drug–microorganism combination. Moreover, our results are quite similar for isolates from other European countries with some differences [27,28]. Overall, there are still good opportunities to treat infections by APP with antimicrobials, but the presence of strains resistant to doxycycline, amoxicillin and enrofloxacin in Spain highlight the importance of monitoring antimicrobial susceptibility and select the most suitable antimicrobial in a case-by-case situation.

In our study, the isolates of PM were highly susceptible for macrolides (tildipirosin, tilmicosin and tulathromycin), florfenicol, enrofloxacin, amoxicillin and ceftiofur. However, the antimicrobial susceptibility was intermediate for sulfamethoxazole/trimethropim and tiamulin, and low for doxycycline. Thus, the antimicrobial susceptibility pattern is different from that described for APP in spite of the fact that both bacteria are respiratory ones. Again, these results highlight that monitoring of antimicrobial susceptibility must be carried out for each drug–microorganism combination. Moreover, the antimicrobial susceptibility pattern described in our study is very similar to the pattern described by Spanish researchers with strains collected from 1987 [29] for macrolides (>97%), ceftiofur (100%), ampicillin (98%), enrofloxacin (100%), tiamulin (50%) and florfenicol (100%), and by European researchers in a multi-country study to determine the antimicrobial susceptibility of PM in pigs for ceftiofur (100%), enrofloxacin (100%), florfenicol (99.3%), tetracycline (65.8%) and macrolides (>90%) [30]. Thus, the antimicrobial susceptibility of PM seems to have not changed significantly across time, at least, in Europe. This result could be surprising taking into account the enormous variability in the consumption of antimicrobials in livestock across Europe and the authors recommend, again, not directly linking the use of antimicrobials with the presence of antimicrobial resistance for any drug–microorganism combination.

Bordetella bronchiseptica causes a mild or non-progressive inflammation in the nasal cavity that usually needs no treatment. However, if the bacterium is co-infecting with toxigenic PM, it can lead to severe progressive atrophic rhinitis [31]. Moreover, BB may cause pneumonia in young piglets in some cases. In our study, the number of BB strains was quite low to precisely define their MIC distributions. Thus, our results of antimicrobial susceptibility for BB must be interpreted with caution. Moreover, there is a lack of approved clinical breakpoints for many antimicrobials with this bacterium, making comparison with other studies extremely complicated. *Bordetella bronchiseptica* has been described to be intrinsically resistant to ampicillin due to production of beta-lactamases [32,33] and our results agree with this affirmation not only for amoxicillin but also for ceftiofur. In our case, the isolates had extremely high MIC values for doxycycline that exclude them as a therapeutic option to treat BB infection. This lack of antimicrobial susceptibility agrees with Speakman et al. [34] who described a plasmid-encoded tetracycline resistance gene, *tetC*, for this bacterium. Finally, macrolides are also the most susceptible family against BB in Denmark [28], and Dayao et al. [35] also reported no resistance to tulathromycin in Australia.

Table 2. *Actinobacillus pleuropneumoniae* (APP), MIC_{50}, MIC_{90}, current recommended clinical breakpoints (CB) and antimicrobial susceptibility. The MIC_{50} and MIC_{90} were determined from the MIC distribution from 162 APP strains isolated from respiratory clinical cases. The antimicrobial susceptibility was calculated as the percentage of bacterial isolates below CB.

Antimicrobial	MIC_{50} (μg/mL)	MIC_{90} (μg/mL)	Clinical Breakpoint (CB) [1] (μg/mL)	Antimicrobial Susceptibility Based on CB
Amoxicillin	0.25	16	0.5 [$]	72.2
Ceftiofur	0.06	0.06	2	100
Doxycycline	1	4	0.5 [+]	35.7
Enrofloxacin	0.06	1	0.25	72.2
Florfenicol	0.25	0.25	2	97.0
Sulfamethoxazole/ trimethropim [&]	0.125	2	0.5	88.9
Tiamulin	16	16	16	98.8
Tildipirosin	4	8	16	99.4
Tilmicosin	8	16	16	99.4
Tulathromycin	32	64	64	100

[1] All clinical breakpoints were obtained from Clinical and Laboratory Standards Institute (CLSI) M100 2018 and CLSI VETO8 4th ed., 2018, with the following clarifications: [$] Schwarz et al. (2008) [36]. [+] Extrapolated from tetracycline. [&] MIC represented in the table is for trimethropin. Sulfamethoxazole/trimethropim ratio tested is 19:1.

Table 3. *Pasteurella multocida* (PM), MIC_{50}, MIC_{90}, current recommended clinical breakpoints (CB) and antimicrobial susceptibility. The MIC_{50} and MIC_{90} were determined from the MIC distribution from 130 PM strains isolated from respiratory clinical cases. The antimicrobial susceptibility was calculated as the percentage of bacterial isolates below CB.

Antimicrobial	MIC_{50} (μg/mL)	MIC_{90} (μg/mL)	Clinical Breakpoint (CB) [1] (μg/mL)	Antimicrobial Susceptibility Based On CB
Amoxicillin	0.25	0.5	0.5 [$]	96.2
Ceftiofur	0.06	0.12	2	100
Doxycycline	0.5	4	0.5 [+]	51.5
Enrofloxacin	0.03	0.06	0.25	98.5
Florfenicol	0.5	0.5	2	100
Sulfamethoxazole/ trimethropim [&]	0.12	4	0.5	74.7
Tiamulin	16	32	16	60.8
Tildipirosin	1	2	4	97.7
Tilmicosin	8	16	16	94.6
Tulathromycin	2	4	16	100

[1] All clinical breakpoints were obtained from CLSI M100 2018 and CLSI VETO8 4th ed., 2018 with the following clarifications: [$] Schwarz et al. (2008) [36]. [+] Extrapolated from tetracycline. [&] MIC represented in the table is for trimethropin. Sulfamethoxazole/trimethropim ratio tested is 19:1.

It is necessary to have valid information about CB to correctly interpret the MIC value obtained in each clinical case. Thus, all the clinical cases with MIC values below CB could be treated with the antimicrobial, at the registered dose, with a high success rate. Unfortunately, there are no clinical veterinary breakpoints available for all the antimicrobials and bacteria for pigs. In our study, we have used well-established CLSI clinical breakpoints for seven out of ten antimicrobials. However, CLSI veterinary breakpoints for sulfamethoxazole/trimethropim and *Pasteurellaceae* have not been set. In this study, the CLSI CB available for *Streptococcus suis* (0.5 μg/mL) have been used. This value exactly agrees with the CB used by El Garch et al. [30] in a study to monitor the antimicrobial susceptibility for sulfamethoxazole/trimethropim of porcine pathogens in Europe, making results directly comparable. These authors carried out this extrapolation due to the high similarity between *Haemophilus influenziae* and respiratory pathogens in pigs. Moreover, The CLSI clinical breakpoint for amoxicillin (0.5 μg/mL) has been obtained from the literature [36]. This CB value for amoxicillin is equal to the CLSI CB for ampicillin that belongs to the same antimicrobial family (beta-lactam antimicrobials). However, Rey et al. [37] proposed that the CB breakpoint (obtained through pharmacokinetics/pharmacodynamic analysis) for amoxicillin, administered by the intramuscular route, could be as low as 0.125 µg/mL for pig respiratory pathogens. If we had used this proposed breakpoint instead of the chosen one (0.5 µg/mL), the percentage of antimicrobial susceptibility for APP and PM would have been 26% and 7% respectively, which is extremely different from the results shown for this antimicrobial in this paper. Thus, there is an urgent need to have CLSI CB breakpoints available for every antimicrobial/bacteria and feedback from swine practitioners when using these antimicrobials at the registered dose [38]. In this sense, the collaboration between microbiologists, pharmacologists and swine practitioners is highly recommended. Finally, CB for doxycycline was extrapolated from CLSI CB available for tetracycline and porcine respiratory pathogens. In general, the percentage of antimicrobial susceptibility determined in our study is comparable with any other study published using CLSI clinical breakpoints. In the case of doxycycline, amoxicillin and sulfamethoxazole/trimethropim, our results must be compared checking the CB used by other authors before making direct comparisons between them. Finally, antimicrobial susceptibility pattern can change with time [28] and this is one of the main reasons to determine it across time in order to select the most suitable antimicrobial, taking into account efficacy criteria and the one-health approach [14].

4. Materials and Methods

4.1. Clinical Samples

Samples were drawn from diseased or recently deceased pigs from farms across Spain showing acute clinical signs of respiratory tract infections that had not been exposed to antimicrobial treatment for, at least, 15 days prior to sampling between the years 2017 and 2019. Thus, the sampled animals were between 3 and 24 weeks old, the pigs had overt clinical respiratory signs with or without depression and/or hyperthermia (>39.8 °C) and the mortality rate increased significantly, versus the previous baseline situation, due mainly to respiratory causes at farm level. For each clinical case, samples of lungs of two recently deceased pigs (<12 h) were submitted under refrigeration to the laboratory (to increase possibility to isolation). If, during the veterinary visit, there were no recently dead pigs suitable for sampling, at least two animals with acute respiratory signs were humanely sacrificed and lung samples were drawn. In any case, only one isolate per animal/herd was included in the study. All experimental procedures were approved by the Ethics Committee for Animal Experimentation of the University of Lleida and performed in accordance with authorization 10343 issued by the Catalan Department of Agriculture, Livestock, Fisheries and Food (Section of biodiversity and hunting).

4.2. Bacterial Isolation and Identification

Clinical specimens were cultured aseptically onto blood agar (Columbia agar with 5% Sheep blood, 254005 BD), chocolate agar (GC II agar with IsoVitaleX, 254060, BD, Franklin Lakes NJ, USA)) and MacConkey agar (4016702, Biolife Italiana Srl, Milano, Italy) and incubated at 35–37 °C in aerobic conditions with 5–10% CO_2 for 24–48 hours. Identification of isolates (APP, PM, BB and GP) was carried out by matrix-assisted laser desorption ionization-time of flight (MALDI-TOF Biotyper System, Bruker Daltonics, Bremen, Germany). Individual strains were stored at −80 °C in brain heart infusion (CM1135, Oxoid, Madrid, Spain) with 30% of glycerol (G9012, Sigma-Aldrich, Madrid, Spain).

4.3. Antimicrobial Sensitivity Testing

MIC values were determined using the broth microdilution method by means of customized 96-well microtiter plates (Sensititre, Trek diagnostic Systems Inc., East Grinstead, UK) containing a total of 10 and 7–8 antimicrobials/concentrations respectively, in accordance with the recommendations presented by the Clinical and Laboratory Standards Institute (CLSI) [21,22]. The antimicrobials tested included amoxicillin, ceftiofur, doxycycline, enrofloxacin, florfenicol, sulfamethoxazole/trimethoprim, tiamulin, tilmicosin, tildipirosin and tulathromycin. This antimicrobial panel was selected to represent common compounds licensed for treatment of pig respiratory diseases in practice.

Bacteria were thawed, cultured on chocolate agar and incubated at 35–37 °C in ambient air (or with 5–10% CO_2 for APP) for 18–24 h. Three to five colonies were picked and emulsified in demineralized water (or cation-adjusted Mueller–Hinton broth (CAMHB) for APP) to obtain a turbidity of 0.5 McFarland standard (Sensititre™ nephelometer V3011). Suspensions were further diluted in CAMHB (for PM and BB) or Veterinary Fastidious Medium (in the case of APP) to reach a final inoculum concentration of 5×10^5 colony forming units (cfu)/mL (Table 4). Then, the Sensititre panel was reconstituted by adding 100 µL/well of the inoculum. Plates containing PM and BB isolates were incubated at 35 ± 2 °C for 18–20 h. In the case of APP isolates, plates were covered with a perforated seal and incubated at 35 ± 2 °C, with 5–10% CO_2 for 20–24 h [21,22]. The antibiotic panels were read manually using Sensititre™ Vizion (V2021) and the MIC value was established as the lowest drug concentration inhibiting visible growth. For each strain tested, a colony count and a purity check were performed following CLSI and manufacturer recommendations. Moreover, quality control strains were also included in all susceptibility testing runs. Thus, *Actinobacillus pleuropneumoniae* (ATCC 27090™) and *Escherichia coli* (ATCC 25922™) were included as quality control [21,22]. The MICs of the quality control strains had to be within acceptable CLSI ranges to accept the results obtained in the laboratory.

Table 4. Details of the conditions used to carry out minimum inhibitory concentration (MIC) determination using the broth microdilution method by means of customized 96-well microtiter plates (Sensititre, Trek diagnostic Systems Inc., East Grinstead, UK).

Microorganism	0.5 McFarland Suspension Medium	Broth	Final Inoculum	Plate Reconstitution	Incubation Conditions
Pasteurella multocida and *Bordetella bronchiseptica*	Water	CAMHB	5×10^5 cfu/mL	100 µL	35 ± 2 °C 18–24 h Non-CO_2 incubator
Actinobacillus pleuropneumoniae	CAMHB	VFM	5×10^5 cfu/mL	100 µL	35 ± 2 °C 20–24 h CO_2 incubator perforated seal

CAMHB—Cation-adjusted Mueller–Hinton Broth. VFM—Veterinary Fastious Medium. cfu—colony forming units.

4.4. Data Analysis

All the clinical cases with MIC values below CB were classified as susceptible because they could be treated with the antimicrobial, at the registered dose, with a high success rate. The results of the sensitivity tests are presented as MIC distributions and these were determined for each species–antimicrobial combination. MIC_{50} and MIC_{90} were defined as MICs inhibiting 50% and 90% of the strains, respectively. Clinical breakpoints from CLSI were used [21,22] to determine antimicrobial susceptibility. However, CLSI veterinary breakpoints for sulfamethoxazole/trimethropim and *Pasteurellaceae* have not been set. Thus, the CLSI CB available for *Streptococcus suis* (0.5 µg/mL) and sulfamethoxazole/trimethropim have been used in this study. The clinical breakpoint for amoxicillin (0.5 µg/mL) has been obtained from the literature [36] and CLSI CB available for tetracycline (0.5 µg/mL) and porcine respiratory pathogens was extrapolated for doxycycline [21,22]. The antimicrobial susceptibility was considered high at levels ≥90% and low at levels ≤60%, as described by Holmer et al. [28].

5. Conclusions

The obtained antimicrobial susceptibility varies between pig respiratory pathogens. *Actinobacillus pleuropneumoniae* and *Pasteurella multocida* were highly susceptible to ceftiofur, florfenicol and macrolides. However, the antimicrobial susceptibility was intermediate for amoxicillin and enrofloxacin in the case of APP and sulfamethoxazole/trimethropim and tiamulin in the case of PM. Both bacteria showed low antimicrobial susceptibility to doxycycline. Finally, *Bordetella bronchiseptica* was highly susceptible only to tildipirosin and tulathromycin and its susceptibility for florfenicol was close to 50% and <30% for the rest of the antimicrobial families tested. These results emphasize the need for determining antimicrobial susceptibility in pig respiratory cases in order to optimize the antimicrobial treatment in a case-by-case scenario and provide a robust criteria to select the most suitable antimicrobials, taking into account the one-health approach. On the other hand, there is an urgent need to have CLSI CB breakpoints available for every antimicrobial/bacteria and feedback from swine practitioners when using these antimicrobials at the registered dose.

Author Contributions: Conceptualization, A.V. and L.J.F.S.; methodology, A.V., E.N., V.E.-T., J.B., S.M. and C.V.; formal analysis, L.J.F.S and C.V.; writing—original draft preparation, L.J.F.S. and A.V.; writing—review and editing, L.J.F.S., C.V. and A.V.; funding acquisition, E.N. and V.E.-T. All authors have read and agreed to the published version of the manuscript.

Funding: This research received no external funding.

Acknowledgments: This study was carried out with the support of the Porcine Sanitation Group of Lleida, Spain (*Grup de Sanejament Porcí*-GSP), in collaboration with veterinary clinicians working in the field. One part of this research was supported by Cost Action CA18217: European Network for Optimization of Veterinary Antimicrobial Treatment. We are very thankful to Dr César B. Gutiérrez Martín for revising the manuscript.

Conflicts of Interest: The authors declare no conflict of interest.

References

1. Brockmeier, S.L.; Halbur, P.G.; Thacker, E.L. Porcine respiratory disease complex. In *Polymicrobial Diseases*; Brogden, K.A., Guthmiller, J.M., Eds.; ASM Press: Washington, DC, USA, 2002.
2. Fraile, L.; Alegre, A.; López-Jiménez, R.; Nofrarías, M.; Segalés, J. Risk factors associated with pleuritis and cranio-ventral pulmonary consolidation in slaughter-aged pigs. *Vet. J.* **2010**, *18*, 326–333. [CrossRef] [PubMed]
3. Fablet, C.; Marois-Crehan, C.; Simon, G.; Grasland, B.; Jestin, A.; Kobisch, M.; Madec, F.; Rose, N. Infectious agents associated with respiratory diseases in 125 farrow-to-finish pig herds: A cross sectional study. *Vet. Microb.* **2012**, *157*, 152–163. [CrossRef] [PubMed]
4. Van Alstine, W.G. Respiratory system. In *Diseases of Swine*; Zimmerman, J.J., Karriker, L.A., Kent, A.R., Schwartz, J., Stevenson, G.W., Eds.; Wiley-Blackwell: Ames, IA, USA, 2012.
5. Maes, D.; Sibila, M.; Kuhnert, P.; Segalés, J.; Haesebrouck, F.; Pieters, M. Update on Mycoplasma hyopneumoniae infections in pigs: Knowledge gaps for improved disease control. *Transbound. Emerg. Dis.* **2018**, *65*, 110–124. [CrossRef] [PubMed]
6. Sassu, E.L.; Bossé, J.T.; Tobias, T.J.; Gottschalk, M.; Langford, P.R.; Hennig-Pauka, I. Update on Actinobacillus pleuropneumoniae—Knowledge, gaps and challenges. *Transbound. Emerg. Dis.* **2018**, *65*, 72–90. [CrossRef] [PubMed]
7. Opriessnig, T.; Giménez-Lirola, L.G.; Halbur, P.G. Polymicrobial respiratory disease in pigs. *Anim. Health Res. Rev.* **2011**, *12*, 133–148. [CrossRef]
8. Colomer, M.À.; Margalida, A.; Fraile, L. Improving the management procedures in farms infected with the Porcine Reproductive and Respiratory Syndrome virus using PDP models. *Sci. Rep.* **2019**, *9*, 1–13. [CrossRef]
9. Khatun, A.; Nazki, S.; Jeong, C.G.; Gu, S.; Mattoo, S.U.S.; Lee, S.I.; Yang, M.S.; Lim, B.; Kim, K.S.; Kim, B.; et al. Effect of polymorphisms in porcine guanylate-binding proteins on host resistance to PRRSV infection in experimentally challenged pigs. *Vet. Res.* **2020**, *51*, 1–14. [CrossRef]
10. Sargeant, J.M.; Deb, B.; Bergevin, M.D.; Churchill, K.; Dawkins, K.; Dunn, J.; Hu, D.; Moody, C.; O'Connor, A.M.; O'Sullivan, T.L.; et al. Efficacy of bacterial vaccines to prevent respiratory disease in swine: A systematic review and network meta-analysis. *Anim. Health Res. Rev.* **2019**, *20*, 274–290. [CrossRef]

11. Fraile, L. *Antimicrobial Therapy in Swine. Practical Approach*; Editorial Servet: Zaragoza, Spain, 2013.
12. Bronzwaer, S.L.A.M.; Cars, O.; Buchholz, U.; Mölstad, S.; Goettsch, W.; Veldhuijzen, I.K.; Kool, J.I.; Sprenger, M.J.W.; Degener, J.E. The relationship between antimicrobial use and antimicrobial resistance in Europe. *Emerg. Infect. Dis.* **2002**, *8*, 278–282. [CrossRef]
13. Aarestrup, F.M.; Duran, C.O.; Burch, D.G.S. Antimicrobial resistance in swine production. *Anim. Health Res. Rev.* **2008**, *9*, 135–148. [CrossRef]
14. World Health Organization. Global Action Plan on Antimicrobial Resistance. Available online: https://www.who.int/antimicrobial-resistance/global-action-plan/en/ (accessed on 1 June 2020).
15. European Surveillance of Veterinary Antimicrobial Consumption (ESVAC). Sales of Veterinary Antimicrobial Agents in 29 European Countries in 2017, Trends from 2011 to 2017. Ninth ESVAC Report. 2019. Available online: https://www.ema.europa.eu/en/documents/report/sales-veterinary-antimicrobial-agents-31-european-countries-2017_en.pdf (accessed on 1 June 2020).
16. Agencia Española De Medicamentos Y Productos Sanitarios. Plan Estratégico y de Acción Para Reducir el Riesgo de Selección y Diseminación de la Resistencia a los Antibióticos, 2019. Plan Nacional Resistencia a Antibióticos (PRAN). Available online: https://www.aemps.gob.es/laAEMPS/planificacion-AEMPS/docs/Plan-estrategico-2019-2022.pdf. (accessed on 1 June 2020).
17. European Commission. Guidelines for the Prudent Use of Antimicrobials in Veterinary Medicine (2015/C299/04). 2015. Available online: https://ec.europa.eu/health/sites/health/files/antimicrobial_resistance/docs/2015_prudent_use_guidelines_en.pdf. (accessed on 1 June 2020).
18. Humphries, R.M.; Kircher, S.; Ferrell, A.; Krause, K.M.; Malherbe, R.; Hsiung, A.; Burnham, C.A. The Continued Value of Disk Diffusion for Assessing Antimicrobial Susceptibility in Clinical Laboratories: Report from the Clinical and Laboratory Standards Institute Methods Development and Standardization Working Group. *J. Clin. Microbiol.* **2018**, *56*, 1–10. [CrossRef] [PubMed]
19. Humphries, R.M.; Hindler, J.A.; Shaffer, K.; Campeau, S.A. Evaluation of Ciprofloxacin and Levofloxacin Disk Diffusion and Etest Using the 2019 *Enterobacteriaceae* CLSI Breakpoints. *J. Clin. Microbiol.* **2019**, *57*, 1–7. [CrossRef] [PubMed]
20. Aguirre, L.; Vidal, A.; Seminati, C.; Tello, M.; Redondo, N.; Darwich, L.; Martín, M. Antimicrobial resistance profile and prevalence of extended-spectrum beta-lactamases (ESBL), AmpC beta-lactamases and colistin resistance (*mcr*) genes in *Escherichia coli* from swine between 1999 and 2018. *Porcine Health Manag. J.* **2020**, *6*, 1–6. [CrossRef] [PubMed]
21. Clinical and Laboratory Standards Institute. *CLSI Supplement VET08. Performance Standards for Antimicrobial Disk and Dilution Susceptibility Tests for Bacteria Isolated from Animals*, 4th ed.; Clinical and Laboratory Standards Institute: Wayne, PA, USA, 2018.
22. Clinical and Laboratory Standards Institute. *CLSI Supplement M100. Performance Standards for Antimicrobial Susceptibility Testing*, 28th ed.; Clinical and Laboratory Standards Institute: Wayne, PA, USA, 2018.
23. Wen, X.; Gehring, R.; Stallbaumer, A.; Riviere, J.E.; Volkova, V.V. Limitations of MIC as sole metric of pharmacodynamic response across the range of antimicrobial susceptibilities within a single bacterial species. *Sci. Rep.* **2016**, *6*, 1–8. [CrossRef]
24. Mouton, J.W.; Muller, A.E.; Canton, R.; Giske, C.G.; Kahlmeter, G.; Turnidge, J. MIC-based dose adjustment: Facts and fables. *J. Antimicrob. Chemother.* **2018**, *73*, 564–568. [CrossRef]
25. Bader, J.C.; Lakota, E.A.; Andes, D.R.; Rubino, C.M.; Ambrose, P.G.; Bhavnani, S.M. Time for Precision: A World Without Susceptibility Breakpoints. *Open Forum Infect. Dis.* **2018**, *5*, 1–6. [CrossRef]
26. Gutiérrez-Martín, C.B.; del Blanco, N.; Blanco, M.; Navas, J.; Rodríguez-Ferri, E.F. Changes in antimicrobial susceptibility of Actinobacillus pleuropneumoniae isolated from pigs in Spain during the last decade. *Vet. Microbiol.* **2006**, *115*, 218–222. [CrossRef]
27. Hendriksen, R.S.; Mevius, D.J.; Schroeter, A.; Teale, C.; Jouy, E.; Butaye, P.; Franco, A.; Utinane, A.; Amado, A.; Moreno, M.; et al. Occurrence of antimicrobial resistance among bacterial pathogens and indicator bacteria in pigs in different European countries from year 2002–2004: The ARBAO-II study. *Acta Vet. Scand.* **2008**, *50*, 1–10. [CrossRef]
28. Holmer, I.; Salomonsen, C.M.; Jorsal, S.E.; Astrup, L.B.; Jensen, V.F.; Høg, B.B.; Pedersen, K. Antibiotic resistance in porcine pathogenic bacteria and relation to antibiotic usage. *BMC Vet. Res.* **2019**, *15*, 1–13. [CrossRef]

29. Lizarazo, Y.A.; Ferri, E.F.; de la Fuente, A.J.; Martín, C.B. Evaluation of changes in antimicrobial susceptibility patterns of Pasteurella multocida subsp multocida isolates from pigs in Spain in 1987–1988 and 2003–2004. *Am. J. Vet. Res.* **2006**, *67*, 663–668. [CrossRef]
30. El Garch, F.; de Jong, A.; Simjee, S.; Moyaert, H.; Klein, U.; Ludwig, C.; Marion, H.; Haag-Diergarten, S.; Richard-Mazet, A.; Thomas, V.; et al. Monitoring of antimicrobial susceptibility of respiratory tract pathogens isolated from diseased cattle and pigs across Europe, 2009–2012: VetPath results. *Vet. Microbiol.* **2016**, *194*, 1–22. [CrossRef]
31. Zhao, Z.; Wang, C.; Xue, Y.; Tang, X.; Wu, B.; Cheng, X.; He, Q.; Chen, H. The occurrence of Bordetella bronchiseptica in pigs with clinical respiratory disease. *Vet. J.* **2011**, *188*, 337–340. [CrossRef] [PubMed]
32. Kadlec, K.; Kehrenberg, C.; Wallmann, J.; Schwarz, S. Antimicrobial susceptibility of Bordetella bronchiseptica isolates from porcine respiratory tract infections. *Antimicrob. Agents Chemother.* **2004**, *48*, 4903–4906. [CrossRef]
33. Prüller, S.; Rensch, U.; Meemken, D.; Kaspar, H.; Kopp, P.A.; Klein, G.; Kehrenberg, C. Antimicrobial susceptibility of Bordetella bronchiseptica isolates from swine and companion animals and detection of resistance genes. *PLoS ONE* **2015**, *10*, 1–14. [CrossRef]
34. Speakman, A.J.; Binns, S.H.; Osborn, A.M.; Corkill, J.E.; Kariuki, S.; Saunders, J.R.; Dawson, S.; Gaskell, R.M.; Hart, C.A. Characterization of antibiotic resistance plasmids from Bordetella bronchiseptica. *J. Antimicrob. Chemother.* **1997**, *40*, 811–816. [CrossRef] [PubMed]
35. Dayao, D.A.; Gibson, J.S.; Blackall, P.J.; Turni, C. Antimicrobial resistance in bacteria associated with porcine respiratory disease in Australia. *Vet. Microbiol.* **2014**, *171*, 232–235. [CrossRef] [PubMed]
36. Schwarz, S.; Böttner, A.; Goossens, L.; Hafez, H.M.; Hartmann, K.; Kaske, M.; Kehrenberg, C.; Kietzmann, M.; Klarmann, D.; Klein, G.; et al. A proposal of clinical breakpoints for amoxicillin applicable to porcine respiratory tract pathogens. *Vet. Microbiol.* **2008**, *126*, 178–188. [CrossRef] [PubMed]
37. Rey, J.F.; Laffont, C.M.; Croubels, S.; De Backer, P.; Zemirline, C.; Bousquet, E.; Guyonnet, J.; Ferran, A.A.; Bousquet-Melou, A.; Toutain, P.L. Use of Monte Carlo simulation to determine pharmacodynamic cutoffs of amoxicillin to establish a breakpoint for antimicrobial susceptibility testing in pigs. *Am. J. Vet. Res.* **2014**, *75*, 124–131. [CrossRef]
38. Burch, D.G.S.; Sperling, D. Amoxicillin-current use in swine medicine. *J. Vet. Pharmacol. Ther.* **2018**, *41*, 356–368. [CrossRef]

antibiotics MDPI

Article

Oxytetracycline Pharmacokinetics After Intramuscular Administration in Cows with Clinical Metritis Associated with *Trueperella Pyogenes* Infection

Rositsa Mileva [1], Manol Karadaev [2], Ivan Fasulkov [2], Tsvetelina Petkova [1], Nikolina Rusenova [3], Nasko Vasilev [2] and Aneliya Milanova [1,*]

1 Department of Pharmacology, Animal Physiology and Physiological Chemistry, Faculty of Veterinary Medicine, Trakia University, 6000 Stara Zagora, Bulgaria; rositsamileva88@gmail.com (R.M.); ts_petkova87@abv.bg (T.P.)

2 Department of Obstetrics, Reproduction and Reproductive Disorders, Faculty of Veterinary Medicine, Trakia University, 6000 Stara Zagora, Bulgaria; karadaev@abv.bg (M.K.); i.fasulkov@gmail.com (I.F.); nasvas@abv.bg (N.V.)

3 Department of Veterinary Microbiology, Infectious and Parasitic Diseases, Faculty of Veterinary Medicine, Trakia University, 6000 Stara Zagora, Bulgaria; n_v_n_v@abv.bg

* Correspondence: akmilanova@gmail.com; Tel.: +359-42-699-696

Received: 23 June 2020; Accepted: 7 July 2020; Published: 9 July 2020

Abstract: Systemic therapy with oxytetracycline is often used for treatment of clinical metritis although data about its penetration into the uterus and uterine secretion are lacking. Uterine secretions and milk from six cows with clinical metritis were collected for microbiological assay. The animals were treated intramuscularly with long-acting oxytetracycline (20 mg/kg) and samples of plasma, milk and uterine secretions were collected for determination of the antibiotic concentrations by HPLC-PDA analysis. Pharmacokinetics of the antibiotic and in silico prediction of its penetration into the uterus were described. *Trueperella pyogenes* with MIC values of 16–64 µg mL^{-1} was isolated (*n* of cows = 4) from uterine secretions. Oxytetracycline showed fast absorption and penetration in the uterine secretions and milk. No change of withdrawal time for milk was necessitated in cows with clinical metritis. Maximum levels in uterine secretions and predicted concentrations of oxytetracycline in the uterus were lower than MIC values. Systemic administration of long-acting oxytetracycline did not guarantee clinical cure and was not a suitable choice for treatment of clinical metritis associated with *Trueperella pyogenes*. The appropriate approach to antibiotic treatment of uterine infections of cows requires knowledge on penetration of the antibiotics at the site of infection and sensitivity of pathogens.

Keywords: oxytetracycline; pharmacokinetics; cows; clinical metritis; *Trueperella pyogenes*

1. Introduction

Among the uterine diseases, clinical metritis is a common complication in dairy farms with financial impact due to increased number of services per conception and decreased milk yield [1]. The costs of treatment and the emergence of resistance to antimicrobial drugs are some serious concerns. Clinical metritis is often associated with mixed infections [2] and isolation of pathogenic bacteria such as *Escherichia coli* and *Trueperella pyogenes* [3].

Broad spectrum antibiotics are used for treatment of these mixed infections of the uterus [4]. Several papers attempted to summarize the knowledge about antibiotic use in treatment of endometritis and metritis in cows and to discuss the efficacy of tetracyclines, macrolides, fluoroquinolones and sulfonamide-trimethoprim combinations [5–7]. A meta-analysis of the published data reveals that application of ceftiofur decreases the prevalence of metritis although some of research studies reported conflicting results [7,8]. Another problem discussed by Haimerl et al. [7] is related to shortage of data that allow making consistent conclusions on the efficacy of the applied drugs. However, the emergence of resistance to antibiotics restricts the use of cephalosporins and fluoroquinolones in veterinary medicine [9,10]. Therefore, more attention is paid to the prudent use of "old" antibiotics and efforts for establishment of clinical breakpoints have been made [11].

Tetracyclines are widely applied in veterinary practice, including in treatment of uterine infections such as metritis [12]. Published studies reported pharmacokinetics of long-acting oxytetracycline formulations in lactating cows based on plasma and milk concentrations after systemic administration of the antibiotic [13]. Its penetration in plasma and milk after intrauterine administration in cows with metritis was described [14,15]. The disposition in the milk was studied for determination of withdrawal time [16]. Concentrations in the uterus after intramuscular administration of long-acting oxytetracycline formulations in calves at a dose rate of 20 mg kg^{-1} were investigated [17]. Concentrations in the uterine tissues and uterine secretion of oxytetracycline were studied by Masera et al. [18] in healthy cows after intravenous and uterine administration of the antibiotic more than 40 years ago. Uterine tissue inflammation results in increased blood flow to the uterus and in breakdown of epithelial barriers [16]. Therefore, we hypothesize that the disposition of oxytetracycline at the site of infection can be affected by the severity of inflammation. No data about the disposition of tetracycline antibiotics in cows with clinical cases of metritis with simultaneous detection of pathogens causing the infection are available. The contemporary approach to the treatment of bacterial infections requires knowledge about pharmacokinetics and pharmacodynamics of the applied antibiotics. Information about the penetration of the antibacterials at the site of action at effective concentrations is crucial for success of the therapy.

Therefore, the aim of the current investigation was to evaluate the pharmacokinetics of intramuscularly administered oxytetracycline as a long-acting drug dosage form in cows with clinical metritis with special emphasis on its penetration in the uterine secretion. As an integral part of the evaluation of oxytetracycline efficacy, a microbiological assay has been performed for determination of the main bacterial pathogens and their sensitivity to oxytetracycline was studied.

2. Results

The animals were diagnosed with clinical metritis, grade 1. The body temperature was within the normal range and only purulent secretion from uterus was observed. The appetite, water consumption and the milk yield were not affected.

2.1. Pharmacokinetics of Oxytetracycline

The pharmacokinetic parameters of oxytetracycline following intramuscular administration are presented in Table 1 and on Figure 1. Analysis of the data for plasma by one-compartmental model showed relatively fast absorption with absorption rate constant k_{ab} 0.87 ± 0.51 h^{-1} and absorption half-life $t_{1/2ab}$ of 0.79 ± 0.46 h. The values of the other parameters such as k_{el} (0.03 ± 0.004 h^{-1}), T_{max} (4.05 ± 1.80 h), C_{max} (6.21 ± 1.27 μg mL^{-1}) and AUC (253.93 ± 34.24 h μg mL^{-1}) were very close to those calculated by non-compartmental analysis (Table 1).

Table 1. Pharmacokinetic parameters in cows ($n = 6$) with clinical metritis presented as arithmetic mean ± SD (Geometric mean ± geometric SD) after single intramuscular administration of 20 mg kg^{-1} oxytetracycline hydrochloride as long-acting drug formulation.

Parameters	Units	Mean ± SD (Geometric Mean ± Geometric SD)
	Non-compartmental analysis—plasma	
k_{el}	h^{-1}	0.03 ± 0.004 (0.03 ± 0.004)
$t_{1/2el}$	h	25.79 ± 3.77 (25.57 ± 4.27)
T_{max}	h	6.17 ± 3.97 (4.76 ± 1.87)
C_{max}	μg mL^{-1}	7.31 ± 1.91 (7.10 ± 0.05)
$AUC_{0\text{-}t}$	h μg mL^{-1}	242.36 ± 31.39 (240.63 ± 33.01)
$AUC_{0\text{-}\infty}$	h μg mL^{-1}	250.43 ± 32.71 (248.62 ± 34.02)
Extrapolation of AUC	%	3.21 ± 0.58 (3.17 ± 0.61)
$AUMC_{0\text{-}t}$	h h μg mL^{-1}	9236.89 ± 1939.66 (9093.71 ± 1707.74)
MRT	h	36.90 ± 5.49 (36.58 ± 5.88)
	Non-compartmental analysis—milk	
k_{el}	h^{-1}	0.024 ± 0.002 (0.024 ± 0.002)
$t_{1/2el}$	h	29.33 ± 2.97 (29.20 ± 2.92)
T_{max}	h	12.00 ± 0.00 (12.00 ± 0.00 *)
C_{max}	μg mL^{-1}	3.43 ± 0.80 (3.35 ± 0.77 *)
$AUC_{0\text{-}t}$	h μg mL^{-1}	144.19 ± 32.07 (141.63 ± 28.40)
$AUC_{0\text{-}\infty}$	Hh μg mL^{-1}	147.26 ± 32.11 (144.73 ± 28.50)
Extrapolation of AUC	%	2.14 ± 0.80 (2.03 ± 0.74)
$AUMC_{0\text{-}t}$	h h μg mL^{-1}	6812.28 ± 1298.36 (6716.54 ± 1219.02)
MRT	h	45.31 ± 3.01 (45.23 ± 2.95)
	Non-compartmental analysis—uterine secretion	
T_{max}	h	12.00 ± 9.29 (9.52 ± 2.78)
C_{max}	μg mL^{-1}	12.50 ± 11.39 (8.06 ± 5.08)

[1] T_{max}, time of C_{max}; C_{max}, maximum plasma or milk levels; k_{el}, elimination rate constant; $t_{1/2el}$—elimination half-life; $AUC_{0\text{-}\infty}$, area under the concentration–time curves from 0 to infinity ∞; $AUC_{0\text{-}t}$, area under the concentration–time curves on the basis of measured concentrations during the treatment; $AUMC_{0\text{-}t}$, area under the moment curve from the time of dosing to the last measurable concentration; MRT, mean residence time on the basis of the predicted data. * Statistically significant difference between plasma and milk at $p < 0.05$.

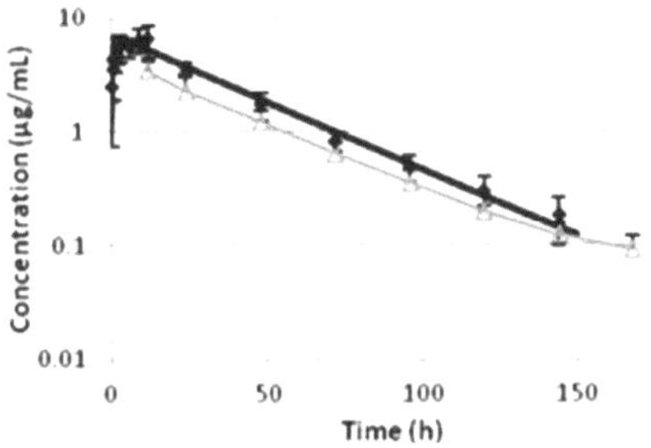

Figure 1. Semi-logarithmic mean ± SD plasma (predicted levels—black line and ♦—observed concentrations) and milk (predicted levels—gray line and Δ—observed concentrations) concentrations of oxytetracycline vs. time curve after a single intramuscular administration in cows ($n = 6$) at a dose rate of 20 mg kg^{-1}.

The levels of oxytetracycline in the milk were below the limits of quantification (LOQ) at the first two sampling intervals, 0.5 and 0.75 h after the treatment. The first measurable concentration was found 1 h after the treatment. They remained lower than the concentrations in plasma during the entire study (Table 2 and Figure 1). Oxytetracycline levels in milk were lower than the LOQ in three cows 168 h after treatment. The maximum concentrations in milk were significantly lower and were achieved significantly later than the levels in plasma. The elimination half-life for milk and plasma had similar values.

Table 2. Milk/plasma ratio (Mean ± SD) of oxytetracycline concentrations in cows (n = 6) with clinical metritis after single intramuscular administration of 20 mg kg^{-1} oxytetracycline hydrochloride as a long-acting drug formulation.

Time (h)	Milk/Plasma Ratio
12	0.54 ± 0.09
24	0.63 ± 0.20
48	0.74 ± 0.24
72	0.81 ± 0.32
96	0.79 ± 0.37
120	0.70 ± 0.17
144	0.80 ± 0.33
168	0.48 ± 0.43

Oxytetracycline was found in the uterine secretion at all sampling intervals (Table 3). High individual variations in the concentrations of the antibiotic were observed between tested cows. The levels of oxytetracycline in the uterine secretion were close to those in plasma 48 h after treatment. The median values of the concentrations in the uterine secretion were twice-lower during the other intervals.

Table 3. Oxytetracycline concentrations in uterine secretion in cows (n = 6) with clinical metritis (Median and range in the parenthesis) and uterine secretion/plasma ratio after single intramuscular administration of 20 mg kg^{-1} oxytetracycline hydrochloride as a long-acting drug formulation.

Time (h)	Cow 1	Cow 2	Cow 3	Cow 4	Cow 5	Cow 6	Mean ± SD
			Concentration (μgmL^{-1})				
6	4.13	2.33	0.66	3.20	8.43	13.67	3.66 (0.66–13.67)
24	1.79	0.38	29.81	2.26	21.86	1.52	2.03 (0.38–29.81)
48	0.90	0.20	5.03	1.48	20.87	0.73	1.19 (0.20–20.87)
72	0.41	0.15	0.48	3.04	8.90	0.41	0.44 (0.15–8.90)
			Uterine secretion/plasma ratio				
6	0.87	0.49	0.12	0.48	1.19	2.88	0.68 (0.12–2.88)
24	0.45	0.10	8.35	0.56	6.17	0.52	0.54 (0.10–8.35)
48	0.64	0.12	2.79	1.03	8.09	0.52	0.84 (0.12–8.09)
72	0.58	0.23	0.57	3.53	8.25	0.53	0.57 (0.23–8.25)

In silico prediction of oxytetracycline levels in the uterine tissue suggested that the antibiotic penetrated in the superficial and deep compartments of the uterus with partition coefficients of $P_{uterus:pl}$ 0.789 and 0.765, respectively.

2.2. *MIC Concentration of Oxytetracycline against Trueperella Pyogenes*

The microbiological assay of uterine secretion revealed presence of *Trueperella pyogenes* (n of cows = 4), *Escherichia coli* (n = 1) and *Vibrio spp.* (n = 1). No pathogenic bacteria were isolated from milk samples. Additionally, the minimum inhibitory concentrations for *Trueperella pyogenes* as a microorganism associated with clinical metritis in cows were determined. Minimum inhibitory concentrations of oxytetracycline against the isolates of *Trueperella pyogenes* were between 16 and 64 μg mL^{-1}.

2.3. *Clinical Outcome after Treatment with Oxytetracycline*

Four of the animals were clinically cured. Three cows (No. 1, 2 and 3) were inseminated and pregnancy was diagnosed by means of ultrasound. Less sensitive *Trueperella pyogenes* strains with MIC value of 64 μg mL^{-1} were isolated from cows No. 4 and 5. These animals showed signs of chronic endometritis during the next oestrus and were subjected to treatment. The last animal demonstrated normal clinical oestrus without signs of chronic inflammation of the uterus but it was not inseminated.

3. Discussion

The prudent use of antimicrobial drugs for treatment of bacterial infections in farm animals is one of the important limitation steps against selection and spread of resistance. The challenge for practitioners in dairy farms consists of implementing an adequate management program for prevention of diseases and in cases of clinically manifested infections of the genital tract, treating them efficiently to maintain the fertility of the cows. Clinical cases of endometritis and metritis are treated by parenteral administration of antibiotics, most often intramuscularly, or locally by the intrauterine route [7,16]. Oxytetracycline is one of the most often used antibiotics in farm animals, including in cases of infections in the genital tract of dairy cows [16].

Pharmacokinetics of long-acting drug formulations of oxytetracycline in cows has been well described but data after its intramuscular administration in cows with clinical metritis are not published. The long-acting formulation of oxytetracycline, administered at a dose of 20 mg kg^{-1} in the current study, showed similar values of elimination half-life to those of dairy cows treated with other long-acting formulations of the antibiotic at a dose rate of 10–11 mg kg^{-1} [13]. C_{max} values were higher because of the double administered dose and were attained slightly earlier in comparison to the results from the cited study [13]. Half-life of absorption was longer (1.03–1.52 h) when the drug was administered at lower doses [13]. Kumar and Malik [19] found similar pharmacokinetic characteristics in healthy calves as in cows with clinical metritis after single i.m. administration of a long-acting oxytetracycline. The cited authors reported C_{max} of 5.34 ± 0.31 μg mL^{-1} at T_{max} of 8.4 ± 0.4 h, $t_{1/2el}$ of 25.63 ± 1.26 h and AUC of 236.63 ± 0.15 h μg mL^{-1}. Altogether these data indicate that the observed pharmacokinetics of long-acting oxytetracycline formulations in cows with clinical metritis is similar to the reported data in healthy dairy cows and calves.

Compared to C_{max} in plasma, oxytetracycline reached significantly earlier twice lower maximum concentrations ($p < 0.05$) in the milk of cows with clinical metritis. Earlier reports show that the observed ratio of free milk to free serum concentration during equilibrium was similar to the calculated ratio in our study [20]. The concentrations in milk between 48 and 144 h after treatment were close to the levels in blood in support of previously reported data [21]. Concentrations in milk in healthy lactating cows after i.m. administration of a long-acting oxytetracycline at a dose of 20 mg kg^{-1} were lower than the values observed by us [22]. The data from our study and previous reports suggest that higher penetration of oxytetracycline in milk can be expected in cows with clinical metritis. Increased blood flow during uterine inflammation can lead to secretion of oxytetracycline into the uterus and to re-absorption of the antibiotic from the uterine secretion into the blood in cows with clinical metritis, especially after administration of long-acting drug dosage forms, and thus to secretion at higher concentrations into the milk [16]. This is a probable reason for high levels of oxytetracycline in the milk, found in the current study if compared to the data in healthy animals. Similar observations, suggesting higher penetration through the blood–milk barrier, were reported for cows with endometritis and cows with metritis after intrauterine administration of oxytetracycline [16]. Nevertheless, the proposed withdrawal time of 7 days by the manufacturer of the used dosage form is long enough and the measured concentrations of oxytetracycline were lower than MRL of 100 μg L^{-1} 168 h after treatment.

Much of the literature is related to investigations in healthy cows and few studies published around 40 years ago present data about the disposition of oxytetracycline after intravenous (i.v.) or i.m. administration in animals with genital tract infection. There is a shortage of evidence for the efficacy of i.m. administration of oxytetracycline for treatment of metritis in cows. The treatment efficacy is highly dependent on the possibility of the antibiotics to reach the site of infection. Penetration of oxytetracycline in healthy cows and in four cows with chronic endometritis after intramuscular administration at a dose of 8 mg/kg as 5% propylene glycol solution has been investigated [18].

In healthy cows, the concentrations in the endometrium were nearly 5 times higher than in plasma 12 h (4.05 ± 1.19 μg g^{-1}) and 24 h (2.1 ± 1.3 μg g^{-1}) after i.m. treatment. These levels were almost twice-lower in the endometrium of cows with chronic endometritis at the same time intervals: 2.3 ± 1.0 μg g^{-1} and 0.96 ± 0.72 μg g^{-1}, respectively. They remained higher in comparison to levels in plasma [18]. The modeling of concentrations in the uterine tissue, performed in our study, predicted comparable penetration in the superficial and deep compartments of uterus. The predicted concentrations in the uterus, based on $P_{uterus:pl}$ coefficient, were between 1.34 μg g^{-1} and 5.0 μg g^{-1} over the first 48 h after treatment. They were close to the measured concentrations reported by Masera et al. [18]. Landoni and Errecalde [17] found 1.1 ± 1.8 to 2.6 ± 1 μg g^{-1} oxytetracycline in the uterus of healthy Hereford calves during the first 48 h after treatment with a long-acting formulation at a dose of 20 mg kg^{-1}. In another study, similarly to our results, the predicted concentrations in the endometrium and uterine wall after simulation of the penetration of oxytetracycline, administered i.v., twice daily at a dose rate of 11 mg kg^{-1}, were lower than the levels in plasma [23]. However, these results require validation with determination of the concentrations after biopsy in cows with clinical metritis. Much higher concentrations were measured in the uterine secretion of individual cows with clinical metritis at different intervals after i.m. treatment with oxytetracycline. In cows No 3 and 5, these levels were between 2 and 9-fold higher than in plasma (at 24 h) which can be related to the severity of tissue inflammation of the uterus. The median values of the uterine secretions/plasma ratio of oxytetracycline, observed in our study, demonstrated twice lower levels in the uterine secretion compared to these in plasma and the range showed that high variations can be expected between individual animals. Masera et al. [18] reported twice-higher mean antibiotic levels in the uterine secretion compared to these in plasma in cows with endometritis. The cited study did not discuss presence of inter-individual variations and absence of the data about the minimum and maximum levels does not allow comparison of the results. Observed concentrations of oxytetracycline in uterine secretion after i.m. administration in cows give evidence for penetration of the antibiotic in the genital tract tissues and secretion through the uterine epithelium which can result in achievement of effective concentrations in the uterus and uterine secretion against some pathogenic bacteria. High inter-individual variation in the uterine secretion levels among the cows in the current study may be attributed not only to the different breeds but also to the different periods for development of postpartum clinical metritis [23]. Altogether these data allow us concluding that oxytetracycline can be secreted through the uterine tissue.

The cited investigations deal with the data for oxytetracycline penetration in genital tissues but do not provide information about the pathogenic isolates from the same cows causing clinical metritis. Contemporary studies proved that bacteriological tests assist the prudent use of antibiotics, resulting in reduction of the number of cases without clinical cure [24]. Microbiological assays for isolation of a specific pathogen and determination of its MIC values are crucial for selection of the proper antibiotic for therapy of uterine infections [4]. Isolated pathogens from the cows with clinical metritis in the current study are among the commonest bacteria causing uterine infections in cows [25,26]. A special attention was paid to *Trueperella pyogenes*, as a pathogen that often causes uterine infections and mastitis at dairy farms. In a study conducted by Galán-Relaño et al., [3] bimodal MIC distribution was detected for oxytetracycline against *Trueperella pyogenes* and MIC_{90} values of 32 μg mL^{-1} were found out. Another study reported MIC values of oxytetracycline within a wide range between 0.25 to ≥128 μg mL^{-1} [27]. MIC values of 16 and 64 μg mL^{-1} of the isolates from cows with clinical metritis were similar to the reported data. Low sensitivity of *Trueperella pyogenes* was associated with overuse of tetracycline antibiotics in veterinary medicine. Although, according to literature data, *Trueperella pyogenes* was isolated from the milk, the pathogen was not detected in milk samples in our study.

The infections, caused by *Trueperella pyogenes*, are usually treated with ceftiofur or with intrauterinely or intramuscularly administered oxytetracycline [28]. Recent studies show different efficacy of oxytetracycline in treatment of endometritis and metritis in dairy cows. Some clinical investigations found higher first service conception rate in groups treated with oxytetracycline compared to other antibiotics [29]. Other authors reported higher efficacy when intrauterine treatment with oxytetracycline was combined with i.m. administration of ampicillin [12], or when only penicillin was used [2]. Successful treatment of clinical metritis depends on the cellular and humoral local immune response which is a prerequisite for less severe consequences of uterine infections in aged animals than in young cows [25]. Correlation between the prevalence of *E. coli* and *Trueperella pyogenes* in cows with uterine infections and balance of uterine microbiota after treatment can be of significance for cure of the animals with clinical metritis [25].

The results from the current study revealed that oxytetracycline penetrated in the uterine tissue and in the uterine secretions at lower levels than MIC values against *Trueperella pyogenes*. Despite that there are no clinical cut-off value and epidemiological cut-off value for *Trueperella pyogenes*, our data demonstrated that intramuscularly administered oxytetracycline was not an appropriate option for treatment of clinical metritis when this microorganism was isolated as pathogen. Clinical efficacy was not observed in two of the cows and they were treated once intrauterinely with 10% povidone iodine solution. Clinical metritis in other two cows was not associated with isolation of *Trueperella pyogenes* and they were successfully treated with broad spectrum oxytetracycline. Other factors such as immune response, balance of microbiota and higher antibiotic concentrations than MIC values (cow No 3) can contribute to the observed cure of the other two animals from which strains of *Trueperella pyogenes* with MIC of 16 $\mu g\ mL^{-1}$ were isolated. A limitation of our study was the number of animals, therefore the conclusion on the efficacy of oxytetracycline in treatment of clinical metritis requires additional clinical trials. Although clinical metritis is associated with isolation of more than one species of microbial pathogens and broad-spectrum antibiotics are expected to be effective, the data from the current study showed that treatment should be based on information about the disposition of the antibiotic at the biophase in the infected animals and the sensitivity of the isolated pathogens.

4. Materials and Methods

4.1. Drugs and Reagents

Tetravet LA (Ceva Sante Animale, France) was used for treatment of the animals. The drug was administered at the dose rate, recommended by the producer. Oxytetracycline was applied at a dose of 20 mg kg^{-1} bw.

The used reagents were HPLC grade. Oxytetracycline hydrochloride ≥95% crystalline and doxycycline hyclate with purity ≥98% (Sigma-Aldrich, St. Louis, MO, USA) were used for analytical tests. Acetonitrile CHROMASOLV®, HPLC grade, ≥99.9% purity (Sigma-Aldrich,), methanol ≥99.8% purity HiPerSolv CHROMANORM® for HPLC isocratic grade (VWR BDH PROLABO®), oxalic acid 98% purity (Sigma Chemical Co., St. Louis, MO, USA), ethylenediaminetetraacetic acid disodium salt dihydrate 99.0–101.0% (Na2H2EDTA × 2H2O, Sigma-Aldrich) and trifluoroacetic acid ReagentPlus®, 99% purity (Sigma-Aldrich) were used for preparation of the mobile phase and for extraction of the studied antibiotics from the biological matrices.

4.2. Animals

The study was conducted between April 2019 and February 2020 according to the rules of Bulgarian legislation (Ordinance No. 20/1.11.2012 on the minimum requirements for protection and welfare of experimental animals and requirements for use, rearing and/or their delivery, License 151/26.09.2016).

Six lactating cows belonging to Training Experimental Farm of Trakia University, Stara Zagora, Bulgaria from different breeds were included in the study. The animals were housed in the experimental farm. They received feed according to the requirements of the species and water ad libitum. The cows were regularly milked twice daily (7:00 h and 17:00 h). The information about the individual animals is included in Table S1. All of them were diagnosed with clinical metritis after observation on days 5, 10, 15 and 21 after parturition for clinical evidence for metritis. The animals underwent a rectal examination to determine uterine health on days 5, 10, 15 and 21 after parturition. During the examination, the uterus was manipulated transrectally to check the uterine contents and confirm the presence of metritis. Cows with abnormal appearance of the vaginal discharge, reported by the vet in the farm, were subjected to rectal examination to confirm the diagnosis metritis. The animals were diagnosed with clinical metritis grade 1 according to the system of Sheldon et al. [26]. The health of the animals was routinely monitored and they were observed for changes in feed intake, condition and udder filling. They did not show clinical signs for other diseases and the body temperature was within the normal range. The animals were included in the experiment after complete medical check, few days after parturition according to the information in Table S1. The clinical status of the animals, included in the experiment, was checked after the end of the investigation. The animals (n = 2) that showed signs of endometritis during the next estrus were subjected to treatment once intrauterinely with 10% povidone iodine solution (Jodouter, Bioveta, Czech Republic).

4.3. Experimental Design

The cows diagnosed with metritis were treated once intramuscularly with a long-acting oxytetracycline formulation (Tetravet LA, Ceva Sante Animale, France) at a dose rate of 20 mg kg^{-1} bw according to the manufacturer instructions. Blood samples (5 mL) from the subcutaneous abdominal vein were collected in heparinized tubes (2.5 mL Lithium heparin, FL Medical, Italy) before the treatment. Milk and uterine secretion samples were collected aseptically in sterile tubes for microbiological assessment (10 mL) before drug administration, at the day of the treatment. Uterine secretion samples were obtained after catheterization with a sterile catheter. The milk and uterine secretion samples were immediately transported to the microbiology lab. Plasma, free from antibiotic, was separated from the blood sample after centrifugation at 1500× *g* for 10 min and was frozen at −25 °C until analysis. The animals were treated between 8:00 and 9:00 h in the morning after complete milking. Blood samples were collected via the *vena epigastrica cranialis superficialis* in heparinized tubes (2.5 mL Lithium heparin, FL Medical, Italy). They were withdrawn at 0.5, 0.75, 1, 1.5, 2, 3, 6, 9, 12, 24, 48, 72, 96, 120, 144 and 168 h after treatment to assess plasma oxytetracycline concentration. After collection, blood samples were centrifuged at 1500× g for 10 min, the plasma fraction was transferred in sterile Eppendorf tubes and frozen at −25 °C until HPLC analysis. Milk samples (10 mL) were collected at the same intervals as for blood samples. The cows were completely milked 12, 24, 48, 72, 96, 120, 144 and 168 h after treatment and only milk samples from these intervals were used for further pharmacokinetic analysis. At the other intervals complete milking was not possible and milk samples were used to evaluate the time of appearance of the first measurable concentration in the milk. Samples from uterine secretion were obtained via sterile catheter 6, 24, 48 and 72 h after oxytetracycline administration. All the samples were immediately stored at −25 °C until analysis.

4.4. Isolation and Identification of Pathogenic Bacteria

The obtained samples from uterine secretion were seeded on Tryptic soy agar (TSA, HiMedia, India) and MacConkey agar (HiMedia, India) and incubated at aerobic conditions for 24–72 h. TSA was used for isolation of aerobe mesophilic pathogenic bacteria causing metritis in cows and was supplemented with 5% defibrinated sheep blood. Primary identification of the isolates was performed with the following tests: Gram staining, Motility test, Catalase test, Oxidase test and Hugh-Leifson oxidative-fermentative test. Additionally, some specific tests were run, according to the characteristics of the isolates, such as Loffler's medium with serum (NCIPD, Bulgaria) and CAMP test for *Trueperella pyogenes*, IMViC test for *Enterobacteriaceae spp.*, including indole detection, methyl red test, Voges-Proskauer test and citrate utilization. The tests were carried out in accordance with the manufacturer's instructions and the general rules for aseptic work in the microbiology laboratory [30]. In addition to conventional biochemical tests, a semi-automated system for phenotypic identification with microplates of generation GenIII (BioLog, USA) was used. The plates were incubated under aerobic conditions at 33 °C for 20–24 h.

4.5. Minimum Inhibitory Concentration Determination (MIC)

Trueperella pyogenes was isolated from most of the investigated cows and its sensitivity to oxytetracycline was tested. MICs of *Trueperella pyogenes* isolates were determined using the micro-dilution method in cation-adjusted Mueller Hinton broth (MHB), according to CLSI Guidelines [31]. Taking into account the growth characteristics of *Trueperella pyogenes*, MHB was supplemented with 2% (vol/vol) lysed horse blood [32]. The plates were incubated for 48 h in a CO_2-enriched atmosphere. The results were read spectrophotometrically at 620 nm wavelength (Synergy LX Multi-Mode Microplate Reader, BioTek, USA). Each experiment was performed in triplicate with 4 independent replications.

4.6. HPLC Analysis

Oxytetracycline concentrations in plasma, milk and uterine secretion were analyzed by HPLC with PDA detection using a method described by Laczay et al. [33] with minor modifications published by Mileva [34]. An aliquot (150 μL) of plasma samples was placed in 1.5 micro-centrifuge tube spiked with 15 μL internal standard (IS, doxycycline 10 μg/mL) and 19.5 μL trifluoroacetic acid (TFA). Samples were vortexed for 1 min and centrifuged at 10,800 g at 22 °C for 10 min. The supernatant was placed in HPLC vials and 20 μL were injected into the HPLC system. The extraction of oxytetracycline from the uterine secretion was performed with 400 μL of sample spiked with 40 μL IS and 52 μL TFA and the explained steps for plasma were followed. The concentrations in the uterine secretion were determined by using the calibration curve for plasma because it was impossible to obtain enough amount of secretion to prepare a separate curve. Four samples of uterine secretion out of 24 had to be diluted and analyzed again due to very high levels of oxytetracycline.

An aliquot of 500 μL milk was mixed with 50 μL IS and 65 μL TFA by vortexing for 1 min. The samples were centrifuged for 10 min at 10,800× g at 22 °C. The supernatant was transferred to another tube and centrifuged again at 10,800× g at 22 °C for 5 minutes. They were filtered through filter paper (pore size 10–20 μm) after the second centrifugation step. The filtrate from each sample was placed in a HPLC vial and 20 μL were injected into the HPLC system (Thermo Fisher Scientific Inc., USA). A Hypersil Gold column (5 μM, 150 × 4.6 mm) was used at room temperature for separation of tetracycline antibiotics. The analysis was performed with PDA detector (Surveyor, Thermo Fisher Scientific Inc., USA) at wavelength of 345 nm. The HPLC system also included a Surveyor LC Pump Plus and a Surveyor Auto sampler Plus. The mobile phase consisted of acetonitrile, methanol, 0.02 M oxalic acid and 0.02 M $Na_2H_2EDTA \times 2H_2O$ (20:15:64:1, *v/v/v/v*). The flow rate was 1.0 mL min^{-1}. The retention times were 2.7 min for oxytetracycline and 5.7 min for doxycycline. ChromQuest Chromatography Data System (Thermo Fisher Scientific Inc., USA) was used for peak area integrations.

The developed method was validated for bovine plasma and milk in terms of linearity, intra-day and inter-day precision, recovery, limits of detection (LOD) and quantification (LOQ). The values LOD and LOQ for plasma were 0.05 μg mL^{-1} and 0.15 μg mL^{-1}, and for the milk 0.026 μg mL^{-1} and 0.086 μg mL^{-1}, respectively. The mean accuracy of the method and mean extraction recovery of oxytetracycline determined in standard solutions in plasma were 95.03% and 97.05%. The same parameters for standard solutions prepared in milk were 95.93% and 91.16%. The mean intra- and inter-day precision (RSD %) values for plasma were 6.38 and 7.55, and for milk: 4.34 and 8.76. The calibration curves for milk and for plasma were built using blank milk and plasma samples, respectively, from untreated cows spiked at 7 different concentrations of oxytetracycline (0.05, 0.2, 0.5, 1, 2.5, 5 and 10 μg mL^{-1}). IS was added during preparation of the samples for calibration curves. The method showed good linearity for both matrices: $R^2 = 0.9987$ for plasma and $R^2 = 0.9996$ for milk. The test for lack of fit for plasma ($p = 0.949$) and for milk ($p = 0.977$) confirmed these results.

4.7. Pharmacokinetic Analysis and Prediction of Oxytetracycline Concentrations in the Uterine Tissue

Oxytetracycline plasma concentration vs time curve was described by one-compartmental analysis with absorption (Model 3) and by a non-compartment model using Phoenix 8.1.0.34 software (Certara®, Cary, NC, USA). The most suitable model for compartmental analysis was selected according to the lowest value of the Akaike information criterion. One-compartmental analysis has been used to characterize the phase of absorption. Non-compartmental approach based on statistical moment theory was applied for analysis of data for plasma and milk. Individual concentrations of oxytetracycline in the plasma and milk used for pharmacokinetic analysis are presented in Table S2 and Table S3, respectively. Cut-off value for goodness of fit was set at $R^2 > 0.95$. A weighting factor $1/y^2$ was used to improve the fit for data of plasma. The area under the curve (AUC) was calculated by the linear-up log-down rule to the last quantifiable drug concentration-time point (Ct) and infinity. Cut-off values for percent of extrapolation of AUC were settled as <20%. Area under the first moment curve ($AUMC_{0-\infty}$) was calculated and mean residence time ($MRT_{0-\infty}$) was determined from AUC and AUMC. The elimination rate constants (k_{el}) associated with the terminal elimination phase following intramuscular administration was estimated by using linear regression of the terminal phase of the log plasma/milk concentration versus time curve. The mean maximum concentration (C_{max}) and time to obtain maximum concentration (T_{max}) for plasma, milk and uterine secretion were calculated on the basis of the observed values.

A model developed by Poulin and Theil [35,36] for non-adipose tissues was used for prediction of oxytetracycline concentrations in the uterine tissue. The following equation describes the relation between drug concentrations in plasma and in tissues:

$$P_{t:p} = (CF_t/CF_p)(fu_p/fu_t) \quad (1)$$

where: fu is the unbound fraction in the plasma (p) or tissue (t), and CF_t/CF_p represents a potential quantitative difference of free concentration between tissues and plasma caused by solubility in lipid and water fractions. Drug specific parameters for oxytetracycline (logPo:w -1.3) [37] and tissue-specific parameters were taken from the literature as described in Haritova and Fink-Gremmels [38]. The values were as follows: fu_p 0.7 and fu_t 0.82; water content in plasma: 0.91; phospholipid content in plasma: 0.0175 and neutral lipid content in plasma: 0.0017. The values for phospholipid content (0.0008) and neutral lipid content (0.0011) in the uterine tissue [39] and the values for water content (0.845 and 0.82 for the superficial and the deep tissue compartments, respectively) were previously published [40].

4.8. Statistical Analysis

The linearity of the calibration curves for milk and plasma was confirmed with test for lack of fit and the curves were linear within the tested range at $p > 0.05$. Pharmacokinetic parameters were presented as arithmetic mean ± SD and as geometric mean ± geometric SD in parenthesis [41]. Normal distribution was assessed by Shapiro–Wilk test. Student's t-test was used to determine statistically significant differences of pharmacokinetic variables between plasma and milk. Differences were considered significant at $p < 0.05$. The concentrations in the uterine secretion were presented as median and range. The analyses were conducted using Statistica for Windows (STATISTICA for Windows 10.0, StatSoft, Inc., USA).

5. Conclusions

Pharmacokinetic study of intramuscularly administered long-acting oxytetracycline (20 mg/kg) in cows with clinical metritis showed that the disposition of the antibiotic at the site of infection does not guarantee achievement of effective concentrations when *Trueperella pyogenes* is isolated from the uterine secretions. The sensitivity of the isolated pathogens should be determined. The choice of the antibiotic and its dosing regimen should be based on analysis of the sensitivity of pathogens and the concentration of the antibiotic in the uterus.

Supplementary Materials: The following are available online at http://www.mdpi.com/2079-6382/9/7/392/s1, Table S1: Information about cows included in the investigation; Table S2: Measured concentrations of oxytetracycline in plasma of each cow ($n = 6$) after single intramuscular administration of 20 mg kg^{-1} oxytetracycline hydrochloride as a long-acting drug formulation; Table S3: Measured concentrations of oxytetracycline in milk of each cow ($n = 6$) after single intramuscular administration of 20 mg kg^{-1} oxytetracycline hydrochloride as a long-acting drug formulation

Author Contributions: Conceptualization: A.M. and N.V.; methodology, R.M., A.M. and N.V.; software, R.M. and A.M.; validation, R.M. and A.M.; formal analysis, T.P.; investigation, R.M., M.K., I.F. and N.R.; resources, I.F. and M.K; data curation, R.M., N.R. and I.F.; writing—original draft preparation, A.M.; writing—review and editing, A.M. and N.V.; visualization, A.M.; project administration, N.V.; funding acquisition, N.V. All authors have read and agreed with the published version of the manuscript.

Funding: This research was funded by National scientific program "Reproductive biotechnologies in breeding in Bulgaria"—REPROBIOTECH, Ministry of Education and Science, Bulgaria.

Acknowledgments: One part of this research is supported by COST Action CA18217—European Network for Optimization of Veterinary Antimicrobial Treatment.

Conflicts of Interest: The authors declare no conflict of interest.

References

1. Sheldon, I.M.; Owens, S.E. Postpartum uterine infection and endometritis in dairy cattle. In Proceedings of the 33rd Annual Scientific Meeting of the European Embryo Transfer Association (AETE), Bath, UK, 8–9 September 2017; Volume 14, pp. 622–629. [CrossRef]
2. Ordell, A.; Unnerstad, H.E.; Nyman, A.; Gustafsson, H.; Bege, R. A longitudinal cohort study of acute puerperal metritis cases in Swedish dairy cows. *Acta Vet. Scand.* **2016**, *58*, 79. [CrossRef] [PubMed]
3. Galán-Relaño, Á.; Gómez-Gascón, L.; Barrero-Domínguez, B.; Luque, I.; Jurado-Martos, F.; Vela, A.I.; Sanz-Tejero, C.; Tarradas, C. Antimicrobial susceptibility of *Trueperella pyogenes* isolated from food producing ruminants. *Vet. Microbiol.* **2020**, *242*, 108593. [CrossRef] [PubMed]
4. Haimerl, P.; Heuwieser, W. Antibiotic treatment of metritis in dairy cows: A systematic approach. *J. Dairy Sci.* **2014**, *97*, 6649–6661. [CrossRef] [PubMed]
5. Smith, B.I.; Donovan, G.A.; Risco, C.; Littell, R.; Young, C.; Stanker, L.H.; Elliott, J. Comparison of various antibiotic treatments for cows diagnosed with toxic puerperal metritis. *J. Dairy Sci.* **1998**, *81*, 1555–1562. [CrossRef]
6. Lefebvre, R.C.; Stock, A.E. Therapeutic efficiency of antibiotics and prostaglandin F2α in postpartum dairy cows with clinical endometritis: An evidence-based evaluation. *Vet. Clin. N. Am. Food A* **2012**, *28*, 79–96. [CrossRef]
7. Haimerl, P.; Arlt, S.; Borchardt, S.; Heuwieser, W. Antibiotic treatment of metritis in dairy cows—A meta-analysis. *J. Dairy Sci.* **2017**, *100*, 3783–3795. [CrossRef]
8. LeBlanc, S.J. Reproductive tract inflammatory disease in postpartum dairy cows. *Animal* **2014**, *8* (Suppl. 1), 54–63. [CrossRef]
9. European Medicine Agency. Committee for Medicinal Products for Veterinary Use (CVMP) and EFSA Panel on Biological Hazards (BIOHAZ), EMA and EFSA Joint Scientific Opinion, RONAFA. *EFSA J.* **2017**, *15*.
10. European Medicine Agency. Categorisation of Antibiotics in the European Union. EMA/CVMP/CHMP/682198/2017. Available online: www.ema.europa.eu/en/documents/report/categorisation-antibiotics-european-union-answer-request-european-commission-updating-scientific_en.pdf (accessed on 14 June 2020).
11. Toutain, P.L.; Bousquet-Mélou, A.; Damborg, P.; Ferran, A.A.; Mevius, D.; Pelligand, L.; Veldman, K.T.; Lees, P. En route towards European clinical breakpoints for veterinary antimicrobial susceptibility testing: A position paper explaining the VetCAST approach. *Front. Microbiol.* **2017**, *8*, 2344. [CrossRef]
12. Armengol, R.; Fraile, L. Comparison of two treatment strategies for cows with metritis in high-risk lactating dairy cows. *Theriogenology* **2015**, *83*, 1344–1351. [CrossRef]
13. Mevius, D.J.; Nouws, J.F.M.; Breukink, H.J.; Vree, T.B.; Driessens, F.; Verkaik, R. Comparative pharmacokinetics, bioavailability and renal clearance of five parenteral oxytetracycline-20% formulations in dairy cows. *Vet. Quart.* **1986**, *8*, 285–294. [CrossRef] [PubMed]

14. Hajurka, J.; Nagy, J.; Popelka, P.; Rozanska, H.; Sokol, J.; Cabadaj, R.; Hura, V. Tetracycline concentrations in blood and milk of cows following intrauterine treatment of acute or subacute/chronic endometritis. *Bull. Vet. Inst. Pulawy* **2003**, *47*, 435–447.
15. Makki, M.; GheisarI, H.R.; Ahmadi, M.R. Effect of different intrauterine oxytetracycline treatment on reproductive performance of dairy cows with clinical endometritis and determination of oxytetracycline residues in milk. *Acta Vet. Eurasia* **2016**, *42*, 80–88. [CrossRef]
16. Gorden, P.J.; Ydstie, J.A.; Kleinhenz, M.D.; Wulf, L.W.; Gehring, R.; Lee, C.J.; Wang, C.; Coetzee, J.F. A study to examine the relationship between metritis severity and depletion of oxytetracycline in plasma and milk after intrauterine infusion. *J. Dairy Sci.* **2016**, *99*, 8314–8322. [CrossRef] [PubMed]
17. Landoni, M.F.; Errecalde, J.O. Tissue concentrations of a long-acting oxytetracycline formulation after intramuscular administration in cattle. *Rev. Sci. Tech.* **1992**, *11*, 909–915. [CrossRef]
18. Masera, J.; Gustafsson, B.K.; Afiefy, M.M.; Stowe, C.M.; Bergt, G.P. Disposition of oxytetracycline in the bovine genital tract: Systemic vs intrauterine administration. *J. Am. Vet. Med.* **1980**, *176*, 1099–1102.
19. Kumar, R.; Malik, J.K. Effects of multiple injections of Escherichia coli endotoxin on the pharmacokinetics and dosage regimens of a long acting formulation of oxytetracycline (OTC-LA) in cross-bred calves. *Vet. Arhiv.* **2001**, *71*, 245–263.
20. Ziv, G.; Sulman, F.G. Analysis of pharmacokinetic properties of nine tetracycline analogues in dairy cows and ewes. *Am. J. Vet. Res.* **1974**, *35*, 1197–1201.
21. Mestorino, N.; Errecalde, O.J. Pharmacokinetic–pharmacodynamic considerations for bovine mastitis treatment. In *A Bird's-Eye View of Veterinary Medicine*; Perez-Marin, C.C., Ed.; InTech: London, UK, 2012; p. 6857. [CrossRef]
22. Longo, F.; Cinquina, A.I.; Anastasi, G.; Barchi, D.; Coresi, A.; Cozzani, R.; Fagiolo, A. Distribution of long acting oxytetracycline formulation in milk samples from lactating cows. In Proceedings of the 8th International Congress of the European Association for Veterinary Pharmacology and Toxicology (EAVPT), Jerusalem, Israel, 30 July–3 August 2000. Abstract No B13.
23. Bretzlaff, K.N.; Ott, R.S.; Koritz, G.D.; Bevill, R.F.; Gustafsson, B.K.; Davis, L.E. Distribution of oxytetracycline in genital tract tissues of postpartum cows given the drug by intravenous and intrauterine routes. *Am. J. Vet. Res.* **1983**, *44*, 764–769.
24. Madoz, L.V.; Prunner, I.; Jaureguiberry, M.; Gelfert, C.-C.; de la Sota, R.L.; Giuliodori, M.J.; Drillich, M. Application of a bacteriological on-farm test to reduce antimicrobial usage in dairy cows with purulent vaginal discharge. *J. Dairy Sci.* **2017**, *100*, 3875–3882. [CrossRef] [PubMed]
25. Földi, J.; Kulcsár, M.; Pécsi, A.; Huyghe, B.; de Sa, C.; Lohuis, J.A.C.M.; Cox, P.; Huszenicza, G. Bacterial complications of postpartum uterine involution in cattle. *Anim. Reprod. Sci.* **2006**, *96*, 265–281. [CrossRef] [PubMed]
26. Sheldon, I.M.; Cronin, J.; Goetze, L.; Donofrio, G.; Schuberth, H.J. Defining postpartum uterine disease and the mechanisms of infection and immunity in the female reproductive tract in cattle. *Biol. Reprod.* **2009**, *81*, 1025–1032. [CrossRef] [PubMed]
27. De Boer, M.; Heuer, C.; Hussein, H.; McDougall, S. Minimum inhibitory concentrations of selected antimicrobials against *Escherichia coli* and *Trueperella pyogenes* of bovine uterine origin. *J. Dairy Sci.* **2015**, *98*, 4427–4438. [CrossRef] [PubMed]
28. Pyörälä, S.; Taponen, J.; Katila, T. Use of antimicrobials in the treatment of reproductive diseases in cattle and horses. *Reprod. Domest. Anim.* **2014**, *49* (Suppl. 3), 16–26. [CrossRef]
29. Manimaran, A.; Raghu, H.V.; Kumaresan, A.; Sreela, L.; Yadav, A.; Layek, S.S.; Mooventhan, P.; Chand, S.; Sarkar, S.N.; Sivaram, M. Oxytetracycline is more suitable antibiotic for clinical endometritis cows. *Indian J. Anim. Sci.* **2019**, *89*, 501–505.
30. Markey, B.; Leonar, F.; Archambault, M.; Cullinane, A.; Maguire, D. *Clinical Veterinary Microbiology*, 2nd ed.; Mosby Elsevier Inc.: New York, NY, USA, 2013; p. 105.
31. NCCLS. *Approved Standard NCCLS Document*; NCCLS: Wayne, PA, USA, 2008.
32. Pohl, A.; Lübke-Becker, A.; Heuwieser, W. Minimum inhibitory concentrations of frequently used antibiotics against *Escherichia coli* and *Trueperella pyogenes* isolated from uteri of postpartum dairy cows. *J. Dairy Sci.* **2018**, *101*, 1355–1364. [CrossRef] [PubMed]
33. Laczay, P.; Semjén, G.; Lehel, J.; Nagy, G. Pharmacokinetics and bioavailability of doxycycline in fasted and nonfasted broiler chickens. *Acta Vet. Hung.* **2001**, *49*, 31–37. [CrossRef]

34. Mileva, R. Determination of free doxycycline concentrations in plasma and milk of sheep and in plasma of rabbits by HPLC method. *Mac. Vet. Rev.* **2019**, *42*, 2. [CrossRef]
35. Poulin, P.; Theil, F.-P. Prediction of pharmacokinetics prior to in vivo studies. I. Mechanism-based prediction of volume of distribution. *J. Pharm. Sci.* **2002**, *91*, 129–156. [CrossRef]
36. Poulin, P.; Theil, F.-P. Prediction of pharmacokinetics prior to in vivo studies. II. Generic physiologically based pharmacokinetic model of drug disposition. *J. Pharm. Sci.* **2002**, *91*, 1358–1370. [CrossRef]
37. Wishart, D.S.; Knox, C.; Guo, A.C.; Cheng, D.; Shrivastava, S.; Tzur, D.; Gautam, B.; Hassanali, M. DrugBank: A knowledgebase for drugs, drug actions and drug targets. *Nucleic Acids Res.* **2008**, *36*, 901–906. [CrossRef] [PubMed]
38. Haritova, A.M.; Fink-Gremmels, J. A simulation model for the prediction of tissue plasma partition coefficients for drug residues in natural casings. *Vet. J.* **2010**, *185*, 278–284. [CrossRef] [PubMed]
39. Henault, M.A.; Killian, G.J. Neutral lipid droplets in bovine oviductal epithelium and lipid composition of epithelial cell homogenates. *J. Dairy Sci.* **1993**, *76*, 691–700. [CrossRef]
40. Breeveld-Dwarkasing, V.N.A.; de Boer-Brouwer, M.; te Koppele, J.M.; Bank, R.A.; van der Weijden, G.C.; Taverne, M.A.M.; van Dissel-Emiliani, F.M.F. Regional differences in water content, collagen content, and collagen degradation in the cervix of nonpregnant cows. *Biol. Reprod.* **2003**, *69*, 1600–1607. [CrossRef] [PubMed]
41. Martinez, M.; Blondeau, J.; Cerniglia, C.E.; Fink-Gremmels, J.; Guenther, S.; Hunter, R.P.; Li, X.Z.; Papich, M.; Silley, P.; Soback, S.; et al. Workshop report: The 2012 antimicrobial agents in veterinary medicine: Exploring the consequences of antimicrobial drug use: A 3-D approach. *J. Vet. Pharm. Therap.* **2014**, *37*. [CrossRef] [PubMed]

MDPI
St. Alban-Anlage 66
4052 Basel
Switzerland
Tel. +41 61 683 77 34
Fax +41 61 302 89 18
www.mdpi.com

Antibiotics Editorial Office
E-mail: antibiotics@mdpi.com
www.mdpi.com/journal/antibiotics